PHYSICK TO PHYSIOLOGY

PHYSICK TO PHYSIOLOGY

TALES FROM AN OXFORD LIFE IN MEDICINE

KEITH DORRINGTON

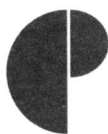

PROFILE
EDITIONS

First published in Great Britain in 2023 by
Profile Editions,
an imprint of Profile Books Ltd
29 Cloth Fair
London
ECIA 7JQ
www.profileeditions.com

1 3 5 7 9 10 8 6 4 2

Typeset in Dante by MacGuru Ltd
Printed and bound in Great Britain by
Clays Ltd, Elcograf S.p.A.

A CIP catalogue record for this book is available from the British Library.

ISBN 978 1 80081 924 5

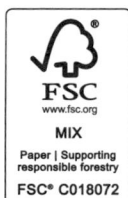

Contents

THE HEAP

"The Medical Libraries are already so full, that adding to the heap may be deemed an unnecessary labour, especially if the new book is little more than a compilation," wrote David Macbride in 1772 in his 700-page tome on 'the theory and practice of physic'.[1] How dare the present author add another book to the heap?

Dr Macbride worked hard to move beyond a 'compilation'; he looked for new discoveries. At the point of discussing how blood poured into a basin gets a 'buffy coat' on the top when left to settle, he turned to "an ingenious modern *physiologist*" (my italics) for a "much more satisfactory" account of why the blood of "patients labouring under inflammatory diseases" gets a particularly thick yellowish coat at the top. The explanation he found (the "red particles" sediment down, leaving "the coagulable lymph" at the top) is still valid today.[2]

This is a book of tales from medical science. I explore lively topics encountered during a professional lifetime in Oxford, which have arisen from my studies and work in seven Oxford colleges and numerous hospitals. An initiative to encourage state schoolboys to consider a university education led me to study engineering at one of the colleges, where I tutored for a decade and learned the nuts and bolts of laboratory science. Dissuaded from helping to dig a tunnel under the English Channel, I found myself instead studying medicine and learning the benevolent practice of anaesthesia. Oxford served up so many awesome lines of discovery and fascination that I have collected some here for the reader to share.

The scientific focus is *physiology*, the study of how living things work. This term physiology has been used over centuries, giving it the historical character of being a 'father faculty' from which offspring have emerged as new ways of studying living organisms. These offspring now include biophysics, biochemistry, genetics and molecular biology. For Lazare Rivière, writing in 1657, his account of the whole of medicine (what he termed the "Body of Physick") consisted of five parts; the first of these was "Physiologie" in which "we consider all those things which are naturally coincident to the constitution of Mans body".[3]

The *Oxford English Dictionary* agrees: physiology is "the branch of science that deals with the normal functioning of living organisms and their systems and organs". What frequently causes heated debate is whether the offspring faculties are still family members or new dynasties. This is not the place to entertain such a debate, but I note a tendency to create names to describe new courses of study, and departments that avoid 'physiology', if only to emphasise their modernity. The University of Oxford taught 'Physiological Sciences' for many years; we now call the course 'Biomedical Sciences'. A new building opposite my office goes by the name 'Nanoscience Discovery' but the word 'Physiology' lives on in the name of the department from which I look out as I write.

A thoughtful "dissection of the meanings" of physiology by two philosophers from Bordeaux in 2018 argues that the key feature of physiology is that it can *explain the function* of the bits and pieces (my words) that you can find in the body.[4] Describing them is not enough, nor is having computers that are able to predict how they behave. At whatever resolution the parts of an organism are examined – from individual molecules up to the whole body – physiology's role is to try to explain what is going on and why.

An example from the work of colleagues illustrates the potential of this explanation. The cause of a rare inherited genetic disease known as 'Chuvash polycythaemia' has been found to be a single mutation in the gene coding for a protein in a biochemical pathway that enables cells to sense the level of oxygen in their environment (I shall note later that the Oxford Nobel Prize of 2019 is part of this story). From an understanding of the physiology of the lungs, my aerospace colleague Dr Tom Smith hypothesised that a patient with this condition would have high blood pressure in the right side of the heart if they were to take a flight in which the level of oxygen experienced by the body would be low. A thirty-year-old Chuvash patient was duly studied by Tom before, during and after a six-hour flight from London to Dubai and the predicted high pressure was observed. Not all the steps in this sequence of events can yet be explained in detail, but many can be, and this example demonstrates the power inherent in the *explanation of the function* of the circulation of blood to the lungs.[5]

In this book we shall meet the medical science of physiology as it bumps into all sorts of things: pioneering surgery, mountains on several continents, the coronavirus pandemic, the laws of thermodynamics, anaesthesia, dog food, poisons, Lord Nuffield's motor works, a lethal hydrogen balloon, and the education of youngsters out of school. We shall meet winners of Nobel Prizes; we look back to seventeenth-century Oxford for some of physiology's origins, and then back further, 400 million years, to the evolution of the heart and lungs.

Scientific discourse is often heavily laden with jargon, graphs, diagrams and equations. Here, I try to keep it simple by using descriptive prose whenever possible, allowing myself some images and portraits. The reader has no need for lots of background scientific knowledge but will be confronted by current as well as past controversies; a row is never far away in scientific work, as in so many other human endeavours. We will take a fresh look at 'ingenious modern physiologists' past and present, and attempt to explain why Oxford provides rich opportunities for encountering them.

CHAPTER ONE

MURDER IN MAIN QUAD

Breathing without the Body:
from Heart Surgery to Covid-19

The first survivor

On the day I nudged my way into the air to use my lungs for the first time, 6 May 1953, something tricky was going on in a hospital in Philadelphia in the United States. Cecelia Bavolek, an eighteen-year-old with a life-threatening hole in the heart, had been offered a surgical repair of this congenital defect while either being immersed in an ice bath or being connected to a device never successfully used in a patient before: a heart–lung machine. She chose the machine, saying, "I couldn't stand the idea of being frozen." She was brave, and so was her surgeon, Dr John Gibbon (Fig. 1). Their decision marked the beginning of a new era of treating heart defects that had previously remained intractable. The heart–lung machine was also to be something that would occupy me for several years of my life. I would see it become an almost casual component of heart operations and then watch a manifestation of it generate huge controversy in the treatment of lung disease. The Covid-19 pandemic was to see a profusion of use like never before.

Almost everything that could go wrong during Cecelia's operation did go wrong.[1] But first let me explain a bit about the machine; only then can the full drama be appreciated. In order to operate inside the heart, it is necessary to open it up. This may not stop the heart beating, but it stops the heart pumping and kills the patient unless another pump takes over. The plumbing around the heart is so complicated that, years before, it had been concluded that you need to combine a mechanical pump with an artificial lung: hence the familiar 'heart–lung' machine. Pumps were easy to devise, relatively speaking; the lung was the big challenge. After twenty years of experimentation, Gibbon and his wife had come up with an answer.[2] Their lung was a plastic box about the size of a large pack of corn-flakes, which contained vertical metal meshes down which blood was made to flow, as if down a waterfall. Oxygen was blown through the box. If the blood didn't clot or gush in rivulets down the screens, it should pick up enough oxygen to keep the patient alive. The term 'oxygenator' was frequently used interchangeably with 'lung'.

The heart in adults normally pumps blood with a flow of about 5 litres per minute from the large veins, through the lungs, and onwards into the arteries. In the veins the pressure of the blood is low; in the arteries it is high. I accuse the plumbing of being complicated because the heart has two sides, each with two chambers. The right side of the heart receives blood low in oxygen from the body tissues and pumps the blood from the veins into the lungs, where oxygen enters the blood; the left side of the heart receives the blood from the lungs and pumps it into the largest artery, called the aorta, from where its high pressure drives it on to the tissues of the body that need the oxygen with which it has been provided. To take over the work of the heart and lungs Gibbon's machine had to be capable of draining blood, in a continuous flow, from a large vein. The blood had to be poured over the metal screens in the oxygenator box, collected safely, making sure that potentially harmful bubbles were removed, and then pumped back across the room via a pipe connected to the patient's aorta. This almost industrial process had to be achieved with complete sterility to avoid infection and run without leaks or clotting of the blood.

The machine was primed with blood and set to circulate it well before the operation; it was no good Gibbon getting started unless the machine was running well. It was made of five pumps, one each for a separate task such as keeping the waterfalls from clotting by having them flowing even when not connected to the patient. Flow from and into the patient started at 12.55 p.m. Full flow was quickly reached at 1 p.m., but soon had to be trimmed back: blood frothed up and began to leak from the oxygenator. Blood was also clotting in the tube leading to the patient, and three of the eight screens lost their smooth film of blood. Too little of the anti-clotting drug heparin had been given, they later found out. The patient's blood oxygen level, acidity and pressure reached values that led to barely controlled panic. Gibbon pleaded "Do something," but kept going. Flow from the machine was stopped at 1.43 p.m., giving a total of forty-eight minutes of artificial circulation, during twenty-six minutes of which the patient was totally dependent on the machine to keep her alive. Such was the rush to finish in the face of these near-catastrophic events that Gibbon closed the heart with a clamp before sewing it up so that the machine could be speedily retired. There was much concern over whether Cecelia's brain could have survived intact, but by the evening she was awake and "completely lucid". She made a full recovery and lived to the age of sixty-five.

In my own career as an anaesthetist, I have known some panicky moments in the operating theatre; this one sounds like a prize-winner. Sometimes the worst moments occur when the blood loss on the floor or in the drapes exceeds how much can be got back in; here, in Cecelia's case, over 2 litres were administered after attempts to stop a "huge leak" from the oxygenator, but these were "to no avail". And bad moments include those when the oxygen levels in the blood drop off the radar, because these are a measure of whether the patient is likely to live; in Cecelia's case they fell to 31.8 per cent, but we usually aim to keep them at over 90 per cent. Knowing well the duties of an anaesthetist, I can imagine that for the nurse anaesthetist, Kitty Rowlands, this must have been a particularly stressful day's work.

Murder: the day someone shot the future cardiac surgeon

In addition to John Gibbon, I have to applaud the achievements of Denis Melrose, who studied medicine at my Oxford college, University College ('Univ'), and survived being shot in the chest by a fellow student, but more importantly helped to evaluate an 'Oxford' heart–lung machine that eventually occupied me for a few years. He was born in Cape Town in 1921. The family moved to Britain and from 1935 young Denis was schooled at Sedbergh in Cumbria, arriving at Univ in 1939. Melrose's niece, in correspondence with Univ's archivist, recounted that Melrose had wanted to study history but the year before his doctor father had made an appointment to see the Master of Univ to enrol his son to study medicine instead; that was the way admissions were done in those days. Melrose is said to have found this irksome, because war had just been declared and he and his colleagues wished to leave university and go to fight and be heroes.[3] But study medicine he did.

The shooting happened on 17 May 1940. There had been a furious argument at the breakfast table about conscientious objectors. John Fulljames was in favour of them, indeed was one, even though he himself was in the Officers' Training Corps and a good shot. He kept a Lee Enfield rifle in his room and lunchtime provided him with a chance to make his feelings clear. He fired out of the window of his room into the college quadrangle towards the set he resented as they went off dressed for tennis. The first bullet brought down Charles Moffat "with blood coming all over the place", according to Norman Dix, the college servant who witnessed it.[4] An attentive Denis Melrose dashed across to look at Moffat and both were hit by bullet number two. This is the one that got Melrose in the chest. He walked a small distance and collapsed. A third shot shattered the nearby doorpost and sent a piece through scout Cummings' foot; damage to the stonework remains visible today. The fourth hit another student in the calf. A trained shot indeed. Poor Moffat succumbed quickly; one bullet had hit him in the head. A view from the very spot where Moffat fell and Melrose was struck is shown in Figure 2 in more recent, calmer times; the appearance of the buildings has remained largely unchanged from 1680 to the present day.

Melrose was saved from death by a ricochet from a large fountain pen in the chest pocket of his tennis blazer (probably assisted by his nearby cigarette case) but was very ill as a consequence and his recovery took weeks in the Acland Hospital. A later master of the college, Sir Robin Butler, remembered Melrose returning for a college gaudy event and raising his shirt to show the wound. College don Peter Bailey had also witnessed a similar undressing at a dinner some years earlier; it sounds as though Melrose, understandably, was rather proud of his exhibit.

Fulljames quietly presented himself to the college chaplain, handing him the rifle and saying, "It's me." Amid much controversy he was found to be guilty of murder but insane, was sentenced to penal servitude, and imprisoned until 1945. He was nineteen when he did his shooting and ninety-one when he died in 2013.[5]

Melrose completed three years of pre-clinical medical studies in Oxford before moving to University College Hospital London (not, alas, owned by the Oxford 'Univ') for his clinical studies. He qualified the year his aspiring assassin left jail. Melrose's Univ record is clean except for an episode of damaging the college's statue of the poet Shelley; he was "punished by a fine of £5, gating [being confined to the college] for the term, and removal of his gramophone".[6] As a tutor at Univ myself, and sometimes involved in disciplinary matters, I like to think that these restrictions on movement and pleasure might have contributed to the scope of his studies, and the remarkable success of his career. On obtaining his full medical degree BM BCh, he joined the Royal Navy, as his father had done, serving in Hong Kong. He returned to the UK in 1947 to an academic post in surgery at the Hammersmith Hospital in London. We shall shortly explore Melrose's innovative approach to building an oxygenator.

Many ways to build a lung

Following John Gibbon's successful surgery in May 1953, his next two patients died and he declared a moratorium on further application of his heart–lung machine.[7] There were to be many alarming events associated with the development of such machines. One summary found a run of eighteen failed attempts to use heart–lung machines in surgery in the years 1952–4 as leading to an attitude of hopelessness.[7] I think that what got them going again was finding that they could conduct heart surgery on children by using human adult volunteers as 'living heart–lung machines' – often a parent, if one with compatible blood was available. The idea here was to use a continuous flow of blood from a large artery of the 'donor' volunteer into the child, with carefully matched, equal but opposite flow back into a large vein in the volunteer. In this way the child was supplied with blood oxygenated by the volunteer and the donor was kept from being depleted of blood. From 1954 Walton Lillehei at the University of Minnesota had success in twenty-eight operations of this kind on forty-five seriously ill children, suggesting that with a reliable machine (in this case, a human) even very sick patients could be helped. The rush was on to make a machine to replace the human volunteers.

The detail of new ways to build a heart–lung machine might be thought as uninteresting as new types of internal combustion engine, but it is in fact fascinating because of the great variety of designs. Engines have only two types of piston, the usual up-and-down (Otto) and the rotary (Wankel). Heart–lung machines have tried lots of ways to get oxygen into the blood. Some found success modifying the Gibbon 'waterfall' of blood screens, adding in a vaporiser to administer anaesthetic and keep the patient soundly asleep. Others found success bubbling oxygen through a container of blood using a simple series of tubes that looked as though they might have been put together in a garden shed (and could be thrown away after single use). A third approach was to use a row of rotating discs on a horizontal shaft partially immersed in blood, looking a bit like something you might see behind a tractor ploughing a field. A fourth approach was to use animal lungs washed of their own blood and suspended in a plastic container: dog lungs and monkey lungs were tried, the former with some success. Then there was a fifth approach in which blood was separated from gas using a plastic sheet or membrane; we shall see later that there have been many ways in which this has been achieved, including flat membranes and round tubes. One state in the United States made heroic progress in two of its hospitals 90 miles apart: the Mayo Clinic in Rochester used a modified version of Gibbon's design and the University of Minnesota Hospital in Minneapolis employed a bubble oxygenator.[7] In addition, in the late 1940s Denis Melrose got going on the same problem and by the year of my birth in 1953 had helped the UK make progress too.[8]

Melrose's boss, Professor Ian Aird, was on a mission: he wanted a heart–lung machine for the same reasons that the Americans wanted one. So far, we have counted five different ways to oxygenate blood; Melrose's became the sixth. Building upon contributions from enthusiasts in Sweden, the Netherlands and France, as well as the United States, he came up with the idea of letting blood slosh down the centre of a hollow rotating cylinder, slightly inclined to the horizontal by 20 degrees, and lined internally with curved battens. Oxygen was fed in too, of course. The system worked well and a prototype was first used in a thirty-two-year-old woman in 1954, initially just to assist the circulation during a repair to an aortic valve.[9]

During this operation Aird wanted to ensure that the blood vessels supplying the patient's brain and the muscle of the heart itself continued to be perfused with blood at sufficient pressure to keep them healthy while performing intricate surgery on the aortic valve by inserting a dilator through the wall of the heart. It was accepted that there would be a lot of bleeding while this was done, and the concern was that this blood loss would lead to a critical reduction in the pressure of blood perfusing the most vital organs, the brain and the heart. Their heart–lung machine was able to provide a flow of blood of 800 ml per minute into the aorta despite the bleeding, so ensuring flow to the brain and heart muscle. A back-up plan was to have the heart–lung machine increase the flow to higher values, even several litres per minute, if the heart stopped completely.[9] In this way it provided an insurance. Its use in other patients progressed "gradually" from this kind of support of the circulation to eventually taking it over completely, in the way Gibbon had used his heart–lung machine.

If this was Melrose's invention number one, his second was arguably even more consequential: stopping the heart from beating during surgery and starting it up again on demand. The 1954 Hammersmith operation on the thirty-two-year-old had been an example of surgeons doing their best *to keep the heart beating* while they operated inside it, using the machine to help keep the heart's own blood vessels perfused so as to prevent damage from lack of oxygen. This was the standard approach at that time. But a beating heart is a moving target and the surgery is intricate. Melrose's team soon got the idea of stopping the heart altogether. In a variety of laboratory experiments in several species, Melrose and his colleagues applied some nineteenth-century knowledge about salts and the heartbeat to show that they could stop the heart within seconds by using potassium salt solution, and start it up at will by washing away the potassium.[10] Not only did their surgical target stop moving, but it also stopped having to work and therefore needing oxygen, a double bonus for "unhurried correction of cardiac abnormalities under direct vision".[10] Over the years, various cocktails of 'cardioplegia' (salt solutions for stopping the heart) have been tried, with or without cooling the heart, and Melrose's giant step forward is now a routine part of thousands of heart operations each year, as are modifications of both Gibbon's and his heart–lung machines. Perhaps it was a good thing that he didn't study history after all.

Oxford's artificial lung

Melrose's work on the heart–lung machine is linked to my own pursuits many years later. After finishing full-time 'house jobs' (as they were then called) as a novice doctor in surgery and then medicine, I started working part-time in the Accident Service at the John Radcliffe Hospital and sought a desk and a laboratory to carry on the research that was by then filling much of my time and interest. This was in 1983. The delightful and generous Brian Bellhouse kindly took me on in his Bioengineering Unit.

Brian Bellhouse was a University Lecturer in Engineering and a tutor at Magdalen College. This sort of joint university–college appointment has been the standard academic post in Oxford for many years; the term 'Oxford don' is sometimes used. In the sciences the norm was for the university to pay two-thirds of the salary and for the college to provide a third. In the university's Department of Engineering Science, Brian had built up a bit of an empire in a large red-brick north-Oxford property not far from the main departmental buildings and gathered people interested in what was called 'medical engineering'. It should perhaps be pointed out that I had previously acquired a doctorate in engineering, as well as my medical degrees, so Brian must have thought that I had something to offer his enterprise.

I remember sitting in the rather luxurious office he allocated to me, with a corner bay window looking out through trees, and wondering how I was going to justify the privilege of this new part-time appointment. Brian was later famous for becoming extremely wealthy by way of inventing something that was never used: needle-free injection of a drug through the skin using an airgun. I knew him as a hugely friendly and supportive engineering don, who carried a lot of people along with his enthusiasm. One of these had been Denis Melrose, with whom Brian had a productive collaboration.

Inspired by Leonardo da Vinci, Brian had by 1968 become interested in swirling vortices being responsible for the efficient closure of the valves of the heart with each heartbeat.[11] The heart–lung people, including Melrose, were by then long convinced of "a general leaning towards the principle of imitation of the normal pulmonary anatomy, where the blood is separated from the gas by a membrane".[12] The trouble with blood flowing smoothly across a plastic membrane was the presence of the 'boundary layer'. This may come as a bit of a surprise, but actually a liquid sticks to any surface, even if most of it is flowing past. This means that blood next to a plastic membrane can pick up oxygen diffusing across the membrane from the other side but has difficulty flowing away to make way for the arrival of fresh unoxygenated blood. Around 1970 Brian's enthusiasm for vortices gave him the idea of building an oxygenator in which the swirling motion of blood was deliberately exploited to disturb the effect of the boundary layer on sheets of membrane;[13] Denis Melrose had been thinking along similar lines, but by using shaking tubes wound into a cylindrical shape (not surprising, considering his earlier large rotating contraption).[14]

By 1981 their interests had merged and their collaboration got under way. A device had been manufactured, tested first by Melrose in calves (weighing 110 kg), and then used in twenty adult patients at the Hammersmith Hospital,[15] and soon in fifty patients in the United States.[16] These were large numbers for a machine that might have seemed like a hairbrained idea, because it involved actively and vigorously agitating the flow of blood to minimise the disadvantages brought about by the boundary layer, but it carried added risks associated with large swings in pressure within the device.

It was called the Interpulse™ membrane oxygenator and was designed in Oxford by Brian and manufactured in the United States. The idea was to have blood flowing across plastic membranes in seven channels and 'pulsed' backwards and forwards as it made its way through, thereby breaking up the boundary layers. The cunning trick was to put furrows across the direction of flow in the membrane, so that thorough mixing occurred with each pulse. (Unless the flow of blood is agitated in some way to minimise the effect of this boundary layer, about 10 square metres of membrane are needed to oxygenate the blood for an adult heart–lung machine; I like to calibrate mentally by noting that this is exactly the area of the floor in my current small office). Having this much plastic surface had been found to cause problems, including damaging the blood cells. With pulsed flow it was possible to make do with about 1 square metre of membrane for the same job. It seemed like a very good idea to get a tenfold reduction, but it did involve some complex pumping equipment, which itself carried the possible risk of traumatising the blood. About the size of a 1980s photocopying machine on wheels, the beast looked a bit of an overkill compared with some contemporary competitors for heart surgery. But it did the job.

Back in Oxford, the technicians' workshop in the Bioengineering Unit was abuzz with the production of new designs of pulsating machines when I arrived in 1983. Roger Lewis, Gerald Walker and John Greenford were Brian Bellhouse's skilled machinists. These three were masters of heavy machinery and fine craftsmanship, working in the undercroft of the Victorian house in which we found ourselves. A new concept caught my eye: it seemed that, if the furrows in the plastic membrane were substituted by deep dimples like those on the surface of a golf ball, even more vigorous mixing could be obtained with an even greater reduction in the area of membrane. So, we entered the phase of "dimple flow".

These new versions of the 'pulsed flow' lung worked remarkably well in laboratory experiments, which I enjoyed conducting with colleagues in Oxford and Geneva; the latter was set in motion by a sabbatical visit to Oxford by Dr Jean-Patrice Gardaz, an anaesthetist from Switzerland. Properly moulded dimples of 1.6 mm diameter and 0.4 mm deep, densely packed across the otherwise flat membranes, seemed to enhance the mixing process to such an extent that the devices improved on a flat membrane by about twenty-five-fold.[17] We assumed that the eddies of blood that formed with each pulse of the flow were quickly ejected from their dimples with the next reversal of flow, but this remained a bit of an article of faith.

Having an efficient oxygenator that could run reliably for hours opened up the possibility of all sorts of interesting experiments, and a big boost to our activities came from the arrival in Oxford of Keith Sykes, our new and dynamic Nuffield Professor of Anaesthetics. Keith came to this chair in 1980 from London and enthused the anaesthetic department with respiratory physiology. He had worked with Denis Melrose, using heart–lung machines in the 1960s, and brought to Oxford the drive to use this technology to support the lungs of patients having breathing problems.[18] It was with his encouragement that Jean-Patrice Gardaz became involved. By 1984 I had also started training as an anaesthetist myself, and found myself barely able to contain the excitement of being surrounded by all this expertise and enthusiasm.

Long-term respiratory support

The new focus of interest was to explore whether any type of heart–lung machine could be used to support patients who were unable to use their own lungs to breathe, in other words to use the lung part of the heart–lung machine to take over somebody's breathing, even if all was well with their heart. Time would be a major factor. Gibbon had managed to keep his patient alive with twenty-six minutes of heart–lung machine flow. By the 1980s it had become routine to have surgery and 'extracorporeal' flow lasting several hours. During the same period serious interest in using the heart–lung machine to maintain life in patients in intensive care units with severe lung disease recognised that it would require an oxygenator working for days or even weeks.

To look at the history of this way of using a heart–lung machine we first need to look back to an event in 1952 when doctors in Cincinnati were confronted with a forty-five-year-old fireman with severe fibrotic lung disease, who presented as breathless and very distressed. The team just happened to be building a heart–lung machine and decided to use it on this patient to see if it could help.[19] The circuit of flow was set up to take blood out of two big veins (in the groin in this case), pass it through the oxygenator and return it to two more veins (in an arm). We might call this 'veno-venous' flow. This enabled the blood arriving at the right side of the heart, from where it was pumped to the lungs, to be partially topped up with oxygen so that the patient's lungs had less work to do in further adding oxygen to the blood. They got the flow up to 1.4 litres per minute. The patient's "apprehension, not adequately controlled before pumping, was relieved … and he remained asleep throughout most of the 75 minutes of partial extracorporeal circulation". His distress would have been lessened by an improvement in the oxygen level in his blood. A dose of codeine helped. All the readings on the monitors improved too, from catastrophically bad to simply bad.

Since nearly all of the oxygen carried in blood is bound to haemoglobin molecules in the red cells in blood, the percentage 'saturation' of these haemoglobin molecules is a good measure of how full the blood is with oxygen. In health, in most circumstances, the blood in our arteries has a haemoglobin saturation of above 95 per cent. We can therefore think of it normally being more than 95 per cent full of oxygen. The values of saturation for this patient were alarmingly low. The saturation of the haemoglobin in his arterial blood had risen from about 40 per cent before running the oxygenator to about 60 per cent while it was running. The blood flowing from the machine had a saturation of over 90 per cent, but there was neither enough of it, nor was it flowing for long enough.

Unfortunately, and as you would expect, the symptoms and monitor readings returned to where they had started when the machine was turned off and the patient died a few weeks later. The investigators had not provided this patient with any long-term benefit but concluded that "this trial of a heart–lung apparatus was apparently without harmful effect on the patient".

Here we need a little more physiology to explore the challenge of this approach. If the aim is to support the lungs, then the focus is on getting oxygen into the blood. It is not necessary also to take on the role of the heart to pump blood from the low-pressure veins into the high-pressure arteries because the heart does not need to be replaced or supported. Indeed, keeping away from tubes with high pressures is a very pleasing strategy if leaks are to be avoided. It follows that it should be possible, as in the fireman from Cincinnati, to use an oxygenator to assist with getting oxygen into a patient's blood using connections only to veins – a veno-venous flow.

Normally, a patient's venous blood arriving at their lungs is about 75 per cent full of oxygen and its passage through the lungs takes it to close to 100 per cent. Because it starts off three-quarters full as it enters the lungs from the veins, each litre of blood can only take up a fairly small amount of oxygen from the lungs. It is consequently necessary to load up the full flow of blood around the body (the cardiac output) of about 5 litres per minute to get enough oxygen into the patient to keep them alive. You cannot overfill a smaller flow of blood because the haemoglobin molecules that carry the oxygen become full, or saturated. Neither can you load up a small flow of blood from 0 to 100 per cent because the body could not tolerate blood close to 0 per cent saturation.

You might therefore spot the problem. Taking out venous blood and returning it back to the tree of veins still needs a large flow of about 5 litres per minute to take over totally from the patient's own lungs. But there is a problem in taking a large flow out of big veins and returning it to big veins: the blood tends to recirculate from one vein to another vein, entering the oxygenator too full of oxygen (well above the normal venous 75 per cent) to take up much more. The reason for this recirculation is that extracting a high flow of blood from a vein causes blood in that vein to be drawn *backwards* against its normal direction of flow towards the right side of the heart. Because the large veins are interconnected this then risks drawing into the oxygenator some of the blood that has just been returned to the patient from the oxygenator.

The Cincinnati doctors had a flow out of and into their patient, on their own estimation, of "one-fourth to one-third of the cardiac output" of fairly well-oxygenated blood; this only raised the patient's arterial blood saturation to 60 per cent. Had they been able to get a much livelier flow, they would have been able to get more oxygen into the patient's body, but recirculation might have set in. We shall see that more recent attempts to oxygenate blood in a similar way have met with the same challenge.

Let us call this 'extracorporeal lung support' (ECLS), whatever way the catheters draining blood out of, and perfusing blood into, the patient are arranged, and look at how well ECLS has progressed since the fireman of 1952. Without a doubt the inspirational drive for this therapy was from the surgeon Robert 'Bob' Bartlett of the University of Michigan, a remarkable innovator who came to visit us in Oxford in 1993. Newborns were the group in which his team developed ECLS, with their first survivor at the Orange Country Medical Centre in California in 1975 being a one-day old 'baby Esperanza', as she was named by staff (her mother having fled the hospital because she thought that her baby would not survive).[20]

Born in 1939, and educated at the University of Michigan Medical School, Bartlett was at the time a young surgical resident on the faculty of the Irvine School of Medicine and responsible for paediatrics. He was busy developing a heart–lung circuit, which was applied to Esperanza for six days and after a further two days she was breathing entirely on her own. As I write, she is alive and well and a mother of three. Bartlett, now in his eighties, has enjoyed introducing her at conferences around the world. "If it wasn't for me there would be no Dr Bartlett," she said at one meeting, then laughed. "I mean, if there was no Dr Bartlett, there'd be no me."

By the end of 1986, 715 newborns had been treated in eighteen centres in the United States. The survival rate was 81 per cent and showed an interesting improvement with experience in individual hospitals during their first twenty cases.[21] This fits with the technical complexity, which requires staff to learn new ways of placing cannulae in blood vessels, manage the flow of blood outside the body, keep the body temperature safe and nurse tiny wriggling patients connected to rather large machines. The babies were treated for a range of problems involving both heart and lungs.

At the moment of birth, the circulation undergoes a near miraculous spontaneous replumbing from that of the foetus 'breathing from its mother', as it were, to the newborn breathing air. Inside its mother's womb, the foetus has very little blood flowing to its own lungs because these contain no air. It picks up the oxygen it needs by pumping blood to the placenta, where oxygen diffuses from the mother's blood into the blood of the foetus. At birth, when the child starts to breathe and inflate their lungs, and the placenta is detached, this needs to change dramatically: the closure of a blood vessel in the foetus called the *ductus arteriosus* helps to force a large flow of blood into the lungs, a process helped by the closure of a hole in the heart called the *foramen ovale*. (Incidentally, the airways of lungs in the foetus are full of liquid, so the first breaths are a sort of 'undrowning' in which they have to be cleared of water and filled with air.)

I myself was fortunate to have achieved this amazing birth transition on the day Gibbon was operating in 1953. However, in some newborns a so-called 'persistent foetal circulation' occurs. It may take days to make the switch to the new circulation, particularly if the birth is premature. In the case of baby Esperanza, despite some surgery while on the ECLS to close a 'patent *ductus arteriosus*' (she had a particular problem with this part of the foetal plumbing that is not needed, or wanted, after birth), she needed six days on extra-corporeal circulation and then two days on a ventilator before being ready to breathe on her own via her own lungs.

In the 715 cases reported by Bartlett and his team up to 1986, problems treated using ECLS included aspiration of meconium (foetal faeces) into the lungs during birth and insufficiency of the normal 'surfactant' secreted to line the inner surface of the young lungs.[21] As the small airways of the lungs (called alveoli) empty of liquid after birth, they have to become coated with a soap-like substance called surfactant for them to stay nicely expanded in the presence of air. This is because surface tension in the tiny lung alveoli tends to make them squeeze shut unless the tension between the air and the inner lining of the alveoli is reduced. Surfactant is secreted by the lungs themselves while they also absorb liquid from the alveoli using a remarkable pumping mechanism we have studied in the laboratory. I shall describe more of those efforts in Chapter Three.

Another problem among the 715 newborns treated using ECLS was a condition called 'diaphragmatic hernia' in which there is a defect in the diaphragm, which normally separates the contents of the abdomen from the contents of the chest. A defect, or hernia, allows the bowel to bulge up into the chest, squash one of the lungs, and prevent lung maturation. It requires surgical repair. A final group among the 715 was those with sepsis, requiring antibiotics as well as support to their lungs.[21]

Survival rates looked impressive, but who was to know whether the babies would have survived without all the tubes, pumps and plastic membranes? The trouble with having treatment that you are convinced works well is that it is not ethical to deny it to anybody who needs it. To take an extreme example, parachutes have not been subjected to a prospective randomised trial because there is good reason to believe that they save lives (even if cases of survival after falling from a great height without one have been reported).

How can we tell whether a treatment works?

Classical medical ethics tells us that the best therapy for a patient is the conventional one until another is shown to be better. The standard approach to evaluating a new medical therapy of unknown efficacy is to ask a patient (or a person responsible for the patient) for permission to enter them into a trial in which they are allocated randomly to either the new medical therapy or to conventional treatment. Avoidance of bias is possible by having both the patient and the medical staff caring for the patient unaware of which group they are allocated to.

Randomisation to one of two therapies is arguably only ethical if those conducting a trial of this kind do not know whether the new therapy is more or less efficacious than the conventional treatment. There has to be genuine uncertainty. But those who expend much time and effort developing a new therapy usually have an expectation of its superiority, so in modern trials there is much emphasis on the involvement of independent adjudicators on the design of a study and its implementation. In the case of something like ECLS, this level of refinement is clearly not usually achievable.

How to assess the efficacy of ECLS therefore became a substantial ethical issue for its developers. They sought a way of conducting a trial that would provide a genuine comparison with the normal therapy while reducing the risk of exposing patients to the less efficacious of the two. Reluctance to do the usual sort of randomisation of babies into two groups, one group getting ECLS and one group getting conventional therapy, led to a rather odd trial being conducted by Bartlett and colleagues in Michigan in 1985.[22] This design was called "randomised play-the-winner". In this method the chance of randomly assigning an infant to one treatment or the other is influenced by the outcome of the preceding patients in the study. This approach had been theoretically possible since 1969 but had never actually been used in a clinical trial.

Bartlett's trial recruited twelve infants. The first patient was randomly assigned to ECLS and survived. The second patient was randomly assigned to conventional therapy and died. The protocol then dictated that the odds of the next patient being randomly assigned ECLS changed to 3:1. This third patient received ECLS and survived. From that point the progressively changing odds of the protocol randomisations allocated ECLS to the remaining nine patients who all survived. Hence the trial led to the rather bizarre outcome of one control patient (the second, who died) and eleven ECLS patients (all of whom survived).[22] Both the design and the result stirred up controversy.

Four years later doctors in Boston published results of a similar trial but with modified design. This first had a small phase of conventional 50:50 randomisation of patients followed by a phase of 'nothing but' what was best after the first phase, and provided more fuel for the fire of controversy. In this trial, twenty-eight of twenty-nine ECLS patients survived (97 per cent) and six of ten who received conventional therapy survived (60 per cent). This seemed to have settled the matter and ECLS has become a standard management for some severely sick newborns, mainly in the United States and some European hospitals.

Interestingly, the type of design used in these small studies has not caught on in other clinical trials; a UK trial using a conventional 50:50 design in 185 newborns found that the relative risk of death in patients allocated ECLS was 0.55, putting the therapy well ahead of its rivals and confirming the experience in the United States.[23]

Grown-ups versus babies

Newborns are a special case because only they have to rearrange their circulation at birth in order to start breathing air. What about other age groups? Here the history is more complicated. Whereas newborns may be beset by particular problems of breathing when born, older age groups face their own characteristic lung problems. One of these has become known as acute respiratory distress syndrome (ARDS) and a version of it became widely familiar during the Covid-19 pandemic. The condition, which may follow all sorts of insults to the body including viral infections, is one of severe failure of the lung to do its job of gas exchange.

What seems to happen in ARDS is that an inflammatory condition in the blood attacks the fine tissue of the lung. One consequence is that the delicate membrane of thin tissue separating the blood in small vessels (or capillaries) from the air in the tiny alveoli becomes leaky, causing alveoli in some parts of the lung to fill with fluid seeping out of the capillaries. Another feature is that the cells lining the alveoli that secrete the surfactant become damaged and a deficiency in surfactant leads to some alveoli collapsing shut and therefore failing to ventilate with air. During the Covid-19 pandemic we have become familiar with hearing about this sort of insult to the lungs: patients have extreme difficulty breathing and despite their best efforts the oxygen level in their blood can become life-threateningly low.

In 1979 a trial of ECLS in ARDS, mostly in patients with pneumonia, put further use in adults under wraps for some years. Ninety patients with severe ARDS were studied in nine centres in the United States and were divided into two groups: conventional mechanical ventilation of the lungs or ECLS. In each group 90 per cent died. A sense of hopelessness set in, like that in the early days of heart–lung machine failures. All sorts of reasons were given for failure, including that of the learning curve of twenty we noted earlier, which was repeated in the many centres.[24]

For the trial of 1979, and other trials that we need to consider, I must make clear what is meant by 'conventional' therapy. If we look at the history of patients being helped to breathe when they had lost the capacity to do so themselves, we find two approaches. These were both introduced during the polio epidemics of the 1950s when it was realised that temporarily helping patients with their breathing gave an opportunity to recover and survive. One approach was called the 'iron lung'. This device surrounded the body below the neck and applied intermittent suction to draw the chest and abdominal wall outwards and encourage air to move into the lungs. It is sometimes called 'negative pressure ventilation'. It became used widely in the United States and Britain.

The second approach, developed in Scandinavia, involved blowing air into the lungs with each breath, via the patient's trachea (windpipe). Access to the trachea was via a tube inserted through the nose or mouth (an endotracheal tube) or via a surgical tracheostomy in the neck. This is termed 'positive pressure ventilation'. Positive pressure ventilation eventually became the mainstay of assisting patients with respiratory failure and so conventional therapy in trials of ECLS in ARDS (and respiratory failure in the newborn) involves intubation of the trachea and mechanical positive pressure ventilation to drive air into the lungs. The sophistication of the ventilators that achieve this has improved dramatically, so the ECLS with which trials make a comparison is facing a moving target as technology develops, a fact that may account for some of the results we shall see below.

Next on this scene was a colourful character, Luciano Gattinoni from Milan, a gruff heavy-smoking intensivist who came up with a new way of not breathing. While visiting Bethesda in the United States, Gattinoni set about showing that you can fully oxygenate the blood of an anaesthetised sheep via its own lungs for twenty-four hours *without it breathing at all.*[25] This work was done with Theodor (Ted) Kolobow who built the experimental lung they used. Kolobow was a refugee from Estonia, born in 1931 to a Russian Orthodox priest. The year 1940 saw Hitler's pact with Stalin that enabled both parties to invade Eastern Europe but from opposite directions. The Kolobow family found relative safety in a refugee camp in Augsburg where Ted stayed until 1949, when he emigrated to the United States with $20 in his pocket. Study of mathematics and physics was followed by medical training and exposure to one of the teams developing heart–lung machines. The product for which Kolobow became most famous was a lung made from a coiled envelope of silicone membrane that could work reliably over long periods of time.[26] His experiment with Gattinoni, in sheep not breathing for twenty-four hours, was a combination of brilliant ideas and good technology.

Let me try to explain why this result was amazing at the time, and why it seized our imagination. What they showed might have been predicted as rather banal from basic physiology but nobody had really thought it through before. We normally breathe *in and out* to take oxygen *into* the body, and breathe carbon dioxide (the gas molecules produced when oxygen reacts with body foods and fuels to generate energy) *out of* the body. This is because, to keep alive, we need every minute to get about 250 ml of oxygen (the volume of a coffee mug) and we have to dispose of about 200 ml of carbon dioxide. If an extracorporeal lung is used not to oxygenate the blood but just to remove carbon dioxide from the blood, it turns out that we no longer need to move our natural lungs at all. The extracorporeal lung does the job of removing the 200 ml per minute of carbon dioxide that our body needs to get rid of while our own lungs can still take up the oxygen the body needs. They do not need to move; they just need to be supplied with oxygen, which can flow freely down the trachea and be taken up from the alveoli by diffusion into the blood, to still give us the 250 ml of oxygen we need every minute. This approach goes by the name 'apnoeic oxygenation', meaning oxygen uptake without breathing.

Blood, whether from veins or arteries, contains a lot of carbon dioxide: about 500 ml of gas per litre of blood. Our artificial lung can easily remove all the carbon dioxide our body needs to get rid of each minute (about 200 ml per minute) from a flow of blood of only 1 litre per minute, well below the high flow of about 5 litres per minute needed for oxygenation of the blood. This means that the blood flow to the artificial lung can be kept low, which in turn means that smaller cannulae can be used in the blood vessels. It also follows that the flow can be from one vein to another, and cannulation of high-pressure arteries can be avoided. In 1984 in Oxford we explored this behaviour in anaesthetised dogs, finding how the gas flowing through the artificial lung set the levels of oxygen in the animal's arterial blood.[27]

So why the fuss over an apparently obscure eccentricity in respiratory physiology? Gattinoni saw that this offered the possibility of easing off mechanical ventilation or completely resting the lungs of patients with ARDS, while using a low flow of blood through an artificial lung from vein to vein. This greatly reduced the complexity of the procedure. It became the Italian brand of ECLS, called 'low-frequency positive-pressure ventilation with extracorporeal carbon dioxide removal' or LFPPV–ECCO$_2$R for short. The Italian team reported survival of twenty-one out of forty-three very sick patients in 1986.[28] They went on to advocate their approach in conferences throughout the world. In 1988 I myself attempted to build some enthusiasm for it in the UK with an editorial in the *British Medical Journal.*[29]

In 1986 our Oxford–Geneva team set to work to explore this

brand of respiratory support further. One emphasis was on whether our pulsing lung would work well for many hours in dogs and was studied by Jean-Patrice Gardaz and his team in Geneva. It did, but we were unclear whether some changes over nine hours in the dogs were due more to barbiturate anaesthesia than the function of the lung itself.[30] Also in Geneva, Mike Sinclair, an anaesthetist from Oxford, led a study of how well an extract of Malayan pit viper venom could stop blood clotting in the plastic circuit.[31] In Oxford we were joined from the United States by student Karen McRae, working on her master's degree, and set about seeing whether human red blood cells rupture when subjected to the very low levels of carbon dioxide that occur where blood flows out of the membrane lung in the 'Gattinoni' technique.[32] This seemed not to be a problem. I am pleased to report that Karen went on to be a thoracic anaesthesiologist in Toronto with expertise in ECLS.

We then got busy in Oxford with an ambitious project to apply the Gattinoni technique to a 'newborn-sized' laboratory model of respiratory failure. This small randomised trial used the 'apnoeic oxygenation' method in anaesthetised rabbits weighing about 2.5 kg to compare a group having the therapy with a group given conventional treatment. We allowed one breath per hour (we thought of it as a 'sigh') for six hours in animals whose lungs had been depleted of surfactant to make them similar to lungs with inadequate development in newborn humans born prematurely. A striking difference was apparent; the animals on ECLS remained stable for six hours, while those having mechanical ventilation deteriorated, four of six dying within six hours.[33] This trial was a bit like a parachute trial because it was known that ventilating surfactant-depleted lungs damaged them further, so it was a no-brainer that not ventilating them would leave them the potential to recover.

Questions arose about how best to look after the sick lungs during the Gattinoni support. Should they be given an occasional sigh, or left totally motionless? I was joined for many happy hours in the laboratory by fellow anaesthetist Fiona Ratcliffe to make some progress in that direction.[34, 35] I look back upon that time as a rare opportunity to both publish with the wife of a future Nobel Prize-winner and (later) with the winner himself.

Conferences provide a lively way of meeting fellow researchers. Jean-Patrice accompanied me to Paris to deliver our results. Keith

Sykes took me to speak in Stockholm, where I was regally entertained because he was so distinguished. With Karen McRae we explored the delights of New York and the American Society for Artificial Internal Organs. Nearer home the Anaesthetic Research Society gave opportunity for Fiona Ratcliffe in Bristol and Karen in London to present their results.

Now, a long way removed from these weeks in the laboratory and the flurry of meetings, I can look back and ask myself whether anything useful was achieved and what subsequent progress has been made. Later topsy-turvy developments in the field make this assessment difficult.

Four trials and then Covid-19

Optimism in the field of ECLS led to experiments in laboratories all over the world. When I presented results from our Oxford study of surfactant deficiency in New York in 1987, Dr Alan Morris from Salt Lake City asked me some details of the experiments and then remarked, "Thank you very much. This is now the second randomised study, both of which suggest that those of us interested in doing clinical trials better hurry up." It turned out that Alan Morris's own trial in patients with ARDS was another big step in the field of ECLS in adults, although perhaps more of a step sideways than forwards.

Morris had designed a randomised trial to compare the best available mechanical ventilation at the time with the Gattinoni $ECCO_2R$ technique. His emphasis was on having similar monitoring in both groups, decisions being made according to computer protocols in order to try to remove human bias from the trial. Limiting the study to a single centre helped to ensure consistency. The results came in 1994: of nineteen patients having conventional treatment, eight survived; of twenty-one patients receiving the $ECCO_2R$, seven survived. Statistical analysis showed no significant difference between the groups but the suggestion was that the overall survival rate of 38 per cent was about four times higher than would be expected from historical data from patients so sick with ARDS. The extracorporeal circulation on its own had not been shown to confer benefit. Dr Morris became an advocate of the protocol-driven decision-making that seemed to have achieved the improvement in survival in both arms of the study, while advocating that ECLS treatments should "be restricted to controlled clinical trials".[36] We shall see similar caution more recently repeated by him.

After a further fifteen years the UK stepped up to provide its own assessment of ECLS in adult patients, the so-called CESAR trial, published in 2009.[37] This was based on patients presenting in the years 2001–6, and as we look further into what happened we shall note the interchangeable use of the terms ECLS and ECMO (extracorporeal membrane oxygenation). Oxygenation of the patient is often foremost in people's minds, so 'ECMO' has reached common parlance. A total of 180 patients were recruited and randomised in equal numbers to conventional management or referral to a single centre in Leicester, which provided veno-venous ECLS. An interesting feature of the design was that patients "allocated for consideration for treatment" by ECLS were not all actually given that treatment; they were first retrieved from the hospital in which they were initially being managed and transported to Leicester. They were then reviewed on conventional ventilation in Leicester, and only then administered ECLS if appropriate according to the protocol. This led to 75 per cent of those allocated for consideration being given the extracorporeal support. Of those initially 'considered' for ECLS, 63 per cent survived. This compares with 47 per cent of those not considered, and consequently receiving conventional management.

This result caused quite a stir. If we look at those who actually received ECLS (sixty-eight patients), we find that forty-three survived to six months (51 per cent). Of those managed without ECLS (112 patients), sixty survived (54 per cent). The detected outcome depends on how it is measured. In assessing the possible merits of ECLS used in the 2009 influenza (H1N1) epidemic, Alan Morris was vocal about the CESAR trial lacking explicit methods. Assessing the three trials to date (his own included), he concluded that "the benefits of ECMO treatment in A(H1N1)-related lung failure are unproven and therefore cannot be considered rescue therapy".[38] It will come as no surprise that this viewpoint was counter to that of Dr Bartlett and his team in a 'for-and-against' debate in the same journal.[39] In the Bartlett piece, an emphasis on progressively improving outcomes in some patients, and the refinements over time in extracorporeal technologies, went with a positive outlook. "The art and the science each have their individual limitations. Taken together, they support inclusion of ECMO as part of a comprehensive algorithm for refractory adult respiratory failure."

Now shift to 2018: it was time for a European perspective and a trial of ECLS was funded by the French Ministry of Health. Again, it was in severe ARDS and veno-venous ECLS was used.[40] Mortality was measured at sixty days. Of 124 patients receiving ECLS, 35 per cent died; of 125 patients given conventional treatment, 46 per cent died. Statistical analysis found this not to be a significant difference. Another huge piece of work had led to a disappointing outcome for those looking to the newer therapy to help these patients.

Move on another four years and we can be astonished at what now happens. The world has a Covid-19 pandemic and the most common cause of death is from a pneumonia that is a type of ARDS. According to the world registry for ECLS in Covid-19 patients, more than 16,000 patients have been (or are being) treated with this therapy and the in-hospital mortality rate is 47 per cent.[41] Various approaches are being used around the world, including many now that are veno-venous (similar to the Gattinoni approach; Figure 3) and some that are veno-arterial, more similar to Bartlett's original therapy in newborns.[42] We ask ourselves: does all this extracorporeal support really work?

Rumination

There are sufficient mortality numbers in this chapter. It is now time to reflect, and I wish to consider two interrelated questions. The first is whether ECLS is a useful therapy in adults with respiratory failure; the second is whether my own long hours in the laboratory were usefully spent. In my early medical career, I, with others, occupied many months developing the methods of artificial lung support for use in respiratory failure. We believed that we were doing something really useful; it was certainly interesting. Much of a book I wrote on mathematical analysis of gas exchange was devoted to work on artificial lungs.[43] However, the large labour-intensive trials of using this technology in adult patients have failed to convince me of benefit, and yet the use of ECLS in the Covid-19 pandemic has become almost routine even in the UK. One might note an astonishing disconnect between the work put in, the evidence of benefit and the widespread application.

Did our work in Oxford help to move the subject along? Citations of publications in the literature are conventionally used to assess research 'impact'. As I write, the CESAR trial of 2009 attracts about 2,500 citations, the Morris trial of 1994 a little over 1,000. My co-investigators of ECLS and I have struggled to make fifty citations from a few modest papers. One contribution that I like to think might have some lasting benefit, if ECLS survives, is a study I enjoyed with my good friend and intensivist Duncan Young. In sheep, we used a sort of kidney dialysis circuit, taking blood from a large artery through a lung and returning it to a large vein to assess how much carbon dioxide exchange could be achieved with and without a pump to assist the flow.[44] The answer was quite a lot, even with a low flow. Others have found this idea attractive. Interestingly, Kolobow and Gattinoni also used the arterio-venous mode of circuit in sheep in their 'alternative to breathing' paper of 1978; it enabled them to make sure that their extracorporeal lung contributed essentially no oxygenation of the blood (arterial blood being already full of oxygen), so that they could show you could stop breathing and still oxygenate your own blood adequately via your own natural lungs.[25]

But 'dialysing out' carbon dioxide is only going to help with a patient's oxygenation of the blood if their own lungs are capable of benefiting from a rest from mechanical ventilation. The whole approach of ECLS is dependent on the concept that the lungs may heal if given the time to do so, and without damage being caused by mechanical ventilation of the lungs, which is unavoidable in conventional therapy. Despite the large numbers of patients with Covid-19 being treated with ECLS, I do wonder whether we shall ever know if it can really be regarded as an efficacious therapy and doing, as Alan Morris reminds us therapies should, "more good than harm".[38, 45]

Given that heart–lung machines are so widely used, whether in the operating theatre or as support for patients with respiratory failure, the question needs to be asked: what is required for their use to be beneficial? John Gibbon dedicated decades to his heart–lung machine and after his single success in 1953 he had two failures leading to patient deaths and gave up further work on it. Despite that halting start, the use of the heart–lung machine for open-heart surgery is now an unquestioned benefit and in daily use. It was never subjected to a prospective randomised trial; it couldn't be, because you cannot open the heart without it.

A retired colleague provides a frequent reminder to me of the efficacy of modern cardiac surgery. He was recently kept alive for over two hours on a heart–lung machine during the repair of cardiac valves. At his follow-up, there seemed to be more concern from the surgeon about the neatness of the scar on his chest than anything else, such has become the routine nature of this remarkable surgery. Clearly, the heart–lung machine is not a cure on its own. It requires the surgeon's hands to reverse the underlying pathology.

Contrast the use of the heart–lung machine, alias ECLS, in the newborn with their various forms of respiratory and cardiac insufficiency. Here some of the underlying disease processes are potentially self-correcting if ECLS can support the patient long enough for this to occur. The immature lung slowly matures and insufficiency of surfactant may be reversed by the lung's own secretion. Alternatively, surgical repairs, such as the closure of the *ductus arteriosus*, as in patient Esperanza, or the repair of a hernia in the diaphragm can deal with the underlying problem. Here again, the heart–lung machine is a means to an end, not a therapy in isolation.

The picture in long-term adult respiratory support seems very different. Since the brief experience in a Cincinnati fireman with lung disease in 1952, there have been four major prospective randomised trials of ECLS in ARDS patients, not one of which has demonstrated clear benefit compared with the more conventional mechanical ventilation of the lungs. Despite this, the Covid-19 pandemic has seen the greatest upsurge ever in the use of ECLS. In Covid-19, as in other causes of ARDS, there are no surgeon's hands; the hope is that supporting life for long enough will provide the opportunity for the lung to do its own healing. Indeed, it is interesting to note that patients who survive ARDS often do show remarkable healing of the lungs, suggesting that such reversal is indeed possible. But how long is long enough?

The Bartlett approach emphasises the mix of 'art and science' to enhance gradually the efficacy of ECLS. The science has indeed moved on. Earlier I listed Melrose's method of oxygenation of the blood sloshing down the inside of a spinning cylinder as version number six and looked to the introduction of a membrane separating blood and gas as number seven. This seventh approach incorporates many forms. Ted Kolobow's introduction of silicone rubber was one such, and a major step forward. He manufactured a 12-metre long envelope of silicone rubber (checked obsessionally to avoid holes) wrapped up into a spiral coil in the style of a large Swiss roll sponge cake.[46] It was so kind to the blood that it was widely used for long-term extracorporeal circulation for many years.

Perhaps the 'capillary membrane lung' is sufficiently distinctive by itself to earn an eighth place in the way of achieving gas exchange. In this arrangement, a dense bundle of very fine capillary tubes is somewhat similar to the natural lung's own vessels. Versions either have blood flowing down the tubes with gas on the outside, or have gas flowing down the tubes with blood on the outside. This latter arrangement is the current fashion for ECLS; an example is shown in Figure 3.[47, 48] So fine are the tubes that the term 'hollow-fibre oxygena-tor' has caught on. The capillaries, or fibres, have a diameter of about 0.5 mm and are made of polypropylene or polymethylpentene. These use a trick that we already had in our Oxford pulsed-flow lung back in the 1980s: micropores; the manufacturing process has made possi-ble thin tears or slits in the material, which provide direct gas-blood contact but which are small enough to prevent blood cells and other constituents from leaking through to the gas side. This is a cunning way of reducing the resistance of the membrane to the passage of oxygen and carbon dioxide.

Technological advances continue but progress in reversing the pathology of the lung in ARDS remains limited. The efficacy of dexa-methasone, which has recently been observed in severe Covid-19, may be a hopeful indicator of some progress in finding the 'sur-geon's hands' in ARDS, or at least some types of this unrelenting disease.[49] The UK's favourite children's author Michael Rosen recently recounted his hospital experience of having to decide whether to be intubated and ventilated for his Covid-19 pneumonia. "I was told as I went under there was a 50:50 chance of survival. And I asked, 'What chance have I got without it?' And they said none. So I said, 'Oh well. That's at least a one in two.'"[50]

Given the results of the ECLS trials, it is worth considering what our response would be to an offer of extracorporeal lung support. The 50:50 keeps popping up there too. I'm still not sure what I would decide.

I need, finally, to answer my two questions: is ECLS a useful therapy in adults with respiratory failure, and did my long hours in the laboratory have any impact? I tend to side with Alan Morris in thinking that the published evidence does not show a convincing benefit of ECLS in adult respiratory failure, but I would like to go along with Bartlett and Gattinoni in assuming that gradual technological development might allow it to be maintained in patients with ARDS for sufficiently long to permit their lungs to recover. I fear, however, that the wind is not set fair for the conduct of a trial in Covid-19 or other causes of ARDS because of the way it has become established in many centres throughout the world. Perhaps a new medical therapy for ARDS needs to evolve first before giving patients longer to recover by using ECLS.

With regard to my 'impact', if a Morris study cited 2,500 times cannot prevent an unproven therapy being used in over 16,000 Covid-19 patients, I'm not sure that counting the few citations of our own work in Oxford can tell us whether any of our efforts were useful. That work was certainly educational for those involved, as we can see from the subsequent careers of participants, including clinical expertise they have employed with patients during their hospital work. Perhaps it is those patients who have been the main beneficiaries of all that effort in the laboratory.

In this chapter we have seen the heart–lung machine as something with both proven efficacy and contested usefulness. The following chapters will expound further examples of where medical science has made real progress and others where the benefits have been illusory or elusive.

CHAPTER TWO

MABEL'S BAROMETER

A Centenarian and a Century of High-Altitude Physiology

Oxford's first woman student of Physiology

The daily hallway stroll to my office inside the building we colloquially call 'Physiology' takes me past Mabel's barometer (Fig. 4). As you might expect from the tendency in universities to meddle with appellations and merge faculties, the current name for the building is much longer (Department of Physiology, Anatomy & Genetics: Sherrington Building), but it is nice to use the name that Mabel herself would have recognised.

Mabel's aneroid barometer is like a piece of jewellery: a circular brass case with a glass face, which you could mistake for a heavy Edwardian pocket watch were you not to take a closer look; this shows only one large 'hand' or pointer. The dial reads in two units: inches and feet. The inches are of mercury, the pointer thereby indicating the atmospheric pressure. These units may seem odd; they hark back to the time when the standard way of measuring atmospheric pressure was to see to what height in inches it could support a vertical column of the heavy liquid metal mercury in a glass tube immersed in a bowl of mercury. The feet indicated on the dial are in thousands and identify the altitude associated with that atmospheric pressure; it can therefore be used as an altimeter.

The barometer belonged to Mabel Purefoy FitzGerald, a remarkable scientist and a strong role model in this time of re-evaluating the contribution of women to science. It sits in a glass display cabinet in which members of the department like to show visitors artefacts from the past of Oxford's Physiology. It accompanied her during the 1911 Anglo-American Pikes Peak Expedition in Colorado as she studied the breathing of 131 mountainside residents at twelve different altitudes; one of the great classic papers on mountain physiology resulted. In 2011, on the centenary of the expedition, I and some colleagues took Mabel's barometer on a pilgrimage to Pikes Peak, in a scientific quest that Mabel herself would probably have liked to join. At the summit (14,100 ft; 4,300 m) it read for us 18.05 inches of mercury, close to the 18.11 inches Mabel herself had recorded in 1911.[1] The barometer was in good shape after 100 years and it got safely back to Oxford. In its present home, on most days, it reads about 30 inches of mercury and agrees perfectly with mete-orological data from the BBC. In that sense it offers an alternative to the internet.

Mabel Purefoy FitzGerald was born in 1872 into a family of country gentry in the village of Preston Candover in Hampshire. The name Purefoy had been preserved within the family since the death in 1847 of a childless George Purefoy Jervoise, said to have been Jane Austen's dancing partner;[2] in his will he had specified that the name be carried on with the inheritance of property, which passed via his brother. Mabel was four generations on from George and the young-est child of seven: two sons and five daughters. Both her parents died when she was twenty-two years old. She spent much of 1896 living with her grandmother not far from Oxford and it was during this time that she seems to have set her mind on a career in laboratory medical science. She moved into Oxford, sharing a house with her sisters at 12 Crick Road. Next door, at number 11, lived a leading phys-iologist of the age, John Scott Haldane, with whom she was destined to conduct her most important science. Ironically, they seem not to have made each other's acquaintance until some years later, by which time Haldane had moved to a larger property some distance away. Perhaps neighbours then could be as dismissive towards each other as they can be today.

Mabel first studied chemistry and biology. By 1897 she was attend-ing university lectures in physiology and soon developed expertise in histology while undertaking research in the Physiological Labo-ratory. Her later work was to lead to twelve scientific papers in the next decade, several under her own name alone.[3] Future Nobel lau-reate Charles Sherrington wrote that he was "greatly struck by the thoroughness, untiring zeal, and truly critical spirit" of her research pursuits. It is perhaps not surprising that Haldane became acquainted with FitzGerald even though they had not done so as neighbours in Crick Road; they both worked in the same building.

Haldane was a 'human physiologist', interested in experimentation related to mining, diving, and the regulation of breathing. Something drew FitzGerald away from her microscope to get her interested in measurements on humans, herself included. She became expert at using apparatus devised by Haldane to measure the pressure of carbon dioxide in the gas in the lungs of human volunteers. This measurement was of great interest as it provided an indirect measure of breathing, or strictly what we call 'ventilation': the number of litres of gas moving into and out of the lungs every minute, a number normally around 5 litres per minute, representing ten excursions of the chest each minute, each one of about 0.5 litre.

Now enters a little more respiratory physiology: one role of breathing is to remove from the body molecules of carbon dioxide which are generated by our body's metabolism. Inspired atmospheric air contains very little carbon dioxide; as a percentage of the air this is around 0.04 per cent (a rising concentration of immense consequence to global heating but too small to be noticed directly by the body). Gas in the lungs of a person close to sea level usually contains about 5 per cent of carbon dioxide. There is consequently a difference of around a hundred-fold between the percentage inside and outside the lungs, allowing the breathing in and out of gas – ventilation – to flush carbon dioxide out of the body.

Metabolism generates a fairly constant number of carbon dioxide molecules each minute unless we are exerting ourselves. If ventilation changes, the percentage of carbon dioxide deep in the lungs changes, thereby keeping what carbon dioxide we breathe out equal to what we generate by metabolism. Thus, for example, if a person doubles his or her ventilation from 5 to 10 litres per minute, we would anticipate the percentage of carbon dioxide in the lungs and the expired gas to halve to 2.5 per cent (after a delay of about fifteen minutes in which a new steady state is attained).

It turns out that the precise relationship between ventilation and the amount of carbon dioxide in the lungs, valid whatever the atmospheric pressure or altitude, is one between ventilation and the *pressure* of carbon dioxide in the lungs. This is why Mabel and Haldane were taking care to measure pressure, and why the barometer was a vital piece of equipment needed for this measurement.

You may wonder why breathing could not be measured directly. It could be, but such measurements of the excursions of the chest involved very cumbersome apparatus suited only to a laboratory setting. Measurements of carbon dioxide pressure could be done with portable apparatus within three or four minutes. They turned out to be remarkably informative.

Haldane had used his apparatus to show that individuals tended to breathe in such a manner as to keep the carbon dioxide pressure deep in the lungs remarkably constant. This had previously been demonstrated in experiments in which he and his co-investigator John Priestley made measurements on themselves on brief visits to the bottom of Dalcoath Mine in Cornwall (2,240 ft below sea level), and the top of Ben Nevis (4,406 ft above sea level), and in a compression chamber at the Brompton Hospital in London where patients were treated with compressed air.

Mabel FitzGerald was acknowledged for help she gave to supplementary experiments in Oxford, notably just one measurement on a woman ("Mrs G") and one on a child, Haldane's ten-year-old son Jack.[4] This small number of volunteers raised the question of how the pressure of carbon dioxide in the lungs might vary between individuals, and it was Mabel's intention to find out.

At a time when human experimentation on healthy women and children was almost unknown, she measured the carbon dioxide pressure in the lungs of 32 women, 27 men, 16 boys and 11 girls. The children included Haldane's son Jack and daughter Naomi (aged seven), some of the children being recruited from Jack's nearby school. The main finding was that the average pressure was about 8 per cent higher in men than in women and children. In other words, men breathe less.[5]

But where does the barometer come into all this, and how did a high mountain in Colorado come to be involved? First, the barometer was a vital part of making the measurements of the pressure of carbon dioxide in the lungs. The reason for this was that Haldane's apparatus gave the *percentage* of carbon dioxide in the gas sample and to calculate the actual *pressure* it was necessary to know atmospheric pressure, very precisely. Second, mountains became relevant because they were being discovered in a new way.

Mountains as a physiology laboratory

The second half of the nineteenth century saw an explosion of interest in mountaineering. Alpine refuges and laboratories were being constructed, like those on the Monte Rosa (4,554 m) and on the summit of Mont Blanc (4,809 m), both built in 1893. Some were accessible by railway (and therefore tourists), such as that on Pikes Peak (4,302 m), on which the cog railway to the summit house was completed in 1891. At the same time interest was forming in the effects of altitude on the human body.

The catastrophe in France in 1875 of two deaths among three occupants during the ascent of the Zenith hydrogen balloon to around 8,000 metres had shown clearly the danger of decompression, which occurs at extreme altitude.[6, 7] Around 1874 the work of Paul Bert in his laboratory in Paris had identified the source of danger as low pressure of oxygen in the lungs, rather than the reduced pressure of the atmosphere at altitude. He used a decompression chamber to lower the ambient pressure in the chamber until the occupant (on one occasion himself) nearly passed out, and found that revival could be achieved by breathing some oxygen delivered at the mouth through a small pipe. This confirmed that it was the oxygen pressure in the lungs that determined how well the low ambient pressure could be tolerated. His experimental volunteers included the two balloonists who were to die in the Zenith a few months later, despite having practised decompression in Bert's laboratory.[8]

For Haldane there were two key questions relating to exposure to high altitude. The first related to why those who stayed at high altitude felt more comfortable as days progressed after the initial ascent. It seemed that humans became accustomed or 'acclimatised' over a number of days or weeks. Haldane wished to measure breathing and other physiological variables over a sufficient duration to explain acclimatisation. If breathing changed during a stay at altitude then his earlier findings down the mine and up on Ben Nevis might not be the full picture of how constant the pressure of carbon dioxide is in the lungs and whether breathing might change with elevation.

The second question related to a particular controversy at the time: a dispute between physiologists in Copenhagen, Cambridge and Oxford concerning whether or not the lungs had the ability to pump or 'secrete' oxygen into the blood from the air inside the tiny alveoli of the lungs to maintain a high blood oxygen level even if the level of oxygen was low in the inspired air. Setting up a laboratory at altitude offered the possibility of settling this dispute.

The Anglo-American Pikes Peak Expedition of 1911 grew from these questions.

Discussions at a conference in Munich in 1910 had raised the possibility of using the hotel on Pikes Peak for a stay of several weeks. This suggestion had come from Yandell Henderson of Yale University while relaxing with Haldane and his Oxford colleague Claude Douglas. Back in Oxford it became apparent that Mabel FitzGerald had useful information. She had visited Colorado twice, and ascended Pikes Peak in 1909. Given her physiological skills and local knowledge, it is not surprising that Haldane invited her to be involved.

Concern about the decorum of Mabel spending five weeks with the four men in confined conditions on the summit was incentive for her to address a third question relating to exposure to high altitude by not staying in the hotel. According to her own account in her 1913 paper:

> Until now, the observations on the changes in the alveolar air and haemoglobin at high altitudes have been practically confined to the various observers and their companions, who were making but a short stay at various heights, and no systematic work has been done on residents, or over a wider range of altitude. For such work Colorado is eminently suitable, as not only are there several readily accessible towns situated at high altitude, but mines, at which the miners both work and live, are to be found up to a height of 13,000 feet.[1]

A third question was therefore: how do long-term residents at altitude breathe? Mabel linked to this question the possibility that the concentration of haemoglobin in the blood might also be affected by living at altitude. In Chapter One we met haemoglobin as the primary means by which oxygen is carried in the blood. Haemoglobin is a protein contained in the red cells in blood. Mabel equipped herself to measure haemoglobin in the blood as well as breathing and her drive for adventure allowed her to explore both in residents at altitude.

While the four male investigators, Haldane and Douglas from Oxford, and Edward Schneider and Henderson from the United States, spent five weeks in luxury at the summit hotel, FitzGerald toured the mountainside, staying in mining establishments where she made measurements on inhabitants who had lived at altitude for months or years. Figure 5 shows Mabel taking a day off her touring in order to be photographed with her male colleagues near the summit hotel on Pikes Peak.

Her trek involved horses and some hardship, though amid spectacular scenery. The apparatus for measuring the carbon dioxide in expired gas had to be light enough to carry on foot and safe when tied to a saddle. At one point it was thought salutary to send it by ropeway to reach miners at Camp Bird Mine while Mabel followed on horseback along a narrow trail on a precipitous incline in landscape that "made the journey most hazardous for the glass gas analyser, to say nothing of human hearts".[9]

The very gas analyser used by Mabel FitzGerald in these altitude studies sits on my desk beside me as I write. It consists of glassware securely fastened in a sturdy wooden box with a height of 31 cm, a width of 20 cm and a depth of 7 cm. When closed, one might mistake it for a bathroom cabinet for housing shaving paraphernalia. On the front door of the box is written one of Mabel's US addresses. It swings open on brass hinges to reveal an impressive row of vertical glass bulbs and tubes furnished with glass taps and linked together with rubber tubing. David O'Connor, our technician, has set about restoring it to its former splendour.

How did this analyser work? A volunteer breathed out gas from the lungs into a tube, from which about 20 ml of gas were drawn into a partially vacuumed glass bulb and captured there by the turn of a tap. Using mercury to manoeuvre the sample of gas around the tubing, the sample was passed to and fro through liquid potash (potassium hydroxide) to remove the carbon dioxide gas. The sample was then returned to the bulb in which it had first been captured and the change in volume brought about by removing the carbon dioxide observed from calibrations on a narrow extension of the bulb, termed a pipette.

The sample was moved around the glassware by the elevation and lowering of a small reservoir of mercury open to the air and connected to the bulb. A vertical brass rack and pinion 'railway' on the inside of the door allowed these movements. For the maintenance of constant temperature, the bulb required a stirred water jacket. Some cunning refinements ensured that the two measurements of sample volume – before and after removing the carbon dioxide – were made at precisely the same temperature, pressure and humidity. In his description of the apparatus in 1901 Haldane alluded to the complex evolution of these refinements going back to 1868 and gave credit to their inventors.[10]

This apparatus has travelled widely. It was taken to the United States by Haldane and Douglas in 1911. Following its use there it returned to Oxford and was found in the house in Crick Road following Mabel's death in 1973. The American physiologist Ralph Kellogg made a request for it to take up residence as a museum piece in the Barcroft Station of the White Mountain Research Center in California, to which it duly travelled back across the Atlantic in 1974. It was unearthed there in a poor state of repair in 2019, and the physiologist Frank Powell kindly returned it to Oxford to rejoin the other equipment once belonging to Mabel. In a nearby laboratory cupboard we still keep the solidly built wooden boxes with White Star Line shipping company labels, in which sit the glass bottles used to transport mercury, potash and other chemicals to Colorado.

What were the results of all this curiosity, transatlantic shipping and precarious travel? Mabel's published chart showed a straight-line relationship between atmospheric pressure and the pressure of carbon dioxide in the alveoli. When the atmospheric pressure high on the mountain was 60 per cent of the sea-level value, the carbon dioxide pressure was 70 per cent of the sea-level value. This indicated that residents high on Pikes Peak had a ventilation of their lungs 43 per cent greater than at sea level. Something must be driving the mountain residents to breathe hard, and that something apparently knew how high they lived. What was seen in the mountain residents did not reflect the earlier measurements of Haldane and Priestley from down the mine and the summit of Ben Nevis.

Mabel's mission was not only to study breathing in mountain residents but also to measure something in the blood, the concentration of haemoglobin. She measured the relationship between atmospheric pressure and the concentration of haemoglobin using blood samples from 128 Colorado residents. Her 'haemoglobinometer' sits next to her barometer in our department's cabinet of curiosities. It involved diluting a tiny sample of blood in a small tube until its colour intensity (judged by holding it up to the light) matched that in a standard tube (Fig. 6). Here another linear relationship was seen; this time a 30 per cent *rise* in haemoglobin concentration was associated with a fall in atmospheric pressure to

60 per cent of the sea-level value. Something appeared to be telling the body to produce more haemoglobin at altitude, and that something also knew how high the body lived. This observation set in motion a century of investigation to find out what might account for this remarkable phenomenon.

Mabel's graphs were later extended by acquiring more data from forty-three residents at lower altitudes (i.e. below 5,000 ft) when she visited North Carolina during the summer of 1913.[11] This confirmed that the graphs showing carbon dioxide pressure and haemoglobin concentration as a function of atmospheric pressure were linear over the whole range of altitudes studied, from sea level up to 4,300 metres. It follows that even residents around sea level have something in their body sensing the altitude at which they live (or something related to it), and not just residents living high in the mountains. Something amazing had been discovered that was functioning in every person on the planet.

Recall that, while Mabel was travelling to mining settlements to study residents of the Colorado mountains, the four male scientists were studying themselves over five weeks after ascending rapidly to 4,300 metres. The results from these summiteers on Pikes Peak complete a picture of the speed and magnitude of human responses to altitude.[12] Measurements over five weeks showed how sensitive the body might be to altitude, and how fast changes in breathing and the blood occurred after the sudden change in altitude. The men measured their own breathing and haemoglobin concentrations, before, during and after their time at the summit. Their measurements of the pressure of carbon dioxide in the lungs showed that breathing changed speedily within the first week of the change in altitude and slowly thereafter. This occurred in both ascent and descent, although in opposite directions of course, breathing increasing with ascent and decreasing with descent. The haemoglobin concentration in the blood followed a similar pattern but changed more slowly, requiring two to three weeks to achieve most of the change.

These changes in both breathing and haemoglobin in the physiologists approached the values that Mabel was also measuring in her highest mountain residents. Overall, the measurements in residents and in visitors gave an indication of both the magnitude and the time course of the effects of altitude on breathing and the blood. What remained to be discovered was the mechanisms that might lie behind these physiological responses. Did the human body have its own internal barometer-altimeter to tell it how high it lived?

Post-war Oxford studies on the control of breathing

Mountains passed me by for the first few years of my life, despite my having been born in the month in which Everest was first climbed, May 1953. But not for long. My father, although having a modest income from the grocery trade, was an enthusiast of family holidays in Switzerland. This was encouraged by having a trustworthy car, which was renewed annually, largely because of his high mileage 'on the road' while visiting retailers. So we enjoyed a brand-new Volkswagen Beetle every year for a decade, not that the car had to make the whole journey unaided; overnight trains from the French channel ports to Lyon made it possible to travel part-way to the mountains with the car on the back of the train. The family photograph album shows me at about the age of four posing in front of serious alps, including the Wetterhorn and the Eiger. Later ski trips as a young adult were not adventurous enough to give one the full experience of the breathlessness of high altitude, though I did notice feeling uncomfortable on getting out of the cable car after rapid ascent to the Klein Matterhorn at nearly 4,000 metres. Interest in the results of the Pikes Peak expedition had to await my appointment to an Oxford university lectureship in 1989, when I started the daily walk past Mabel's barometer.

I had the great fortune to be appointed to succeed the respiratory physiologist Dr Daniel Cunningham in the Laboratory of Physiology (as it was called at that time). I could not help but be intimidated by succeeding someone who both had a distinguished war record in the Royal Army Medical Corps (RAMC) and was a physiologist of international repute. Taking over some of his duties in Physiology and his teaching responsibilities in University College was a huge step forward for me as an aspiring scientist and tutor.

Dan Cunningham was born in India in 1919. He undertook his pre-clinical medical studies at Worcester College in Oxford, completed his clinical studies in Edinburgh in 1943, and became a house physician at the Royal Infirmary there.[13] He joined the RAMC and in the dark of night of D-Day, 5–6 June 1944, he parachuted into Normandy as part of the operation that captured the Pegasus and Orne

Bridges north of Caen. Landing with the chaplain (whose company he did not particularly enjoy), by noon that day he had helped to set up a main dressing station at a farm at the Le Mesnil crossroads, right at the eastern end of the Normandy landings and a mere 300 yards from German positions. Here and over weeks at several other locations he faced enemy gunfire and bombing and had to deal with some dreadful injuries. Even in the relative remoteness from the front line in a camp at Riva Bella by the coast nobody was safe. On 10 August a Junkers 88 German transport plane, which had been shot down, crashed into the camp, killing thirteen and wounding twenty. The dangers of 'friendly fire' were also very real; on 13 June the Le Mesnil dressing station was attacked by two RAF Typhoon aircraft: "They circled round before attacking and completely disregarded the two 20 foot square Geneva Crosses which were prominently displayed".[14] The farmer's wife was killed. On 19 August Lieut. Cunningham was at a casualty collection point near Dozulé when "casualties were coming in rapidly and there was insufficient transport to evacuate them".[14]

Through 1944 and into 1945 Dan continued to serve in the RAMC. Following the armistice, and while still in the army, he contributed to the Oxford Nutrition Survey in Germany and in 1947 returned to Oxford to complete a first-class degree in physiology. He was appointed Radcliffe Medical Fellow at University College in the same year. Years of human respiratory research followed, including learning from Claude Douglas of Pikes Peak fame. His tenured university post as Lecturer in Physiology began in 1952; this separation of college and university appointments is a reminder that these were, and remain, independent institutions within Oxford's educational establishment; they often collaborate but are as frequently in dispute.

Dan Cunningham's research focused on metabolism and the regulation of breathing. The emphasis was on studying how, in fairly short-term experiments, stimuli such as high levels of carbon dioxide (hypercapnia), low levels of oxygen (hypoxia) and exercise worked together to control ventilation. His experiments were in a sense a continuation of those of Haldane and Priestley from the mine and Ben Nevis, except that his laboratory breathing apparatus was built so that it could mimic changes in the pressure of oxygen that occur with changes in altitude and could also force changes in carbon dioxide pressure in the lungs to see how sensitive ventilation was to these stimuli. Dan and his physiologist colleague Brian Lloyd rather shocked the establishment by fitting some mathematical equations to the ventilatory responses of human volunteers to hypoxia and hypercapnia; students to this day are not always grateful to them for the complexity of the 'Lloyd–Cunningham equations'.[15]

A visitor to Oxford in 1959 reminded Brian Lloyd and Dan Cunningham that Haldane had been born in 1860 and suggested that they arrange a centenary symposium in his honour. Being a bit late off the mark for 1960, they managed a jamboree of scientific and social events for 1961. It was in the flurry of organising this conference in Oxford that Dan found Mabel FitzGerald's name in the telephone directory and he was presumably rather surprised that she was both still alive and living nearby in Crick Road.[2] Accordingly, she was a guest of honour at the symposium. Photographs of her appear in the volume of proceedings published in 1963, in which, perhaps not surprisingly, a particularly lucid presentation of those slightly scary Lloyd–Cunningham equations appears alongside many contributions from among those in a spectacular photograph of 101 of the great and good of respiratory physiology of the time.[16] As I look through this 591-page treasure-chest of contributions, I feel sorry for not having attended because I recognise so many names from the history of my subject. (I was, however, only eight years old at the time and more focused on the physiology of safely riding a bicycle than breathing.)

The re-emergence of Mabel FitzGerald from the obscurity of Crick Road into the limelight at the international symposium led a few years later to the university degree she had been unable to obtain earlier in life because until 1920 the University of Oxford did not award degrees to women. She was proposed for an honorary Master of Arts by Richard Doll, Professor of Medicine, and she received this at a special Congregation on 14 December 1972, at the age of 100. On that day Mabel's barometer would have been reading 30.3 inches of mercury. It was windy, raining on and off, and 12 degrees Celsius. The Old Congregation House was not known for warmth. She arrived by ambulance, turned down the offer of brandy before the ceremony, entered the building in her wheelchair, was lauded in Latin, and became the first centenarian to receive an Oxford MA.

Dan Cunningham retired in 1987. It took until 1989 for me, his replacement, to be appointed, and the reason for the delay is revealing of the way these things sometimes work in academia. In short, there was no money, or at least the expectation had developed that college fellowships needed a capital sum from which the interest would support the relatively modest salary of the appointee.

The way the money was found is both partly alarming and also heart-warming. A post-lunch aside at a 1988 summer gathering of current and previous members of University College at the home of Sir David Miers, who had recently been ambassador to the Lebanon, brought up that the college did not have funding to replace Dan Cunningham. Dr Christopher Bateman, a haematologist, recounts that he "put the information to the back of my mind". Towards the end of the year, Christopher Bateman was one of a group who started a hospice in Chichester. There was a church service to celebrate the opening of the hospice around Christmas and as attendees were leaving the church a new trustee of the hospice, Kay Glendinning, approached Bateman and said that her family trust (the Dunhill Medical Trust) had to spend £4 million by the end of the financial year, asking if he had any ideas.

The trust had got into this pleasant dilemma in a round-about way. It had been set up by Kay Glendinning's uncle, Herbert Dunhill, for research into tuberculosis, the disease of which he died in 1950. Management of the trust passed to Kay's mother, Mary Dunhill, who retained all the assets as shares in the family company, Alfred Dunhill. These had multiplied over the next twenty years but had never paid a dividend. When Mary died in 1988, Kay took over looking after the trust and she and her son, Tim Sanderson, decided that it was crazy to have all their eggs in one basket. So they sold most of the shares and put the money on deposit – hence the sudden arrival of lots of income. They were very much aware that charities are meant to spend their income.

Christopher Bateman and George Cawkwell, senior fellow of the college and a classicist, drew up a proposal for a fellowship to be named after Mary Dunhill to submit to Kay Glendinning. She took one look at it and said of course she would support it as her son Tim had been at the college, a fact not previously known to the applicants. At that time, she basically ran the trust on her own and so her word was all that was needed to fund the replacement (me)! Subsequently, as links between medical charities and the tobacco industry became no longer acceptable, the complete diversification of the trust's holdings away from tobacco has been both advisable and pleasing.

The history of this funding is a reminder of the extent to which teaching and research are dependent upon charitable giving. I like to think that 'Uncle Bertie' would approve of our current respiratory physiology as fitting well with his intention for us to better understand tuberculosis. The trust has gone on to fund several of Oxford's medical research projects as well as other appointments.

Dan Cunningham spent thirty years probing the short-term responses of human breathing, and also the circulatory system, to stimuli such as high carbon dioxide, low oxygen, exercise and adrenaline. Some of his experiments were designed to change stimuli within the duration of a single breath. The interest here was to probe the remarkable speed with which breathing can change at the onset of exercise and the way breathing is so closely linked to the severity of exercise. Other responses to stimuli were studied over periods of a few minutes, during which time slower mechanisms have the potential to be involved. Dan notably studied the breathing of Roger Bannister (later Sir Roger) during treadmill exercise in the laboratory. In 1954 they published two papers in the *Journal of Physiology* and on 6 May 1954, the day on which I was appreciating a birthday cake with a single candle, Roger Bannister ran his sub-four-minute mile around the university running track in Oxford and into history. It was clearly a good year for exercise physiology.

So perhaps we might think of Dan as a *'four-minute'* physiologist, intensely preoccupied by acute breathing responses to brief stimuli. Contrast Mabel FitzGerald's findings from her participation in the Pikes Peak expedition in 1911: she wanted only data from mountainside residents who had been at altitude for *one year* and "in the case of a change of abode within the range of high altitudes, *six weeks to two months* was usually taken as the minimum time".[1] What is perhaps so striking from these two approaches to research is how little the later experiments achieved in explaining the earlier ones. Indeed, to try to find some connection between the two we need to explore something first well identified in the 1920s: the smallest organ in the body.

The body's oxygen barometer

In 1743, one Hardovicus Taube presented his *Theses Physiologicae* on intercostal nerves in Göttingen. He included mention of a *Ganglion minutum*, clearly something tiny, close to the carotid artery in the neck at a point where it divides into two arteries, the internal going to the brain and the external going to the face.[17] There is good reason to believe that he was describing what we might call our body's own internal 'oxygen barometer' or, to use its best-known name, the 'carotid body'.

The carotid body did its best to hide its identity for 200 years, aided by two tricks. The first is to be very small and in hiding. It is only about 4 mm in diameter and is tucked into a notch at the division of a large blood vessel in a part of the body crowded with nerves and other vital structures. The second is to sit next to a major player doing something different. Its neighbour is a part of the same blood vessel: a bulging section of the internal carotid artery, the carotid *sinus*, which detects arterial blood pressure by the degree to which it is distended. It was patient, persistent, microscopic work from 1926 by the Spanish researcher Fernando De Castro in Madrid that led him to conclude that the nerve endings in the carotid body have a different sensory function from those in the nearby sinus detecting pressure. He saw the carotid body as a detector of chemical changes in the blood, even identifying the individual 'glomus' cells that 'taste' the blood.

The complexity of the investigation that eventually sorted out the distinctive roles of the carotid *body* and the carotid *sinus* is worthy of the plot of a ghoulish historical drama series.[18] The first episode would start with a scene in 1920s Weimar Köln in Germany, Heinrich Hering demonstrating dramatic slowing of the heart in dogs administered electrical shocks to the neck: the 'sinus-*reflex*'. In Belgium we would find the head of one (chloralosed) decapitated dog ('*la tête isolée*') connected via tubes to the trunk of another dog in a 'parabiosis' experiment in which Jean-François Heymans and his son Corneille demonstrate that the sinus reflex is conducted via the brain and that breathing is affected by the chemical composition of carotid blood.

The drama would now move to Madrid to embrace the Spanish Civil War. The laboratory of the Cajal Institute is crowded with tissue samples from humans, monkeys, cows, cats, rabbits and rodents; the city is a battlefront where Republicans face Franco's army, but physiology continues. In the face of wartime privation in the laboratory, some remarkable experiments are under way: De Castro surgically rewires nerves in the necks of cats to manufacture new reflexes that elucidate structures and pathways. One such rewiring results in stimuli to the carotid body being observed as a widening of the pupil

in the cat's eye on the same side of the body: an artificially manufactured *external* readout in a contented resident of the laboratory of
internal chemical change in the blood during experiments, such as
lowering the oxygen in inspired air. This gives the scientists a way of
seeing the activity of the carotid body by looking in the eye!

As tensions rise throughout Europe, convivial visits take place
between scientists of different countries, including two by De Castro
to Heymans in Ghent, where they undertake parabiosis together.
The final episode sees the younger Heymans eventually awarded the
Nobel Prize in Physiology or Medicine in Ghent in January 1940, just
before the German army marches into Belgium. The Nobel lecture,
in Stockholm, would wait until 1945, after the capitulation, its title:
'The part played by vascular presso- and chemo-receptors in respiratory control'. It barely mentions De Castro, who "opened the
way" to Heymans' discoveries but did not receive due credit, even
at the moment when the latter was awarded the Nobel Prize.[19] The
drama would portray scientific progress as teamwork in which some
members of the team are more fortunate than others. Our closing
scene might have climbing enthusiast Ferdinand De Castro among
the snowy Andes on a visit to Chile, contented to be among the
mountains, the immensity of his scientific contribution being better
recognised by future generations.

Eventually it became clear that the carotid body, however small, is
indeed the body's 'oxygen barometer'. It is stimulated by low oxygen
pressure, but also by high carbon dioxide pressure, and the acidity
of arterial blood arriving in the carotid artery. It sends signals to the
brain via a branch of the glossopharyngeal nerve, the ninth of the
twelve cranial nerves. The neighbouring carotid sinus has the role of
detecting arterial blood pressure, beat by beat, and sends messages
to the brain via the same branch, appropriately enough named 'Hering's nerve'. Dan Cunningham's Oxford experiments were, in part, an
elucidation of the pattern of the responses of this mysterious little
organ to stimuli.

On my arrival in the Laboratory of Physiology in 1989 I felt the
brisk current of the Oxford tradition of human respiratory physiology sweeping me along. This mostly came from Dr Peter Robbins,
formerly Dan's graduate student and by the time of my arrival
a young lecturer in the department. Peter had spent his doctoral
studies with Dan developing the laboratory hardware and computer

software needed to apply rigorous 'systems control engineering' to the assessment of rapid breathing responses to varying levels of oxygen in inspired gas. To account for why such experiments can be challenging, I need to explain more about breathing and chemo-receptors. The Pikes Peak expedition had already shown that changes in breathing change the pressure of carbon dioxide in the lungs and in the blood. When ventilation goes up the carbon dioxide pressure goes down, and vice versa. Things get complicated because the body has chemoreceptors that respond to these changes in carbon dioxide. We have already noted that the carotid body is one of these systems. What we haven't allowed for so far is that the brain itself also contains chemoreceptors that respond vigorously to carbon dioxide pressure and alter ventilation. A further loop-within-a-loop, as it were, is that all the chemoreceptors respond to acidity, and changes in carbon dioxide pressure themselves alter blood acidity. So, we have a complex network of interconnected phenomena involved in the regulation of breathing. It comes as no surprise, therefore, that students of phys-iology frequently find the control of breathing impenetrable; those Lloyd–Cunningham equations are rarely congenial.

Dan Cunningham and Peter Robbins had wanted to observe the breathing response to isolated low oxygen pressure in the body. They knew that responses to low oxygen would alter the carbon dioxide pressure (and acidity) in the body. So they devised a way of fooling the control system so that it could only 'see' changes in oxygen. The trick was to modify the inspired air by adding carbon dioxide, breath by breath, at an amount that would force the level of carbon dioxide in the lungs (and therefore the arterial blood) to remain constant *whatever changes in ventilation occurred* in response to changes in the oxygen level in the body. To this trick they gave the name 'end-tidal forcing', and it has become a powerful tool for unravelling how the body responds to low and high oxygen levels and other stimuli. The term 'end-tidal' relates to detecting the pressures of carbon dioxide and oxygen in the alveolar gas breathed out at the end of a breath (and therefore a good sample of gas from the lungs). 'Forcing' refers to using speedy sampling of alveolar gas to alter the composition of subsequent inspired breaths of gas to try to keep the alveolar gas composition constant. Engineers call this a feedback control. Physi-ologists prefer the term 'clamp'.

If Dan had been a 'four-minute physiologist', early in his research career Peter became a *'thirty-minute physiologist'*, unravelling how humans breathe in response to a dip into what was called 'pure hypoxia' for half an hour. Volunteers were exposed to a degree of hypoxia that took the oxygen pressure in the lungs to about half normal, which is similar to that experienced on the summit of Mont Blanc (4,809 m). In the laboratory this was achieved by breathing air enriched breath-by-breath with nitrogen as well as carbon dioxide. The result was a pure stimulus for thirty minutes of constant low oxygen with 'clamped' carbon dioxide pressure, ensuring that no changes in the latter could interfere with the response to sustained exposure to a constant level of hypoxia.

An unexpected response to this pure sustained hypoxia had been noted by others a few years earlier: ventilation rose rapidly to a peak at about three minutes into the hypoxia (as would be expected) and then fell off gradually over the rest of the thirty minutes (as was not expected). No clear explanation was apparent for this fall after the initial rise. Peter's technical wizardry was able to investigate this 'hypoxic ventilatory decline', and found that the carotid body itself (or its connections to the brain) seemed to account for the behaviour.[20] The body's oxygen barometer was showing some unaccountable up-and-down behaviour.

In 1988, the year before I joined the Laboratory of Physiology, Oxford's young New Zealand physiologist David Paterson took a lead in establishing an appropriate home for Mabel's barometer, and other curiosities from the Pikes Peak expedition, in the display cabinet I was to walk past daily. At a modest ceremony to unveil the cabinet he was captured on camera with Dan Cunningham, Roger Bannister and Peter Robbins (Fig. 7).

On my arrival in Physiology, Peter Robbins and I soon became jointly interested in the effect of hormones and drugs on the response of the carotid body to low oxygen. We administered a range of agents to volunteers, the aim being to choose molecules that might inter-act with biochemical pathways known to send signals between cells. One of these molecules, dopamine, was known from microscopy to be present in the glomus cells of the carotid body, the cells that De Castro had identified as 'tasting' the blood. We found that dopa-mine decreased (and its antagonists domperidone and haloperidol increased) the vigour with which breathing responded to hypoxia.[21, 22] Somatostatin, another hormone that lurks in parts of the body where dopamine is found, also decreased the response.[23] Midazolam and its antagonist flumazenil had no effect, possibly ruling out the involvement of a cell membrane receptor called 'GABA'.[24] Perhaps the finding of most immediate medical importance was to confirm something alarming which had been noted by Canadian researchers, that even low or 'sedative' doses of inhalational anaesthetics can profoundly decrease the ventilatory response to hypoxia, on which a patient may be reliant during and following surgery.[25-27] The intravenous anaesthetic propofol, increasingly used for 'total intravenous anaesthesia', behaved similarly.[28]

This tinkering with drugs and hormones tended to have rather abstruse scientific objectives, as with other studies Peter and I worked on in the 1990s; the fine details of the signals between cells of the carotid body were of interest to only a few scientists. The findings with anaesthetic agents were more relevant to the anaesthetic community. Added to their practical importance in obtunding the breathing responses of patients, the findings have recently provided colleagues in Oxford with an insight into the precise cell membrane proteins in the glomus cells that may be a site of action of both hypoxia and the vapours, the so-called 'TASK' channels by which potassium can enter and leave cells.[29]

Possibly frustrated that no thirty-minute experiments seemed to be shedding much light on the phenomena that had occupied Haldane and FitzGerald nearly a century before, Peter Robbins came up with a really bright idea. The 'end-tidal forcing' technique of changing the composition of inspired gas breath by breath, trying to keep the composition of the gas in the lungs clamped however much ventilation changed, worked really well in thirty-minute experiments. Could we go on for much longer? The trouble with that idea is that volunteers cannot tolerate breathing through a mouthpiece with their noses occluded for much longer than thirty minutes; it is simply too unpleasant. Peter extended the end-tidal forcing to periods of hours by building a small chamber in which the ambient air (the inspired gas) was modified every five minutes to provide constant levels of oxygen and carbon dioxide in the lungs without the need for volunteers to breathe through a mouthpiece. Their expired 'end-tidal' gas was sampled via a small tube taped close to a nostril. Measurements of the composition of this gas in the lungs were made over several breaths and then used to regulate changes every five minutes to the ambient air in the chamber.

When built, the chamber was large enough to accommodate a volunteer with a desk, chair and couch, and a little space to move around. This made it possible to do a curtailed Pikes Peak-like expedition simulation to examine the body's gradual acclimatisation to a fixed level of hypoxia. As in the thirty-minute experiments with end-tidal forcing, in these longer experiments we could avoid confounding changes in carbon dioxide pressure in the lungs, and acidity in the blood, which complicate the responses of the chemoreceptors. We could have hours of pure hypoxia with nothing else. We now had the means to address a big controversy in mountain physiology.

The dominant hypothesis for explaining why the Pikes Peak summiters found a gradual increase in breathing during their sojourn at the top had been for many years that it was a change in carbon dioxide pressure itself that was responsible. The hypothesis went as follows: the hypoxia of altitude stimulates the carotid body to make you breathe more; the increase in breathing lowers the carbon dioxide pressure and makes the blood less acidic (more alkaline); the carotid body and the brain's chemoreceptors see this alkalinity and limit the increase in breathing; over hours and days, the body gradually corrects the alkalinity of the brain and the blood, and thereby releases the brake on breathing that results from it. Breathing progressively increases as a result: problem solved.

Knocking dogma on the head was led by Gerry Bisgard in the United States, whose studies with goats suggested otherwise. Bisgard had the good fortune to acquire as his laboratory a farm donated to the University of Wisconsin. Veterinary earnings were directed to research and added to the resources. In a magnificent series of experiments with goats, Bisgard and his team made a major contribution to understanding the behaviour of the 'caprine oxygen barometer' (if we may be permitted this term to refer to the goat's carotid body). Using strategies to prevent chemoreceptors from being exposed to changes in carbon dioxide pressure or acidity, he and his co-workers showed that hypoxia alone led gradually to a fourfold increase in breathing ('ventilatory acclimatisation') over hours.[30, 31]

Without knowing about the Gerry Bisgard farmyard, Peter Robbins had built the Oxford chamber to perform the 'goat experiment' on human volunteers. Eleven adults spent eight hours in the chamber on three occasions: once to breathe air (control), once to have hypoxia with the carbon dioxide level drifting down freely (as it would have done on Pikes Peak), and once with hypoxia and carbon dioxide added to the chamber air to keep the levels of both constant (the 'clamping' experiment with low oxygen and normal carbon dioxide pressures). The results were astonishing, and consistent with Bisgard's. When changes in carbon dioxide pressure were prevented by the clamping method, breathing increased to about four times its normal volume each minute over eight hours showing that the tiny *Ganglion minutum* tucked up close to the carotid artery takes full charge of the breathing response to low oxygen in the carotid blood.[32]

Eight hours did not, of course, approximate to the five weeks spent by those on Pikes Peak. Peter Robbins wanted to know more about the time course of the stimulus to breathe coming from the carotid body, so experiments were extended to forty-eight hours.[33] Tolerant volunteers offered to spend this prolonged period in isolation, somewhat beset by heavy breathing and the possibility of altitude sickness that can occur even in a sea-level laboratory. Indeed, one of ten in the study withdrew after developing "headache, nausea and general discomfort", classic symptoms of acute altitude sickness (see Chapter Three).

The conclusion has been that for those on the top of Pikes Peak in 1911, the increase in breathing over the first two days or so would have been attributable largely to the carotid body sending a progressively more intense 'low-oxygen' message to the brain. After that time, further increases in breathing would have been mainly due to the kidneys gradually correcting the acidity of the blood back towards normal from the alkalinity that the heavy breathing was creating. In short, the carotid body was doing some two-day speeding, and the kidney some two-week speeding of breathing. Together they built up the long, slow rise in breathing on the summit. And together, both these phenomena would have driven the breathing of the Colorado mountain residents visited by Mabel and her pony.

The connection we have been trying to make here is between the way breathing varies with altitude in residents and the way breathing changes over minutes, hours, days and weeks when humans change altitude rapidly. The 'oxygen barometer' that provides the link is that smallest organ in the body, the carotid body. In everyone, at whatever altitude they live, it constantly signals to the brain to regulate breathing. It has very rapid responses to alterations in oxygen, but also has some very slow responses: 'ventilatory acclimatisation'. These slow responses can be studied in experiments lasting eight hours (which conveniently fit into the laboratory working day), but they continue for several days.

To double-check that this acclimatisation was active in people living at sea level, not just at high altitude, Peter Robbins did the equivalents of Haldane's Dalcoath deep mine and Ben Nevis experiments, but each of them over an ambitious six days in the Oxford chamber with the 'clamping' that allows observation of the effects of 'pure' changes in oxygen pressure, respectively *up* and *down*.[34] The *slightly high* oxygen experiment used a lung oxygen pressure 10 per cent higher than the normal value at sea level, equivalent to being down a mine just a little deeper than Dalcoath. The *slightly low* oxygen experiment used 10 per cent lower than normal, equivalent to being about two-thirds of the way up Ben Nevis. Ten volunteers gave up their time to spend 12 days each in the chamber, and a large team of researchers was recruited to monitor them day and night.

These 'close to sea level' chamber experiments and the earlier Oxford studies mimicking the hypoxia of greater altitudes generated a very beautiful graph of the relationship between the activity of the carotid body and the changes in oxygen pressure that occur with ascent (and descent). On a plot of the sensitivity of the 'acclimatised' carotid body against oxygen pressure a straight 'Robbins line' beautifully replicated the straight 'FitzGerald line' on her graph of her measure of breathing (the lowered carbon dioxide pressure in the lungs) against the ambient pressure of different altitudes. Both lines tell us about breathing all the way from around sea level up to quite high altitude. The 'Robbins line' suggested that the carotid body has a slowly adapting sensitivity to oxygen that varies with altitude by about 3.5 per cent for each 1 per cent change in the atmospheric pressure. The Pikes-Peakers would have experienced a ~140 per cent increase in the activity of their carotid bodies associated with the ~40 per cent lower atmospheric pressure and oxygen pressure at the top of the mountain. This natural oxygen barometer turns out to be quite a lively little organ.

Haldane and Priestley's short Dalcoath mine and Ben Nevis experiments were published in 1905. Peter Robbins' prolonged six-day recreation of them appeared in 2005. The 100 years between the two had revealed the carotid body to be a kind of barometer telling the body how high it lives by measuring the pressure of oxygen in the blood and then telling the body how hard to breathe. Careful probing of its behaviour found it to respond slowly to the changes it detects (in addition to its rapid up-and-down responses that had diverted us researchers for so long). But no work in the 100 years had come up with an explanation for this slow adaptive behaviour. What lay ahead was a Nobel Prize associated with unravelling the mechanism of this slow component of the response to oxygen. It would turn out to be a biochemical mechanism present not just in the carotid body but in every cell of the body. And it would be a mechanism almost as old as animals themselves.

The ancient molecular oxygen barometer inside all of the body's cells

I missed biology at school. The O level in biology that I eventually took at the age of twenty-five in order to become a medical student did not prompt me to think about the history of life. Neither, perhaps surprisingly, did my five years as a medical student. The emphasis was on what (for example) the anatomy of the limbs looks like *now*, not on how other vertebrates perambulate, or how our ancestors might have slid out of the oceans and onto their primitive legs. I will admit that a small part of our embryology made us reflect on how we shared the three layers of a tube with other 'bilaterian metazoans': ectoderm on the outside forming skin and brain, mesoderm in the middle making muscles, and endoderm forming the inner viscera. I think I owe it to Richard Dawkins' (and co-researcher Yan Wong's) *The Ancestor's Tale: A Pilgrimage to the Dawn of Evolution* of 2004 to have made me seriously aware of deep time relatively late in life.[35] In its original hardback version this beautifully illustrated and weighty volume takes the reader back in time over around forty points of evolutionary history. This made me think 'tree of life' for understanding the relationship between all living organisms and prompted me to hunt for 'trees of life' elsewhere.

All the emotive stuff one hears about natural selection, religion and whether evolution is a 'theory' can be bypassed in general conversation by asking people whether they think they are literally related to the cat on their lap or the geraniums in the window box: related, that is, in the same way that they are to Auntie Elsie or Marilyn Monroe, by having a common ancestor. I find it surprising how few

people have ever given the matter a moment's thought or are prepared to assent to being relatives of all living organisms. The 'trees
of life' I have looked for are revealed in natural history museums
around the globe, or, rather disappointingly, sometimes they are not.
I recall disappointment when I went looking in London, New York
and Berlin. In Berlin I did find an electronic interactive version well
away from the main hall of spectacular Tanzanian dinosaurs, but it
was not functioning.

Today, I popped next door to the Oxford Museum of Natural
History to check there. It is a most wonderful airy building of Victorian neo-gothic iron and glass. I always experience a child-like
excitement as I enter this hallowed space with its thousands of biological and geological specimens and exhibits. I walked around looking
for a tree of life, even checking for the more technical term 'philo-
geny'. I asked the staff at 'enquiries', who denied any knowledge
of a 'tree-of-life' exhibit. There was a radio check to a more senior
level and an email to a curator: nothing doing. One member of staff
thought there might have been a poster in the past but that it was now
long gone. In the museum shop there were cuddly dodos and books
on fossils. There was no evidence of the most fundamental concept
in the history of life on earth. I put it to the reader that the first thing
you need to meet on entering such a museum, after the notice about
the cloakrooms, needs to be some kind of display inviting the visitor
to reflect on the unity underlying all living organisms before directing
them to the immense diversity on display.

And a time scale is needed too. How old are all these specimens?
We have been introduced recently to the revival from Siberian permafrost of a ½-mm-long rotifer animal, which had been frozen for 24,000
years. You can see the video of it moving around to feed (perhaps not
surprising after such a long fast).[36] Clearly, not everything that is old
has to be dead. In human history, we have recently been reminded of
how a child burial was conducted in Africa 78,000 years ago, helping
us imagine people with some of our own preoccupations living tens
of thousands of years ago.[37] Even these periods of time are tiny
compared with the full stretch of that tree of life that would have a
junction at the beginning of the metazoa (animals) some 760 million
years ago, ten thousand times older than the African burial.

Enter 'HIF' into the tree of life. Mabel FitzGerald's barometer was
an essential component of the physiological research that led to the

discovery of that oxygen barometer, the carotid body, in goats, dogs and man. We now know that the cells that make up living organisms have had the capability of detecting oxygen for most of the history of multicellular animals. Had there been a tree of life with a time scale in the Museum of Natural History, our visit would have enabled us to trace the metazoa back to multicellular marine organisms called *Placozoa*; these were the earliest we currently know to have evolved a system for sensing oxygen pressure in their environment, called 'HIF', short for hypoxia-inducible factor.[38] The date was around 680 million years ago. A little further back in the evolutionary tree are comb jellies and sponges, also regarded as metazoa but apparently lacking this HIF system.[39] The elucidation of how this primordial system enables cells to sense and respond to oxygen resulted in the award of the 2019 Nobel Prize for Physiology or Medicine jointly to William Kaelin, Gregg Semenza and Peter Ratcliffe.

Of the three, Sir Peter Ratcliffe FRS is the best known in Oxford. As a registrar in renal medicine here, he set out to unravel the mystery of how and why the kidney can sense the level of haemoglobin in the blood and use that information to secrete a hormone, erythropoietin, which causes the body to regulate the production of new red blood cells in the bone marrow. The sequence of events had been known for some years but how the kidney sensed the concentration of haemoglobin in the blood was a mystery. Mabel's observation of the increasing concentration of haemoglobin with altitude was suggestive that perhaps the kidney could also sense oxygen pressure rather than the concentration of haemoglobin itself.[40]

It was Peter Ratcliffe's persistence in the field that led to his and his team's contribution to the HIF story. This was the discovery of a sequence of biochemical reactions that sense oxygen pressure and regulate manufacturing processes in cells.[41] In conditions of normal oxygen pressure, the molecule called HIF is constantly produced and broken down rapidly, within minutes, by nearly all cells of the body. This recycling of HIF is made possible by a a chemical reaction that takes one of two oxygen atoms from an oxygen molecule and, in the presence of an iron atom and vitamin C, uses the oxygen atom to add a hydroxyl group (OH) to HIF, thereby 'labelling' it as ready for 'degradation'. When oxygen becomes sparse (as oxygen pressure becomes low) this breaking down of HIF is slowed and HIF enters the nucleus of the cell where it can regulate the manufacture of many molecules.

What molecules are manufactured depends upon the tissue in which the cells find themselves. It may seem a waste of resources for cells constantly to produce and recycle the HIF molecule, but that is after all how the body renews a lot of its components.

Here at last was the explanation for Mabel FitzGerald's graph of increasing haemoglobin concentration with altitude in the residents of Colorado and New England. Here too (although it is taking longer to unravel the detail)[42] is the explanation for the acclimatisation of the carotid body to low oxygen that results in breathing varying with altitude, all the way from the bottom of a mine up to high peaks.

At this point we may pause to clarify why this discovery is the one that explains the gradual responses to oxygen (and altitude) that have been the theme of this chapter. HIF is what is known as a 'transcription factor'. This means that it is a molecular mechanism for regulating the way codes written within genes are converted into the equipment with which cells undertake their activities. HIF controls the manufacturing process. The items of equipment manufactured are usually proteins. They serve all kinds of roles from structural materials like the collagen in bones to messenger hormones such as the kidney's erythropoietin. A key point is that this manufacturing process is relatively slow and the time course of the process varies according to what is being manufactured. Thus, for example, erythropoietin is secreted by the kidney within one to two hours of the body being made hypoxic,[43] but the resulting generation of red blood cells by the bone marrow tends to take days, as can be seen from the Pikes Peak measurements. To achieve the slow response of the carotid body to hypoxia, the HIF system appears to lead to the generation of new components of the small intracellular organelles called mitochondria, where some of the responses to oxygen take place.[42]

I intimated earlier in this chapter that Mabel might have liked to join us in 2011 on our centenary visit back to Pikes Peak on a scientific quest as well as a pilgrimage for her barometer. My thinking was based in science. We were using the journey to study a response of the human body to low oxygen pressure that Mabel would not have known about at the time. She studied two acclimatisation responses that we now know to be associated with HIF: the slow rise in the haemoglobin concentration and the component of breathing that increases gradually over hours and days. A third response, now known to be of importance in determining how adversely people respond to high altitude, is constriction of blood vessels in the lungs. This can make it difficult for the heart to pump blood through the lungs at altitude, and is even a cause of death from 'high altitude pulmonary oedema' in some cases (oedema being the accumulation of water in the airways of the lungs, making breathing difficult). The time course of this constriction, like that of breathing, has both fast and slow components. The slow component of the time course we term 'acclimatisation' but its effect may be the opposite of the positive association that this word carries. It is a harmful response in this setting, even though it may have benefit in other settings (such as in a patient with Covid-19 pneumonia). We call the response 'hypoxic pulmonary vasoconstriction', vasoconstriction referring to the narrowing of blood vessels. This narrowing in the lungs has good and bad effects.

Our team's plan was to examine for the first time a bad side of this vasoconstriction. In modern passenger planes there is a low cabin air pressure that is similar to that experienced on ascending to about 2,000 metres, even though the plane is actually flying at about 10,000 metres. The reason for this design feature is that a low cabin air pressure reduces the stresses to which the cabin walls are subjected as the aircraft is exposed to the very low atmospheric pressure at its flying altitude. The low air pressure experienced by the passengers has the potential to expose some patients to a harmful level of hypoxia. No one had previously evaluated, in the actual environment and for the duration of an intercontinental flight, the extent to which the vasoconstriction leads to a rise in the pressure in the pulmonary artery against which the heart has the extra work of pumping.

We set out to observe passengers on a transatlantic flight to Denver, Colorado, while on our way to a conference and the visit to Pikes Peak. British Airways gave permission for eight healthy volunteers, including our physiologists Tom Smith and Nick Talbot, to occupy the back row of passenger seats in a Boeing 777 for the nine-hour flight.[44] With them was an echocardiograph machine with which the pressure in the pulmonary artery could be measured. Mabel FitzGerald would have been amazed at the capability of a machine somewhat smaller than her bathroom-cabinet-sized breathing apparatus being capable of measuring the pressure in an artery by bouncing soundwaves off moving blood.

Our measurements found the (anticipated) rise in pressure to be

20 per cent. Denver itself, being at an altitude of 1,610 metres, simulates a commercial airliner environment and provided another week for measurements. In a later flight, this time from London to Dubai, Tom Smith was able to establish for the first time that the inherited condition 'Chuvash polycythaemia' put patients at an especial risk in the cabin environment by increasing the pulmonary artery pressure by 50 per cent.[45] Mabel FitzGerald would have found meeting patients with Chuvash polycythaemia in the laboratory particularly fascinating. The genetic mutation they have in their HIF system (of which she would, of course, have been in awe) gives them very high concentrations of haemoglobin in the blood and makes them breathe hard, to an even greater extent than the residents she studied high in the Rockies of Colorado, and this despite the fact that they live around sea level. Indeed, were patients with this condition to try to add high-altitude ascent to their condition, they would be unlikely to survive.

The century of research that followed Mabel's travels with her barometer in Colorado and New England has shed much light on the way the low oxygen pressure of altitude stimulates breathing and the production of haemoglobin. Only in the most recent half of that century has the effect of low oxygen pressure on the blood vessels in the lungs come to light and been widely studied. I will show in Chapter Three what life-and-death consequences are associated with this third physiological effect of low oxygen.

It has been exhilarating to be involved in research on all these topics. What one misses is the opportunity to discuss developments with Mabel herself, imagined over a coffee in the Physiology common room close to where her portrait is displayed. Her contributions to physiology were celebrated afresh when NASA astronaut and physiologist Jessica Meir unveiled a plaque in Oxford in honour of Mabel's role as 'Physiologist and Scientific Explorer' in 2021 (Fig. 8).

When Mabel FitzGerald died in 1973 a small hand-held barometer was found in her home with an inscrutable inscription on the back: 'J. Haldane from P.C.M. & G.E.C.P 1891'. It sits in a small padded, green-felted receptacle and reads 32 inches of mercury, strangely reminiscent of being *below* sea level (Fig. 9). In 2011, shortly before he died, Bob Torrance, lecturer in physiology, had handed it on to my present head of department, David Paterson, who encouraged Peter Ratcliffe to make it an Oxford donation to the Nobel Museum in Stockholm, which he duly did.[46] I would like to think that this was a treasured gift to Mabel FitzGerald from Haldane shortly before he died in 1936. Whether this smaller barometer travelled to Pikes Peak, and in whose pocket it might have done so, remains to be clarified. Alternatively, one might wonder whether it was a gift associated with Haldane's marriage in Edinburgh in 1891 to Kathleen Trotter, with whom he had a perhaps equally famous son: J. B. S. Haldane, the geneticist. This barometer may perhaps have accompanied Haldane on visits deep into collieries, which were frequent in the 1890s as he investigated mining disasters. If only a barometer could speak, this one, like the one in our departmental hallway, might have a fascinating story to tell.

CHAPTER THREE

ILLS OF THE HILLS

Medicine and Mountains

A sick climber on Mont Blanc

The weather turned to a howling gale as we settled into the tightly packed accommodation of the Refuge du Goûter, some 200 enthusiasts hopeful of a pre-dawn departure for the six-hour ascent to the summit of Mont Blanc, and all of us trying to get a few hours of sleep amid the snoring and the odour of human exertion. It was 1 September 2000, a time of year when the cold bites hard at that altitude, 3,835 metres. The refuge lay peeping over the precipitous cliff of granite that we had climbed from the refuge beside the Tête Rousse glacier nearly 700 metres below. The Goûter refuge is the most popular hut for a 2 a.m. departure to see the sunrise from the icy ridge of the summit at 4,809 metres. But this makes it high enough for visitors to get sick.

At midnight I was called to assist in the care of a French climber. I found a middle-aged man slumped and barely responsive, in an upper bunk. His facial colour suggested lack of oxygen in the blood and coarse breath sounds indicated fluid in his lungs: this was high-altitude pulmonary oedema. His poor mental state suggested the double insult of high-altitude cerebral oedema as well, a swollen brain making him unable even to ask for assistance. I was dismayed to find no medical facilities available at the refuge. It promisingly had a small room designated as the infirmary, but sadly this served as a store and bedroom and contained nothing to help. Some aid was at hand from other visitors; we administered some nifedipine tablets under the tongue to help with those wet lungs and acetazolamide tablets to stimulate some urine output of the fluid. We monitored this output, improved his posture and issued reassuring words. I called the rescue helicopter from Chamonix but this was able to land only five hours later because of poor visibility and high winds.

It was a relief to hear some days later that our climber colleague had survived and later still to receive a letter of gratitude from the patient himself, a French radiologist, thanking me for what I had done to help. I'm not sure that he realised how little had been possible with such limited facilities.[1] Some oxygen would have been particularly useful.

Later correspondence with the Club Alpine Français, I am sad to say, drew no response. A new refuge was built in 2013. I hope that its stunning new architecture has been matched by appropriate medical supplies for the life-threatening illnesses that can occur at altitude.

The Urquhart chalet, altitude and health

Both the delights and hazards of visits to the mountains took on a personal note for me when I started to help run alpine reading parties for students from University College soon after being appointed Tutor in Physiology and Medicine there in 1989. My college had participated since 1952 in a tradition of annual summer retreats going back to 1891 at a chalet located at 1,685 metres (5,530 ft) on the western edge of the Mont Blanc massif in the French Alps, above the village of St Gervais-les-Bains. Jointly with academic colleagues this venture became an important personal commitment, taking me away from my other duties for two or more weeks each summer and occupying other parts of the year with fundraising, reunions, and other responsibilities linked with running an educational trust.

There is perhaps a little irony in the fact that the builder of the chalet where these retreats have taken place was a firm believer in high altitude being *beneficial* to health. It was the eccentric British diplomat David Urquhart who sought out a site for a summer home around 6,000 feet above sea level. A Turcophile following his government appointment to Constantinople in the 1830s, Urquhart became a leading UK advocate of Turkish baths, making an association between cleanliness and virtue, and between clean bodies and minds.[2] A similar association between high altitude and better functioning of the brain led him and his wife Harriet, then living in Geneva, "on the ground of health" in a challenging six-month search for a site with flat ground and a water supply at sufficient altitude. They found this on the Prarion mountain, one of the foothills of Mont Blanc, where they raised their chalet in 1865. Urquhart explained the project in a letter to a friend of July 1865:

This plan is based on the observations we both made during our excursion of last summer, on the effect produced on us of high altitudes. This was so often repeated … that there remained no ambiguity or doubt. The point at which this relief was experienced we separately fixed at five thousand feet. Suffering from very different maladies, though originating in the same source – excessive mental labour – the symptoms of both were lessened or relieved almost as soon as the limit of five thousand feet was attained. We then experienced in addition renewed physical and mental energy, as shown by increased speed and flow of conversation; a sense of enjoyment in lieu of depression or exhaustion, appetite for food, readiness to sleep, and the power of sleeping longer.[3]

The resulting two-storey hybrid stone-wood chalet had four bedrooms, later extended to six (Fig. 10). It was to be their family home during the summer months. A distinctive feature was that the main living area, or salon, was designed to be entered through a Turkish bath. It may be common practice to expect guests to remove muddy shoes on arrival; a less frequent expectation is that they take a Turkish bath! The chalet soon acquired the name 'Chalet des Anglais', by which it has been known henceforth. In 1906 it was destroyed by fire and rebuilt on a much larger scale, allowing it the use for students it has today.

David and Harriet Urquhart married in 1854 and had four children before the construction of their mountain residence. Their fifth, Francis, was born in 1868 and was due to become the Francis Fortesque Urquhart known by hundreds of Oxford students from summer reading parties at the chalet. This link came with Francis' admission in 1890 to Balliol College, Oxford. He graduated in 1894 and went on to make his career within the college, being elected a fellow in 1896.

In 1891, at the end of his first year as a student, Francis invited six guests to join him for a summer party at the family chalet. The tradition of vacation 'reading parties' was well established among Oxford dons and students: usually a retreat to a location at the coast or elsewhere scenic and involving study and modest exercise. During one such UK party, in Minehead, Francis was given his famous nickname 'Sligger', by which he was known throughout his life and after his

death in 1934.[2] Although Sligger regarded reading as largely exclud-
ing climbing, his friend Cyril Bailey "induced" him in that first year
"to try a climb, and starting at two from the chalet – there was no
Tête Rousse hut in those days – we got to the top of the Aiguille du
Goûter, no further, and even then we were out over eighteen hours".[4]

The chalet party of 1891 marked the beginning of the long-lasting
tradition in which I became involved with my first reading party in
1990, by which time the summer season was divided between three
colleges: Balliol, New College and Univ. During most summers since
then I have participated in running reading parties for students from
Univ. The chalet is managed by a board of UK trustees on which each
of the three participating colleges maintains three members. The
institution is affectionately remembered by hundreds of old-member
'chaletites', many of whom continue to support its educational
mission and upkeep.

Mont Blanc disasters of 1892

Two events in the year following the first reading party, 1892, showed
that mountain life might not be as conducive to health as the Urqu-
harts thought when surveying for their mountain home thirty years
before. First, the *Catastrophe de St Gervais*. The Tête Rousse glacier is
a relatively small icefield some 400 metres in length and ascending
about 150 metres vertically, at the bottom of the 700-metre cliff below
the Aiguille du Goûter. During the night of 11 July 1892 the deadliest
ever flood from an intraglacial lake broke out from deep inside the
Tête Rousse glacier, devastating the valley below the glacier, sweeping
away the thermal baths and part of the town of St Gervais-le-Fayet.[5]
The water was released when a massive tongue of glacial ice broke
away, fragmented, and accompanied the water into the valley. Some
175 people died. Estimates suggest that 100 million litres of water
were discharged from the glacier and generated a flood of 800 million
litres of ice and sediment into the valley. Charles Mathews, author of
the most readable of accounts of Mont Blanc and its fatalities up to
1898, recounts following the course of the devastation on foot a few
weeks after the event:

> I climbed to the glacier of Tête Rousse and was let down into
> the empty lake; then following the track of the avalanche, I

walked along its whole course to the site of the Baths, and on to Le Fayet. Utter ruin was everywhere. The once lovely gardens were five or six feet deep in mud, fine trees had been snapped like reeds, and enormous blocks of stone were strewn over the dreary waste.[5]

Mathews furnished his account with a photograph of the vast hole through which the water had found its exit from the glacier (and into which he allowed himself to be 'let down'); given scale by two tiny figures peering into the abyss, we can estimate that it is about 40 metres in diameter.[5] Figure 11 shows the same view by Coutet from the St Gervais archives.

Tunnels were built into the base of the glacier in 1899 and 1904 to prevent a re-accumulation of the lake but were found, mysteriously, to drain little over subsequent years.

However, on 13 July 2010, scientists monitoring the glacier using radar, surface magnetic resonance and bore holes announced an emergency. They had detected a subglacial lake approaching the size of that of 1892. Immediate action was taken and nearly 48 million litres of water were drained from bore holes over the following two months. The reasons for this peculiar risk remain unclear. They may include that the glacier sits in a bowl-shaped ledge abutting the massif and has a glacial tongue that is colder than the body of the glacial ice and therefore acts as a barrier to drainage of meltwater.[6]

The *Catastrophe de St Gervais* prevented Sligger from running a Balliol reading party in 1892 but did not stop one Balliol don from climbing on Mont Blanc. The Reverend Richard Lewis Nettleship had been an undergraduate at Balliol, was made a fellow on graduating in Classics in 1869 and rose to being Tutor in Classics in 1871. In August 1892 he spent ten days at the Montanvert hotel above Chamonix, attempting ambitious climbs, and then set himself the objective of climbing Mont Blanc via the western aspect of the massif.

With his two guides, Alfred Comte and Gaspard Simond, the ascent was started at 4 a.m. on Wednesday, 24 August, from the Pavillon de Bellevue on the Col de Voza at about 1,800 metres. They ascended to the vast cavity in the Tête Rousse glacier from the month before and reached the Aiguille du Goûter at 11.30 a.m. – a time suggesting considerable delay. Their aim was to strike higher to the Dôme du Goûter, the enormous ice field above the Aiguille, and head for a small cabin on the Roches des Bosses at 4,362 metres, two hours distant from the summit.

They made the mistake of leaving the Aiguille du Goûter (where the then-tiny cabin could have provided refuge) in deteriorating weather and pushed on. On the Dôme a situation described by the guides as *"un orage épouvantable"* (a terrible storm) struck them and they lost their bearings in the *"tourmente"*. From 5 p.m. they spent the night in a snow-hole and the morning of Thursday, 25 August, found them still unable to find their directions. They disputed what to do. Nettleship wanted to move on. He was confrontational, behaved irrationally, was scarcely able to walk, then staggered and fell. Following confused conversation in French and English, he closed his eyes and died.[7] The guides' account suggests that Nettleship was suffering from cerebral oedema and unable to think clearly.

It seems remarkable that a body could be recovered from such a remote location after heavy snowfall, but it was and a post-mortem examination was conducted in Geneva by Dr Pavey of London and Dr Wisard of Geneva. A reason given for these efforts was that "it was thought at first the manner of death was not what would ordinarily result from cold". The examination "found every organ practically sound", which led to the conclusion that nothing but cold was left to explain the death.[7] At that time the changes in the brain we now associate with high-altitude cerebral oedema were unknown.

Today Nettleship's body rests in the small graveyard of the English church close to the main railway station of Chamonix. If he were alive, from here he would see the Aiguille and Dôme de Goûter clearly against the skyline, and might just be able to make out his intended destination, the cabin of the Roches des Bosses. This is now an aluminium box that glistens in the sunlight and is known as the Refuge Vallot.

Following my eventful night of 1–2 September 2000 in the Goûter hut, the Refuge Vallot turned out to be the furthest my own small party reached in our attempt on the mountain. I had previously reached the summit in 1997 but this time the wind on the final ridge was regarded by our guides as too hazardous. We retreated to the valley, taking refuge in a café only a few metres distant from Nettleship's grave.

These events of 1892 raise the question of what we might include as 'ills of the hills'. For many visitors to the mountains the most

obvious risks to their wellbeing are fatal falls, rock slides and ava-
lanches. The *Catastrophe de St Gervais* serves as an extreme example.
Dangers to physiology may be less prominent concerns. Nettleship is
a reminder that even if accidents are avoided the mountain environment offers serious risks to health.

Ernest Starling: the dropsy explained

What is this 'oedema' of the lungs and of the brain at high altitude?
The concept is one of tissues of the body swelling with an excess of
water. The human body comprises around 60 per cent of its weight as
water, an average of about 40 litres in an adult. Some of the water is
in the liquid form of blood (~5 litres) or much smaller liquid volumes
such as the cerebrospinal fluid around the brain and spinal cord (~0.15
litre). Much of the rest is within individual cells or in the sponge-
like tissue surrounding cells. The term 'oedema' is applied to tissues
that have an abnormally high content of water. To understand how
oedema, including types associated with exposure to high altitude,
can form we need to consult Ernest Starling, one of the best-known
names in physiology. The appropriate distribution of water to the
various compartments of the body is maintained by what have
become known as 'Starling's forces', and the 'ills of the hills' are to a
large extent a disturbance of his forces.

Ernest Starling became a medical student in 1882 at Guy's Hospital
at the age of sixteen. He soon fell in with company more interested in
the scientific basis of medicine than in speedy progression to practise
in Harley Street. Among these was Leonard Wooldridge, a physician
and lecturer in physiology some nine years Starling's senior, with
whom Starling became a close friend. At that time Germany offered
more favourable conditions for physiological research because of
tighter legal constraints in Britain. Wooldridge had undertaken
research in Leipzig and returned to London with increased enthusiasm. Soon Starling himself took the opportunity of a summer of
research (with the intention of improving his German) in Heidelberg
in 1885 in the laboratory of Willy Kühne, professor of physiology.

Starling became indebted to Wooldridge for more than this
encouragement. Wooldridge died suddenly of ulcerative colitis in
1889, aged thirty-two.[8] Not only did Starling succeed Wooldridge
as the developer of physiology at Guy's, but he married his widow

Florence in 1891. Florence became a great supporter of Starling's work and helped to provide him with financial security during a relatively poorly remunerated career.[9]

It was a second research visit to Germany, to Breslau in 1893, that may be key to my topic. There, with Rudolf Heidenhain, Starling investigated how lymph forms. As blood flows through the tiniest blood vessels of the body, the capillaries, a very small proportion of the water in the blood filters through the wall of the capillary and leaks away through similarly tiny vessels called lymphatics, which lie close to the capillaries. This fluid is termed lymph. It finds its way back into the bloodstream via a channel called the thoracic duct, which drains into a vein in the upper chest.

By 1896 Starling had come to appreciate that the forces in the formation of lymph are the *hydrostatic pressure* of blood in the capillaries and the *oncotic pressure* of the proteins in the blood. It is these two pressures that constitute Starling's forces (which would be more helpfully called Starling's 'pressures') and these are the basis of keeping water where it ought to be in the body, and in the right quantities.

Hydrostatic pressure is the pressure at the bottom of a column of water, which is why historically it has often been measured in centimetres or inches of water. If we are not divers we may rarely experience the bottom of a column of water directly, but we are all familiar with the gush of water from a tap that is a consequence of the pressure in our domestic plumbing. I live in a rather old house with a water tank in the roof. The water coming from the bathroom tap in the floor below is a vertical distance of about 3 metres below the open surface in the tank. The pressure behind the jet from the tap is thus ~300 cmH$_2$O, equivalent to about one-third of an atmosphere of pressure, and quite a driver for filling a bath. In the setting that Starling was considering, the difference between the hydrostatic pressure of blood in a capillary and the fluid in the lymph in a lymph vessel is around 30 cmH$_2$O. We know that there are pores through which water can move out of capillaries and into lymph vessels, and this pressure would be enough to produce a sizeable flow through such pores were it not for something in blood that prevents a rapid flow: this is the presence in blood of large protein molecules, which cannot pass through the pores.

The presence in blood of protein molecules that cannot accompany any water that leaves the blood through pores in the capillary wall leads to water being retained in the blood by a phenomenon that has been named 'oncotic pressure'. This refers to the tendency of water to 'diffuse' from a compartment where its concentration is high into a compartment where its concentration is low. The blood contains a high concentration of proteins. It is the presence of these large molecules that reduces the concentration of the water around them in the blood compared with the concentration of water in the neighbouring lymph vessel and thereby provides a *difference in concentration of water*, which tends to drive water back into the blood.

Putting these factors together, we can see that there is a hydrostatic pressure acting to drive water out of blood in capillaries and into lymph vessels. Acting in the opposite direction is a tendency for water to move down a concentration gradient from the lymph vessels, where there are few protein molecules, into the blood where there are many: oncotic pressure. Does one of these win over the other? The usual state of affairs is that only a small imbalance exists, which allows a flow of water from the capillaries into the lymph vessels of a few litres each day. When this small imbalance becomes a large imbalance oedema forms in tissues because the lymph vessels cannot drain water away fast enough.

By 1896 many experiments by Starling and others had shown the importance of hydrostatic pressure in driving lymph formation. Experiments in anaesthetised dogs were used to measure the flow of lymph along the thoracic duct, via which lymph collects before returning to the bloodstream. One way of achieving this was to increase the hydrostatic pressure of blood in capillaries using clamps or ligations on the veins downstream from the capillaries. That half of the story was clear. The second half only became clear to Starling when he conducted ingenious experiments in which water was able to move *from tissues* into blood.[10] In his key experiment he measured the oncotic pressure of the proteins in the blood and found that it was "comparable to that of the capillary (hydrostatic) pressures". His conclusion was that "at any given time, there must be a balance between the hydrostatic pressure of the blood in the capillaries and the osmotic attraction of the blood for the surrounding fluids". The implication for the formation of lymph was that normally these two pressures are almost in perfect balance but that to a small degree hydrostatic pressure dominates over the oncotic pressure and allows a tiny flow of lymph: something like 5 litres per day in an adult human – small compared with the large flow of blood around the body of around 8,000 litres per day.

For many in the medical world these rather abstruse reckonings had little meaning until they became applied to a common and visually striking medical problem: *dropsy*. This is what Starling did in his lectures and in his textbook *The Fluids of the Body*, published in 1909.[11] 'The dropsy' is a historical term applied to swelling of the soft tissues of the body due to accumulation of excess water. In a sense it is the same as what we now call oedema but it came to have a particularly strong association. This was the often gross swelling of the feet, ankles and calves seen in patients with heart failure.

Starling's lecture VIII on 'The causation of the dropsy' in his text of 1909 takes us through what we can now understand as causes of excess water in the tissues. In the fifteen "factors" he lists, we can recognise three groups: abnormal hydrostatic pressures, abnormal oncotic pressures and derangements of the barrier between blood and tissue. In heart failure the dominant feature is the high venous back-pressure from a failing heart, exacerbated in the dependent lower limb by gravity, hence the swelling of the legs.

It is not often that the oedema of high altitude is described as 'dropsy'. However, in Starling's day a disease of cattle at altitude in Colorado in which the 'brisket' area of the upper chest and neck became grossly swollen with water was referred to as "brisket disease, the dropsy of high altitudes".[12] Conventionally we retain the word 'oedema' (noting the American spelling 'edema') and apply Starling's insights to try to understand why a number of people who ascend to altitude experience pulmonary oedema, others are struck down by cerebral oedema, and some have the double misfortune of both at once.

High-altitude pulmonary oedema

My French climber's appalling night on 1 September 2000 was actually a stroke of bad luck. The chance of getting pulmonary oedema shortly after ascent to the Goûter Refuge is probably well below 0.1 per cent. Marco Maggiorini, an intensive care doctor in the University Hospital in Zürich, has published much on the topic, including a review of various studies that try to pin down the incidence.[13] Patients present with breathlessness, coughing, pink frothy sputum, and then the signs of the lungs becoming overloaded with water: blue lips, fast breathing and a noisy chest. The condition usually takes two or more days to develop, but not always. I recall ascending to the Capanna Margherita refuge on the Monte Rosa at 4,559 metres, the highest alpine refuge. Of a group of five one, became distressed by his breathing and a cough soon after arrival, so we did not delay our descent long after a bowl of hot soup. At that refuge, in the years 1980–4, Hochstrasser and colleagues identified one of 588 overnight residents needing to be air-rescued because of pulmonary oedema.[14] Like my French climber, about a third of the fifty patients they observed being rescued from throughout the Alps with pulmonary oedema also had cerebral oedema.

Pulmonary oedema is the abnormal accumulation of water in the airways of the lungs. To consider how ascent to altitude might predispose the airways of the lungs to fill with water, we need to consider the tiny blood vessels of the lungs. We also need a trip back in time, some 400 million years, to when evolution permitted sea-dwelling animals to take to the land.

Our lungs receive blood from the heart through the pulmonary artery. Many divisions occur downstream from the pulmonary artery and as we follow the flow of blood the arteries become smaller until they give way to tiny lung *capillaries*. Across the very thin walls of these the blood is able to receive oxygen from the air in the adjacent alveoli of the lung and also eliminate carbon dioxide.

A lung alveolus has the appearance of a single polygonal chamber, having six to eight straight sides, stacked with other alveoli in a honeycomb (Fig. 12 and Fig. 13). We call the sides *septa*; each *septum* separates two alveoli and carries a row of about five capillaries. In the adult human there are about 300 million of these alveoli, each about 0.25 mm in diameter, just visible to the naked eye.[15]

Fibres of *collagen* and *elastin* provide the structural support for capillaries in the septa, winding their way like the strands of a wicker basket past alternate sides of capillaries lying in a row. Along with the fibres run channels which link to lymph vessels so that any leakage of water from the side of a capillary next to the fibres can be drained away (Fig. 14). On the other side of the capillary things are more precarious. Here, a remarkably thin capillary wall only 0.5 micrometres thick has no channel through which any leaking water can flow away into lymph vessels.[16] Because it is so thin it is the side best suited for gas exchange between alveolar air and capillary blood, but leakage of water on this side is directly into the alveolar air and risks producing pulmonary oedema.

Here we come to a serious consequence of being a mammal breathing air. The area of the lung is about 50–100 square metres, often likened to that of a tennis court, and certainly our biggest window on the world (the surface area of our skin being only 1–2 square metres). It follows that over much of this area our blood is contained by a remarkably thin membrane. We might feel vulnerable. The membrane might rupture and fill our alveoli with blood or, less catastrophically, leak and produce pulmonary oedema.

You may think that the next important question is: what is the pressure of blood in these precariously exposed capillaries? After all, this will determine how likely it is that the Starling forces might precipitate alveolar flooding with water, or blood leaking across a damaged capillary wall. It is here that we need to think about the pressures involved in pumping blood around the circulation.

Blood pressure: horse, man and fish

To consider pressure we need to be quantitative. Here we confront the problem that there are different units of measurement. We earlier met a pressure of 30 cmH$_2$O in some capillaries while noting the term *hydrostatic* as referring to a column of water. The use of a column of the liquid metal mercury instead of a column of water goes back to the year 1643 when the Italian Evangelista Torricelli filled with mercury a metre-long tube, one end of which was sealed, set it vertically in a basin of mercury, and found that a column of mercury about 760 mm high remained in the tube. This demonstrated that the pressure of the atmosphere air was 760 mmHg. Had the experiment been conducted with a tube of water, which is 13.6 times less dense than mercury, a column height of about 10.3 metres would have been needed, illustrating the practical convenience of using mercury rather than water for such a purpose. But are the pressures of blood in the body sufficiently high to justify using mercury rather than water?

Of note is the first ever measurement of arterial blood pressure. From around 1714 the Reverend Stephen Hales used a vertical column of blood to measure the arterial blood pressure of three horses (Fig. 15). A detailed account from 1733 involved a brass cannula in the carotid artery of a restrained mare (lying down), connected via the excised windpipe of a goose to a glass tube 12¾ feet high and with a bore of ¹/₇th inch.[17] This was a delicate operation. On the release of a carotid ligature (a tie in the vessel) blood rose in the glass tube to 9½ feet (290 cm). The equivalent pressure measured in mmHg would be about 200 mmHg. The unit of mmHg has become well established for the measurement of pressure in medicine, meteorology and aviation, so we shall accustom ourselves to it here. It has another name that gives credit to Torricelli: one mmHg is identical to one *Torr* for all practical purposes.

Having settled on using the unit mmHg for pressure, we can consider pressures in the circulation. The horse we have seen – at least the horse under some degree of distress – has an arterial blood pressure of 200 mmHg. We are used to a normal human mean arterial blood pressure of 100 mmHg. Why do we have such a high pressure of blood in our arteries? A short answer seems to be that it is because we live on land. For the heart and vascular system to be able to perfuse a body under the influence of gravity, it is necessary for it to generate a sufficiently high pressure to lift blood to the head against the force of gravity. With this in mind, it is not surprising that arterial blood pressure increases with body mass in mammals, reaching very high values in the giraffe.[18]

A high arterial blood pressure may be good for perfusing tall bodies on land but presents a challenge to the lungs, which have to avoid high pressures because of the risk they carry of leakage and rupture. To see how this problem found a solution we need to think back about 400 million years to the challenges of evolving from life in the seas to life on land, breathing air.

First, we need to realise that an aquatic environment for a body provides buoyancy and removes any marked effect of gravity on the circulation of blood. Fish therefore have a low arterial blood pressure. It needs to be sufficient to drive blood around the body but not to lift blood against gravity. Fish therefore manage with an arterial pressure of about one-third of that of humans.

Second, we think about the demands of an organ for taking up oxygen from the environment. The organ for oxygen uptake from water – the *gill* in current species – has water on both sides of its gas-exchange surface: on one side, sea or river water; on the other side, water in blood. There is no risk of oedema disabling the exchange of

gas. The circulation of blood in fish takes the simple form of having
a heart that pumps blood first to the gills to pick up oxygen from the
surrounding water and onward to the tissues of the body, which can
use that oxygen.[19] A relatively low pumping pressure from the heart
is sufficient to perfuse this single-circuit arrangement.

In animals dependent upon air-breathing on land, the needs of the
lungs are very different from those of the gills of the fish. A separate
low-pressure circulation of blood has evolved in which the pressure of
blood in the capillaries, which exchange oxygen and carbon dioxide,
can (usually) be kept low enough to avoid rupture and to prevent the
accumulation of water in the airways. This has freed the main circulation to operate at much higher pressures capable of overcoming the
challenge of gravity. The circulation to the lungs is termed the *pulmonary circulation*. The pump for this is the *right* side of the heart. The
circulation to the rest of the body is the *systemic circulation* and this
is perfused from the *left* side of the heart. The needs of living under
gravity and air-breathing were therefore responsible for the evolution
of a heart with right and left sides, each supplying its own circulation
at a different pressure.[20]

Dr Maggiorini's studies at altitude

In humans the pulmonary circulation has a perfusion pressure about
one-fifth of that in the systemic circulation: a mean pressure of around
20 mmHg in the pulmonary artery supplying the lungs, in contrast to
the 100 mmHg in the arteries of the systemic circulation. The Swiss
intensivist Marco Maggiorini and colleagues conducted a fine study
in 2001, which gave us measurements both on healthy volunteers and
on climbers who developed high-altitude pulmonary oedema. Their
elegant study identified a pressure for the capillaries in the lung that
is a threshold above which the alveoli begin to fill with water.[21]

The technique used by Maggiorini is an illustration of scientific
cunning aided by modern technology. A sterile catheter about 1 metre
long passed via a large vein in the right arm reaches the right side of
the heart and can be passed onward into the pulmonary artery. The
catheter is a hollow tube filled with sterile salt solution. The pressure
at the end of the catheter in the pulmonary artery is measured by a
transducer connected to the end of the catheter outside the body. The
catheter width is 2 mm, small enough for it to be advanced further

into one of the second or third divisions of the main pulmonary artery. In one of these small divisions, the flow of blood can be halted by occluding the artery by inflating an elastic balloon of 5–10 mm diameter close to the end of the catheter. The pressure measured at the end of the catheter then suddenly drops from the pulmonary artery pressure to the capillary pressure; it then drops further, more slowly, to reflect the pressure in the veins of the lungs beyond the capillaries. This 'pressure-decay curve' needs a little mathematical analysis to cope with minor delays over the two-second period following occlusion, but the principle is simple and sound.

Maggiorini's study recruited thirty volunteers, sixteen of whom had a history of high-altitude pulmonary oedema on one or more occasions. The other fourteen volunteers acted as healthy controls. They were all studied first in the laboratory in Zürich (altitude 490 m) and then they ascended on foot to the Capanna Regina Margherita on the Monte Rosa (4,559 m). Further catheter studies were made after a night at the top. Among their many data, let us be selective and focus on the capillary pressures. In the healthy controls in Zürich the pressure was 10 mmHg. At the Margherita hut this rose to 13 mmHg. However, the capillary pressures in the volunteers who had a history of oedema went from 9 mmHg in Zürich to 19 mmHg at the hut and something very interesting happened in this group. Of the sixteen climbers who were vulnerable on the basis of their history, nine actually developed oedema; in these the capillary pressure averaged 22 mmHg; the five who did not develop oedema had an average capillary pressure of 16 mmHg. The key threshold value for the onset of pulmonary oedema was identified as 19 mmHg.[21] If capillary pressure exceeded that value, the alveoli began to fill with water. Below that value, the water in the capillary blood was contained.

These findings might seem to confirm Starling's hypothesis about the balance of hydrostatic pressure tending to cause water to leak from a capillary with the oncotic pressure working in the opposite direction to retain water in the blood. Perhaps the threshold of 19 mmHg is where the former overpowers the latter and water leakage occurs across the thin capillary wall. We shall see that, although this simple conclusion may seem persuasive, there is an elephant in the room in the shape of an alleged *watery film* in the alveolus: this has provided a century of controversy about what keeps the alveoli aerated as well as keeping it free from flooding with water. However, I would like to shelve for the present this question of whether the alveolus is lined by a watery film in favour of first thinking about the capillary pressure.

Hypoxic pulmonary vasoconstriction: cow, rabbit and man

Let us turn here to the question of why ascent to high altitude should cause a rise in capillary pressure. For me this is a scientific cause célèbre. It first occupied me in 1991 when Dr Niels Vejlstrup, a young Danish physician, came to work in the Oxford Laboratory of Physiology for his doctorate.[22] He has now long been a consultant paediatric cardiologist in Copenhagen, but our team in Oxford continued up to 2020 to chip away at the topic, sometimes in the mountains themselves.[23]

Altitude is associated with a low pressure of oxygen in the air we breathe and therefore in the alveolar gas in our lungs, and hence in the blood circulating in the body. We know from experiments extending back to the 1940s that low oxygen pressure in the alveoli stimulates nearby small arteries in the lung to constrict. These small arteries are the vessels that carry blood towards the capillaries. This reflex is known as hypoxic pulmonary vasoconstriction (HPV). It occurs as a local effect of low oxygen on small arteries, within small regions of lung tissue, and therefore does not necessarily involve the whole of both lungs unless those lungs jointly experience a low oxygen pressure.[24] Unfortunately, it is indeed the case that at high altitude both lungs are exposed to low oxygen pressure in the inspired air and so the 'local' reflex becomes a 'global' reflex, one to which all of the lung is subjected. Since the whole of the output of the right side of the heart has to be pumped through the lungs, this global constriction of the vessels through which it has to pass obstructs the circulation.

This reflex, which obstructs the circulation in the mountains, actually has an established benefit nearer sea level. The benefit comes from the need for the flow of blood in the lungs to be well matched to the flow of gas into and out of the lungs and to be so at the level of quite small areas of lung. To illustrate the importance of this matching, a situation can be imagined in which one of our two lungs is well perfused with blood but all the ventilation entering the body goes to the other lung: no exchange of oxygen into (or carbon dioxide out of) the blood could then take place – a state of affairs incompatible with life. Diseases such as pneumonia are characterised by creating areas of lung that are poorly ventilated because of the alveoli filling with inflammatory debris or liquid, or becoming collapsed, and survival depends upon effective gas exchange in the less affected areas of lung. It is consequently beneficial to divert the flow of blood to the healthier parts of the lung from the poorly ventilated areas by using the low levels of oxygen in these areas to constrict the blood vessels there. This is the job of HPV.

The Covid-19 pandemic has enlivened interest in HPV because this virus shows an ability to switch off the HPV reflex and leave blood flowing freely to areas of lung that are poorly ventilated.[25] The unoxygenated blood from these areas then mixes with the rest, lowering the overall saturation. The profoundly low levels of oxygen in the blood of many Covid-19 patients even early in the illness appears to be associated with this ability to damage this potentially life-saving reflex.

One of the limitations in finding how the lung responds to days at altitude (or days of pneumonia) is that laboratory experiments have tended to fit into a nine-to-five working day, and many of those hours can be required to get an experiment set up. It follows that we know a lot about how lung blood vessels respond to around thirty minutes of low oxygen and what cellular events might be involved, but not when subjects are exposed over many hours or days.

A second factor to consider is the relative ease of studying lung tissue from sacrificed animals compared with the challenges of exploring how lung behaves in intact animals or humans. Many studies are therefore on pieces of tissue, which of necessity do not survive long.

A third factor is the challenge of studying the effect on the lung of one stimulus at a time. Low oxygen is usually accompanied by other factors, which cause their own changes in the lung. If we take someone to altitude (or study them with simulated altitude in a laboratory chamber with low oxygen pressure) their breathing is stimulated by the low oxygen. The increase in breathing decreases the level of carbon dioxide in the blood and makes the blood alkalotic. Each of these three factors has its own effect on (inhibiting) HPV, and so it is very difficult to define the effect of low oxygen separately on the behaviour of the lung blood vessels.

In 1979 Jack Reeves, a leading Colorado expert on altitude physiology, and his colleagues reviewed the effects of low oxygen in the laboratory and also during high-altitude exposure, using ten animal species. They found the cow to have the most vigorous HPV reflex and the rabbit to have little or no HPV.[26] I have already noted that the cow can get into difficulties in the mountains.

The lowly status of the rabbit in the ranking came as a surprise to Dr Vejlstrup and me in the light of some fascinating experiments published in 1948 by two dextrous Dutch researchers, who seemed at that time to have become lost to history. Marinus Dirken and Hiepke Heemstra worked in the Physiological Institute of the University of Groningen. Dirken had taken a doctorate on the control of breathing in 1937 and Heemstra was writing his in 1948. They devised an arrangement where the two lungs of an anaesthetised rabbit could be separately ventilated with gases containing different fractions of oxygen, while at the same time they were able to measure how much oxygen each lung was allowing into the blood. These differential oxygen uptakes were used as measures of the blood flows to the two lungs.[27, 28] Office hours were no limitation to the length of their experiments; many were nine or ten hours in length and their papers show that several ran through the night. Maintaining a small anaesthetised animal stable, warm and healthy over such long periods, was a remarkable achievement.

They found that when one of the two lungs was ventilated with air containing very little oxygen the blood flow "may be gradually reduced to less than half of the original value, while the circulation of the other lung shows a corresponding increase". This was HPV observed over many hours. In some experiments it became more intense and was still getting stronger after eight hours. Some commentators dismissed their findings as "bizarre" and insisted from short experiments that the rabbit was "a notorious non-responder".

Here was a controversy. In Oxford we dutifully set about revisiting the work of these distinguished predecessors, noting a few imperfections in their methods; these included rather poor control of levels of carbon dioxide in their preparations (which we know can affect HPV), and their failure to consider any component of the HPV response that may have occurred in the first ten minutes (which most researchers took to be enough time for most of the response). We were not keen all-nighters, so we limited our measurements to six hours. We observed anaesthetised animals that had either nitrogen gas or saline liquid in a stationary left lung (keeping the oxygen level low in that lung) while the right lung was ventilated with oxygen. We were astonished to find that even within six hours the HPV response became so vigorous that it was capable of diverting nearly all of the blood flow away from the low-oxygen lung over to the ventilated lung. The rabbit was confirmed as having the strongest HPV ever seen, provided one waits long enough.[22] However, the underlying mechanisms remained a mystery.

The reader may insist at this point that, although a case might be made for the importance of knowing how cattle respond to altitude, the response of the rabbit to the mountain environment is not of practical concern. But our findings quickly led to the question of whether humans might have the slow, rabbit-like response of lung blood vessels to low oxygen, which had not been detected previously simply because it had not been looked for. So we set about investigating. Oxford lacks mountains, but we had the facility built by Peter Robbins of a chamber in which volunteers may be exposed to a low-oxygen environment for many hours while relaxing or working at a desk. We have seen in Chapter Two that it had the added feature that the air in the chamber could be modified every five minutes to achieve 'end-tidal forcing' of the gas in the lungs to have a constant (low) pressure of oxygen and a constant (normal) level of carbon dioxide, however vigorously the volunteer's breathing responded to the low-oxygen environment. This was achieved by frequently changing the composition of the gas in the chamber to 'clamp' the composition of expired alveolar gases measured at the nose at the values required for the experiment, regardless of how vigorously the volunteer breathed. We decided to set the low oxygen pressure in the lungs at half the normal value (50 mmHg instead of 100 mmHg); this is approximately the level experienced high in the Alps.

We therefore had a suitable environment in which to mimic altitude ascent with the added benefit of keeping the low-oxygen stimulus constant and not having the HPV response compromised by changing levels of carbon dioxide. The next issue was that of designing the experiment itself. It was not possible to mimic the rabbit experiments by having each of the two lungs of the volunteer exposed to a different concentration of oxygen (though this can be done in anaesthetised patients through separate endobronchial tubes). For our measure of the intensity and time-course of HPV we decided to use the catheter adopted by Maggiorini to determine how pressures in the pulmonary artery (and, from these, the resistance of the pulmonary circulation) change over time during eight hours of low oxygen.[29]

Six healthy medical colleagues volunteered and completed the study. We found that the HPV response at thirty minutes was apparent as a ~40 per cent rise in the resistance of the pulmonary circulation. It then changed little until at one hour it rose dramatically to reach a high point rise of ~130 per cent after a further hour, and then changed little thereafter. Another similar study on human volunteers found an even more continuous 'rabbit-like' intensification of the human HPV response up to eight hours.[30] By way of comparison, in the Maggiorini study of 2001, the resistance of the pulmonary circulation on ascent to the Margherita hut rose by ~140 per cent in the volunteers with no history of oedema and by ~160 per cent in those who did have a history.

These approaches all show that low oxygen induces a vigorous HPV response in pulmonary vessels and that this leads to pressures that are sometimes high enough to overwhelm the normal Starling balance of forces and hence lead to flooding of the alveoli. But is there not something that appears to make no sense here? The small pulmonary arteries that have a lively contractile response to low oxygen are *upstream* of the capillaries that have their thin walls exposed to the air in the alveoli. If the upstream arteries constrict in response to low oxygen, you would expect the pressure in the downstream capillaries to *decrease*, not to increase. You might therefore expect HPV to *protect* the alveoli from oedema, not predispose them to it. Here we find ourselves in the middle of a dispute that has occupied researchers in the field for a long time. How can one explain the opposite of what we would expect from the basic plumbing characteristics of blood vessels in the lungs?

There are two common hypotheses. The most widely advocated explanation for the leakage of water from *some* capillaries is that HPV varies throughout the lungs. This means that in some parts the capillary bed is not well protected from the pressure of blood in the pulmonary arteries, which is high enough to cause leakage, while in other parts a more intense HPV response protects the capillaries.[31] Some, including Marco Maggiorini and his colleagues, are less convinced by this explanation. They comment that "it is difficult … to conceive that the tip of the pulmonary catheter *always* went to pulmonary arteries perfusing edematous lung regions" (my italics).[21]

Here they draw attention to the fact that, if the HPV response was very variable throughout the lung, sometimes the tip of the study catheter would end up in a part of the lung with intense HPV and *low* capillary pressure. This appeared never to happen. The explanation they prefer is that the pulmonary veins, which lie *downstream* of the capillaries, also have a degree of constriction and that this may be enough to cause the rise in capillary pressure seen in their study. Many experiments support this (to me) more appealing possibility, but I suspect that we can anticipate many more studies before the matter is settled.[24] Perhaps the final result will be that both the hypotheses are true: it is possible both to have variability in the strength of HPV throughout the lung *and* a role for the constriction of veins in response to the low oxygen.

The alveolar 'watery film': does it exist?

We have been considering how the lungs may find themselves filling with water when exposed to high altitude. I would like to return now to the lining of the alveoli. Readers may be surprised to find that schoolboys and girls arriving to study biomedical sciences or medicine over many years have almost invariably been taught in their biology lessons that the lungs are normally *lined with water*, and that without this lining they cannot function properly.[32] The standard teaching is that "the inner surface of the alveoli is lined with a watery film which exerts a surface tension" and that "it is essential that these membranes do not dry out, otherwise gases would not be able to diffuse across them".[33] It would be easy at this point to get immersed in what can be described as a 'dogs' dinner' of a topic, inner contradictions of which pervade not just the school textbooks but university teaching as well. But a brief crash course on the 'watery film' may help us understand high-altitude pulmonary oedema.[34]

Contrary to the claim of school texts, we do not need a layer of water on our thin capillary walls to enable gases to diffuse between the capillary blood and the alveolus: myth number 1. The blowing of soap bubbles is enough to remind us that the only stable liquid–gas surface has the shape of a sphere (unless gravity upsets this with really enormous bubbles). It follows that the polyhedronal honeycomb-like alveolus cannot be lined with a thin layer of liquid water (or liquid anything else), which follows its fairly flat sides and sharply

curved corners: myth number 2. We ask how these misunderstand-
ings may have arisen.

Some smart experiments in 1929 by Kurt von Neergaard, a
German-born physiologist working in Zürich, showed that the air
passages of isolated animal and human lungs could be inflated with
a watery solution (gum arabic) using only about half the pressure
needed to inflate the lung with air in the normal way.[35] This, correctly,
led to the notion that the inner surface of the alveoli has a surface
tension that tends to collapse the alveoli. However, it led, incorrectly,
to myth number 2, that there must be a continuous layer of liquid
responsible for this surface tension.

It was realised that if this (hypothetical) liquid were pure water,
which has a very high surface tension, then its presence would cause
all alveoli to collapse. With the discovery of a frothy soap-like material in the lungs in the 1960s, the idea was born that this *surfactant*
(much of which is dipalmitoyl lecithin) floats on top of a lining of
water and serves to reduce the surface tension of the water to a value
compatible with the alveoli staying inflated.

Expert microscopists of the lung have shown us that healthy lung
has surfactant lying directly on the alveolar epithelial cells and only
tiny amounts of liquid sitting in corners of the alveoli or clefts between
adjacent capillaries in the alveolar walls.[36] Pulmonary oedema provides a striking contrast. Here an excess of water may be sufficient
to flood alveoli partially or fully.[37] In this context, it is interesting to
note that if spherical surfaces of pure water were to be present in
alveoli with a diameter of ~0.2 mm, then the surface tension of the
water would apply a suction to the capillary wall of ~10 mmHg. This
would unbalance the Starling forces in favour of drawing more water
into the alveoli and flooding the lung; we can think of it as being
equivalent to raising the hydrostatic pressure in the lung capillary by
10 mmHg, a doubling of the normal value from Maggiorini's measurements and a sure way to induce pulmonary oedema.

Before I complete this crash course on the 'watery lining' (or
absence of it), I need to address a final widespread misunderstanding
in its teaching. Myth number 3 is that unaided 'passive' Starling forces
alone are normally sufficient to keep the alveoli free of flooding. A
major step in correcting this myth was made by Christian Crone of
Copenhagen who travelled to Paris to work with colleagues on the
question of whether the capillary wall in the lung might use an active

pumping process in its efforts to keep the alveolus clear of water. Active use of fuel molecules (adenosine triphosphate – the body's equivalent of battery power) has been known since the 1950s to be responsible for the pumping of molecules across the wall of the intestine for the absorption of food and across the tubule of the kidney to regulate the composition of urine. Crone suspected that a similar sort of pumping might be present in the alveoli of the lungs (which are derived embryologically from the intestine during development) and that this might help to keep the lungs from flooding. In a masterly set of experiments using rat lungs and published in 1987, Crone and his French co-workers showed that some of the epithelial cells that sit on the air-side of the alveolar wall actively pump sodium ions, glucose and water from the air-side of the alveoli into spaces next to capillaries, and therefore onward into the blood.[38, 39] Crone was on the way to finding out more about this mechanism when he died at the age of sixty-four in 1990.[40]

In Oxford, Niels Vejlstrup and I set about investigating whether the same active pumping process played a role in clearing water from the lungs of the anaesthetised rabbit. We made a model of extreme pulmonary oedema by filling the left lung of the rabbit with salt solution and observing it over six hours. We found that the lung was able to pump into the blood about 1.5 ml per hour of water over a range of alveolar pressures (2–7 mmHg). When we applied drugs that inhibit the pumping mechanisms (which Crone and colleagues had identified: amiloride and phloridzin), we found that water moved in the reverse direction; it leaked from the blood into the alveoli when the alveolar pressure was below 3 mmHg, which it is during normal breathing (when it is ~0 mmHg). When the alveolar pressure was higher than 3 mmHg, there was still an uptake of water into the blood but at a rate below the normal value.[41] These experiments offered the astonishing suggestion that without the active pumping process our lungs would slowly fill up with water from the blood. When we extrapolated to an adult human weighing 70 kg, we concluded that the rate of filling would be ~1.5 litres per day. Crone and his colleagues extrapolated data from their rat experiments and came to exactly the same estimate.[38]

Another way of interpreting the data from these experiments is to go back to thinking about Starling's forces. We can think of the active pumping mechanism as providing a boost to the Starling force (or rather pressure) of about 5 mmHg acting to counter the efforts of the hydrostatic pressure of blood in the capillaries, which causes water to leak out of the blood. In other terms, the active pumping of solutes adds ~5 mmHg to the oncotic pressure acting to keep water in the blood stream.

Studies in various species, including patients in hospital, have confirmed the presence of active pumping of solutes and water from the alveoli of the lungs. The extent to which we depend upon this pumping to stay alive in health remains somewhat uncertain.[42] One possibility for high-altitude pulmonary oedema is that inhibition of this pumping mechanism is triggered by the low-oxygen environment of the mountains allowing water to accumulate in alveoli. Of note here is that the drug salmeterol may be used to stimulate the pumping and thereby reduce the risk of the high-altitude pulmonary oedema by 50 per cent.[43]

We have met three myths. A summary of the likely state of affairs may help. The healthy alveolus of the lung contains very little water, but what there is has the potential to have a high surface tension, which can act in two unwelcome ways: it can collapse the alveolus or it can draw more water to enter the alveolus from the blood. The lung has two mechanisms for reducing these risks. The first involves surfactant. This coats the whole surface of the alveolus, including the surface of any pools of water that may be present. The surfactant reduces the surface tension of the pools and thereby reduces the tension in the whole of the alveolar surface. The second protective mechanism is the pumping of water from pools of water to minimise their size and thereby concentrate the surfactant on their surface. Gas exchange between alveolar air and capillary blood benefits from alveoli remaining open and free of excess water.

Angelo Mosso and 'mountain sickness'

It may be that preoccupation with some recent science has led to some discourtesy in ignoring the contributions of Professor Angelo Mosso, Italy's historic contributor to both the infrastructure and the science of mountain physiology. The experiments of Maggiorini measuring the capillary pressure of the lungs, and those mentioned in the section above using salmeterol (by Sartori and colleagues from Lausanne), were undertaken in the Capanna Margherita on the Monte Rosa massif. We owe this remarkable facility largely to Mosso, professor of physiology in Turin from 1879 (Fig. 16). His proposal to construct a very high hut for scientific research went before the Italian Alpine Club in 1889. Widespread support was received, including from Queen Margherita who made an arduous ascent on 18 August 1893 to inaugurate the new refuge.[44] It sat (as its successor sits) in Italy, a few metres from the Swiss–Italian border, on a rocky peak known both as the Signalkuppe and the Punta Gnifetti, at 4,559 metres (Fig. 17).

Mosso led his first scientific expedition there in the summer of 1894, having asked the Minister for War for permission to take ten soldiers and an army surgeon.[45] The studies were interrupted by life-threatening pulmonary oedema in one twenty-two-year-old soldier, Pietro Ramella, who became ill soon after arriving on 12 August. On that day, his "violent headache" was treated with cocaine and Masala wine. From early the next day lung "inflammation" developed and persisted for four days and made the four doctors concerned that "we should perhaps have had to witness the death of our comrade, and to the summit of Monte Rosa would cling to-day the sorrowful recollection of a fatal case … similar to that which caused the death of Dr Jacottet on Mont Blanc". (This is a clear example now of fatal pulmonary oedema, Jacottet dying in the Vallot refuge on 2 September 1891.) Mosso adds a hint of a friendship with Oxford's professor of physiology, Burdon Sanderson, to whom he dedicated by hand my department's author-signed copy of his *Life of Man on the High Alps*, and reminds us of the uncertainty at the time about the cause of the "alarming dyspnoea" of altitude:

> Dr. Burdon Sanderson tells me that on a visit to Zermatt many years ago, a well-known German professor who had attempted a high ascent was brought down by his guide in a state of intense and alarming dyspnoea. His case was recognized as one of pneumonia, and treated accordingly. In a couple of days he was convalescent. Dr S. thinks it probable that this case was of the same kind as that of soldier Ramella.[45]

Perhaps it is the "violent headache" that needs some thought before closing a chapter that has focused on an infrequent, albeit dangerous, form of altitude sickness to the neglect of the more common form, 'acute mountain sickness'. A large proportion of people who ascend to above 4,000 metres experience headache. This is commonly accompanied by nausea, vomiting, loss of appetite, dizziness and fatigue. Mosso spent most of his book describing cases of mountain sickness and reviewing the dozens of opinions about its possible causes, including exhaustion from insufficient air pressure to keep the hip joint from dislocating , "anaemia of the brain", alighting from (rather than remaining on) one's mule, cold wind blowing on the skin, standing in a hollow rather than on a ridge, and being in rocky terrain rather than on snow.[45] Quite a selection.

Mosso had a particular interest in detecting pulsatile blood flow to the brain by finding subjects with holes in their skulls. In 1877 he had studied two boys with traumatic holes in the head, which enabled direct examination of the pulsating brain: one was a fourteen-year-old who had fallen from a balcony and was studied in a decompression chamber; the other was a thirteen-year-old who had been struck on the head by an axe, who was studied breathing air with a low concentration of oxygen. Mosso's conclusion was that these two forms of mimicked ascent led neither to "cerebral anaemia" nor "congestion" and that "the blood circulates in a sufficient quantity through the brain and in a manner little differing from the normal as far as an altitude of 5,520 metres".[45] He was disappointed not to be able to undertake further experiments in the mountain setting. "It was my wish to find some man with a hole in his skull who would have been willing to come with me on the Monte Rosa expedition, but I was not successful in my search."[45]

One of the sad things about Mosso is that he has gone down in history as the man who got things wrong despite great efforts. We now know that blood flow to the brain increases substantially at high altitude, at least in the first few days after ascent and sometimes by about 50 per cent. What we do not know is whether these changes are related to development of acute mountain sickness.[46] More certain is that acute mountain sickness can progress to the devastating condition of high-altitude cerebral oedema, in which swelling of the brain leads to decline of cognition, unsteadiness, lassitude, confusion and coma. My French climber in 2000 at the Goûter refuge ticked off some from the list. Our knowledge of why only a few are affected by this progression remains minimal; it is not surprising that Mosso could make little progress by looking into the head in his day.

The misunderstanding that Mosso is perhaps best known for is captured in the title of his Chapter Twelve: 'Explanation of mountain-sickness – acapnia'.[45] He coined the term 'acapnia' from the Latin word meaning 'without smoke', capturing his view that reduction of the amount of carbonic acid, or carbon dioxide, in the body "plays some part in" the symptoms of mountain sickness. In experiments on his "servant in the laboratory", and on himself, he became convinced that symptoms were worse when the carbon dioxide level was lowered even if the "weight of oxygen breathed" remained unchanged. Sadly, his chapter title rather overstated the case by suggesting that oxygen played *no* role, although I think this was not what he intended. We now know that reduction in the level of carbon dioxide in the body, which arises from the increase in breathing at altitude, plays a major role in the regulation of breathing, and in the responses of blood vessels both in the lungs and in the brain, aspects of which have kept many of us busy in the laboratory.[47]

A demonstration of the importance of carbon dioxide in regulating the blood flow to the brain is the fact that you can rapidly make yourself feel (or actually) faint by voluntarily over-breathing for less than a minute; this is a response to the reduction in brain blood flow that follows the fall in carbon dioxide in the blood as you breathe out more than usual. Given that the level of carbon dioxide in the blood in a climber breathing air on the summit of Everest is *less than one-fifth* of normal, we should be in no doubt of its importance in affecting the body's response to ascent.[48] Mosso was partially correct.

Dexamethasone and friends

I began this chapter thinking about what little medication was available to help a seriously ill climber at the Goûter refuge on Mont Blanc. The drug I really needed (apart from oxygen) was dexamethasone, of which sadly none was available that day. This is only one member of an armoury of medications that can help prevent or treat the various forms of altitude illness, but it has quite a reputation.[49] In fact, it is so efficacious in preventing altitude illness that physicians are reluctant to recommend it for that purpose because it can encourage overambitious rates of ascent. Nevertheless, I administered it to myself as prophylaxis for a trip to Mount Kenya in 2004.

Our team in Oxford became intrigued as to why dexamethasone

was such an effective drug in the mountain setting, as was shown in a fine study at the Capanna Margherita by Maggiorini.[50] Making do with our Oxford low-oxygen chamber as our substitute mountain (although with pictures of mountains on its walls), graduate student Chun Liu set about exposing eight healthy volunteers individually to four separate eight-hour stays in the chamber, breathing either air or low oxygen, and taking tablets of either dexamethasone or a placebo.[51] Angelo Mosso would have been pleased to see us keeping the carbon dioxide concentration in the lungs constant when the oxygen was low by supplementing the air in the chamber with carbon dioxide. We measured breathing and the HPV response of the blood vessels in the lungs.

Our most striking finding shed light on the reputation dexamethasone has for efficacy and on my own previous experience of taking the drug. On its own, it was a marked stimulant of breathing, more than doubling the ventilation of gas into and out of the lungs. When volunteers had a day with dexamethasone combined with low oxygen, breathing was even greater than with either stimulus alone. I was reminded of how desperately breathless I had felt traversing to Mackinder's Chimney at around 5,000 metres on Mount Kenya. It is a very steep section and on the longest route I had tackled. On reaching the Nelion summit (5,188 m) and sitting for a rest, measurements of the oxyhaemoglobin saturation of my blood (S_pO_2) with a pulse oximeter on a finger provided us with the sort of clinical trial that Mosso would have liked in his book:

Volunteer on Nelion (17 January 2004)	S_pO_2
Author (dexamethasone 4 mg 12 hourly)	86 per cent
Guide Charles Mathenge (control)	75 per cent

Increase in breathing stimulated by dexamethasone may well be beneficial in increasing the level of oxygen in the blood, but it induces disabling dyspnoea on exertion! It may be satisfying to shed light on how an old medication might work, and the promising role of dexamethasone in Covid-19 has brought it more recent fame.

We also wanted to explore something more innovative that might help with altitude exposure. Mosso had considered the merits of smelling salts. We thought to try doses of intravenous iron, based on the role of iron in the molecular response to low oxygen throughout the body, which was uncovered in recent years in the 'hypoxia-inducible factor' pathway that we visited in Chapter Two. A team visit to Peru in 2008 studied healthy volunteers ascending from sea level in Lima to the mining town of Cerro de Pasco at 4,340 metres. A dose of iron on the third day at altitude reduced the HPV response to altitude by 40 per cent, raising the possibility that this could help to prevent pulmonary oedema.[52] With the same team we examined the effects of prophylactic iron on the common symptoms of acute mountain sickness and found in those receiving iron a smaller increase in a score of mountain sickness after the first day at altitude.[53] In a later Himalayan study by a combined Oxford–military team, climbers ascending to 5,100 metres on Dhaulagiri were given prior administration of intravenous iron in London and had a rather striking 5 per cent increase in oxyhaemoglobin saturation in their blood when they were in the higher parts of the climb; this level of benefit means a lot when S_pO_2 falls towards 80 per cent.[23] The studies jointly suggested that making volunteers replete with iron (but not overloading them) may diminish the unhelpful excess HPV response that occurs at altitude.

So, what have we learned about high-altitude pulmonary oedema? It occurs when low atmospheric oxygen pressure at altitude leads to the hydrostatic pressure of blood in the lung capillaries exceeding a threshold. This threshold is determined by the oncotic pressure of blood, the vigour of a pumping mechanism at the alveolar wall, and the surface properties of the alveolar wall. The hydrostatic pressure of blood in the capillaries is influenced by the phenomenon of HPV whereby the small arteries and veins respectively upstream and downstream of the capillaries constrict in response to low oxygen. Fortunately, drugs are available that can reduce the risk of oedema by modulating these factors.

No such help was available a century ago. I return now to Sligger to follow mountaineering events at the turn of the twentieth century.

Sligger (Francis Urquhart) and mountaineers

Balliol College lost its tutor, the Reverend Richard Nettleship, to altitude exposure in 1892, the year of the *catastrophe*, in which Sligger was unable to convene a reading party at his family chalet. From 1893 the reading parties continued, that year's consisting of himself and five of his peers. We can note that the chalet was supported by servants so that a domestic existence of relative comfort, similar to that enjoyed in an Oxford college at the time, prevailed in the mountain environment.[2] The following year, 1894, was the year of Sligger's graduation. A total of sixteen party members visited during a season extending from June to September, setting a pattern of numbers and diversity of age for the decades to come. A tradition of long hours of silent study was established; days of reading were interspersed with outings on the mountainside, which were often very vigorous, sometimes lasting several days, with glacier crossings and overnight stays in mountain refuges on both the French and Italian sides of the Mont Blanc massif.

Increasingly, Sligger's reading parties collected visitors with distinguished careers in public life, including two generations of prime minister Herbert Asquith's family and later the future prime minister Harold Macmillan. The year 1900 saw a remarkable group of visitors, which induced Sligger to make his one and only ascent of Mont Blanc. Sligger's brother-in-law, William Tyrrell, was a diplomat at the Foreign Office, a family connection that broadened Sligger's network. This link seems likely to have been responsible for the invitation to the chalet of two historic figures: the climber-explorer Gertrude Bell and Roger Casement, who was to collaborate with Germany in supporting the Irish rebellion of 1916, and consequently was executed for treason.

The party of 1900 also included the German Count Gebhard Blücher, another friend of Tyrrell, whose fabulously wealthy family owned palaces in Silesia and Berlin, one of which became for many years the US Embassy next to the Brandenburg Gate. In one of the strange twists of British–German relations of the early twentieth century, it was to visit Count Blücher's English wife Evelyn, holed up (though in relative luxury) through much of the First World War in the Berlin Esplanade Hotel, that Casement went on 4 April 1916, shortly before his return to Ireland and arrest in May. Realising that he was regarded as a traitor by the British and an enemy spy by the Germans he "came into the room like one demented", fearing that they might be overheard. "You were right a year ago when you told me that I had put my head into a noose in coming here. ... I realised from the moment I landed here what a mistake I had made," she recounted him saying. "And at these words he sat down and sobbed like a child. I saw the man was beside himself with terror and grief."[54]

The horrors of this conflict were a world away in 1900 when

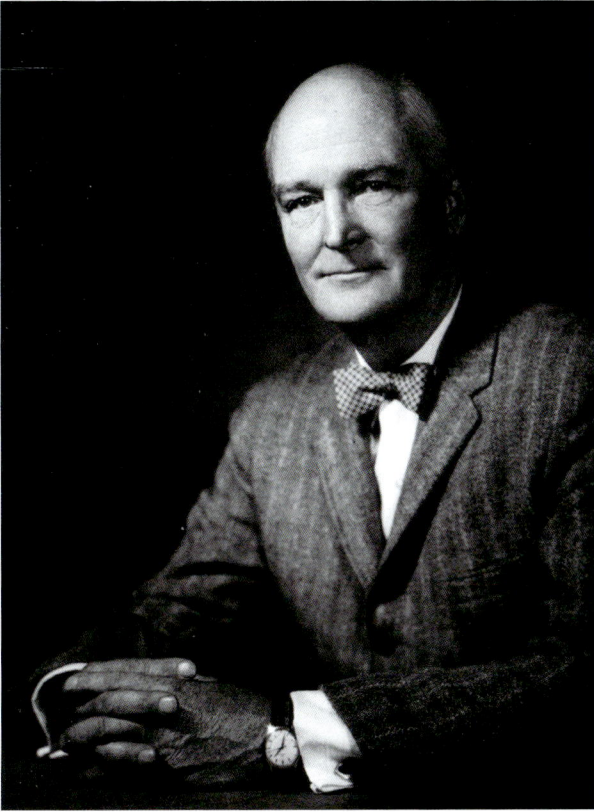

Figure 1. John H. Gibbon (1903–73), originator of the first successful heart–lung machine, photographed in 1968.

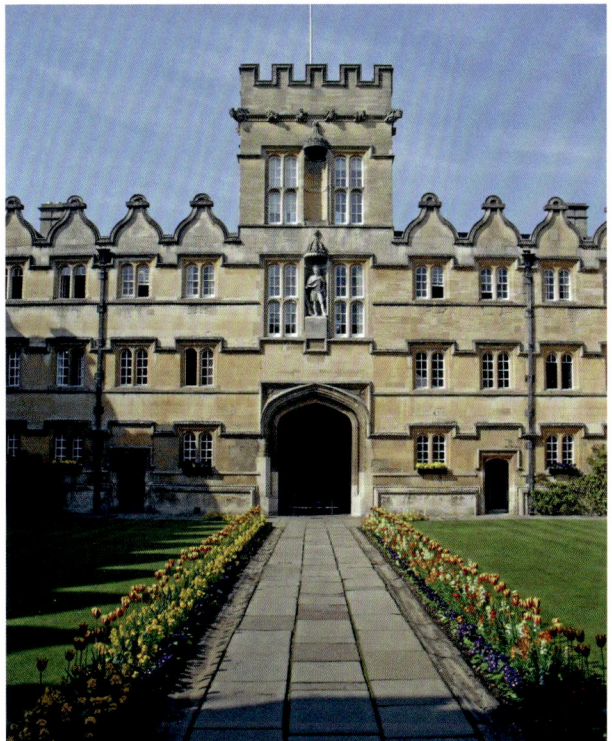

Figure 2. University College, Oxford, Main Quadrangle ('Front Quad') completed around the year 1680, seen from the spot where Charles Moffat fell mortally wounded and Denis Melrose was struck in the chest on 17 May 1940 as they were targeted by a fellow student John Fulljames with a rifle from a window close to the tower.

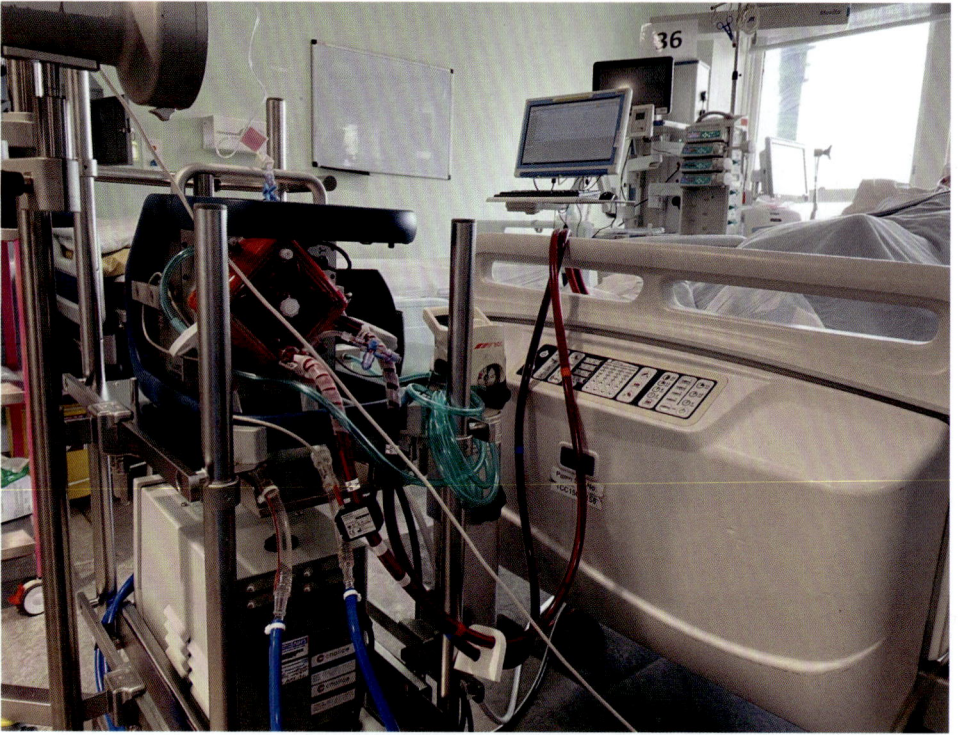

Figure 3. Extracorporeal membrane oxygenation equipment in use at Guy's and St Thomas' Hospital in London during the Covid-19 pandemic. Visible is the Maquet–Quadrox microporous capillary oxygenator (red square frame), to which leads a tube carrying deoxygenated dark-red blood from the patient, and from which a tube returns oxygenated bright-red blood to the patient. Pumping is provided by a centrifugal pump which sits behind the oxygenator. The patient's bed is on the right.

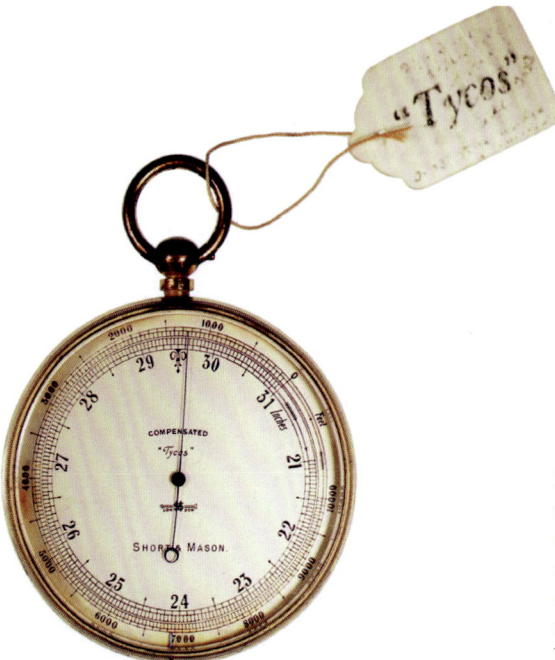

Figure 4. Mabel FitzGerald's barometer accompanied her on her expedition to Colorado in 1911 and provided measurements of atmospheric pressure against which she could compare measurements of breathing and of haemoglobin concentration in the blood of high-altitude residents.

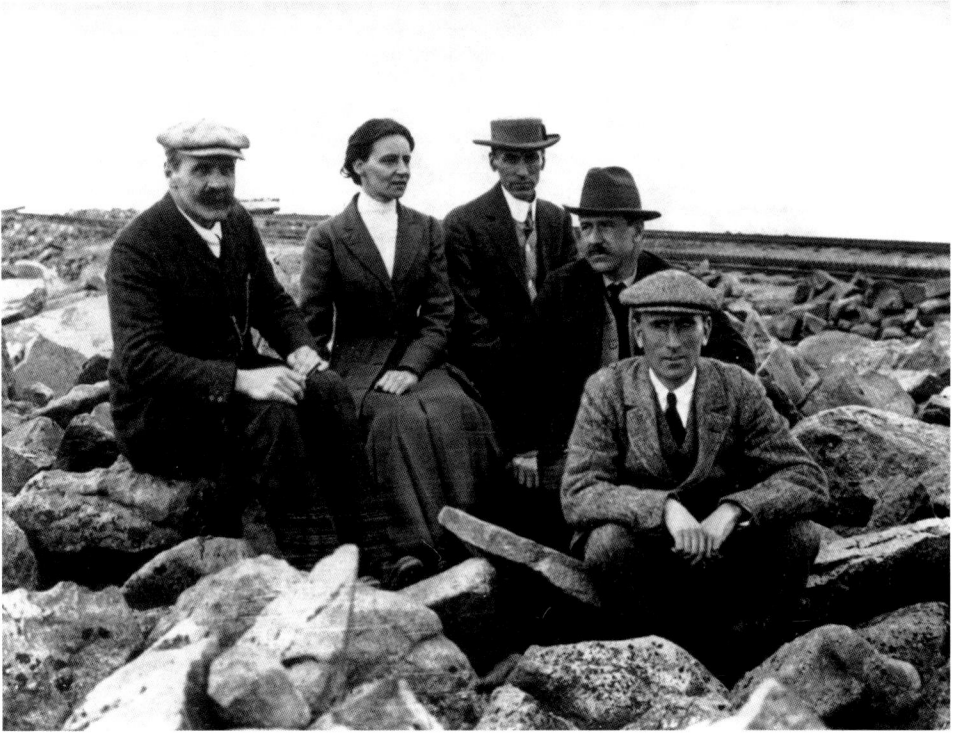

Figure 5. Members of the Anglo-American Pikes Peak expedition of 1911 seated close to the summit station at 4,300 m. From left: John Scott Haldane, Mabel FitzGerald, Edward C. Schneider, Yandell Henderson and Claude G. Douglas.

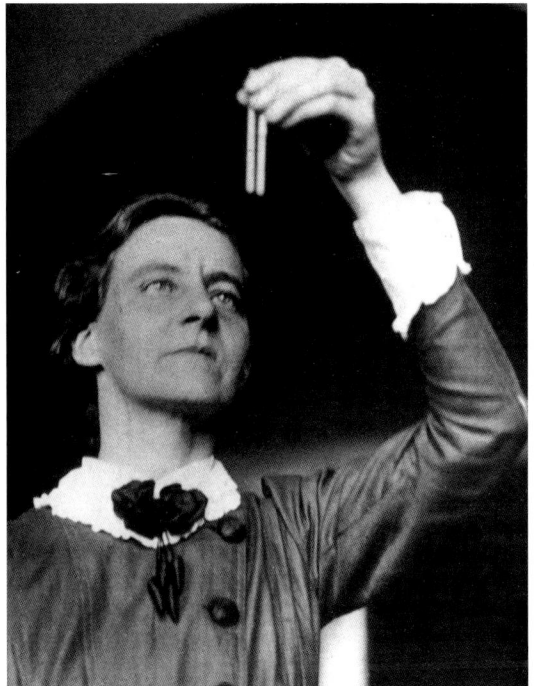

Figure 6. Mabel FitzGerald, measuring the haemoglobin concentration in blood. This was achieved by diluting the blood sample in one of two tubes until it matched the colour of a standard in the other tube.

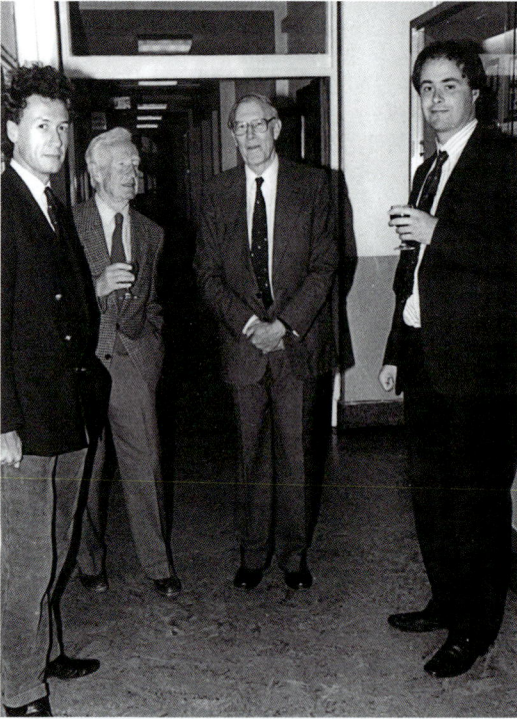

Figure 7. The unveiling of a new display cabinet for Mabel FitzGerald's barometer in 1988. From left: David Paterson, Dan Cunningham, Sir Roger Bannister and Peter Robbins (by the cabinet).

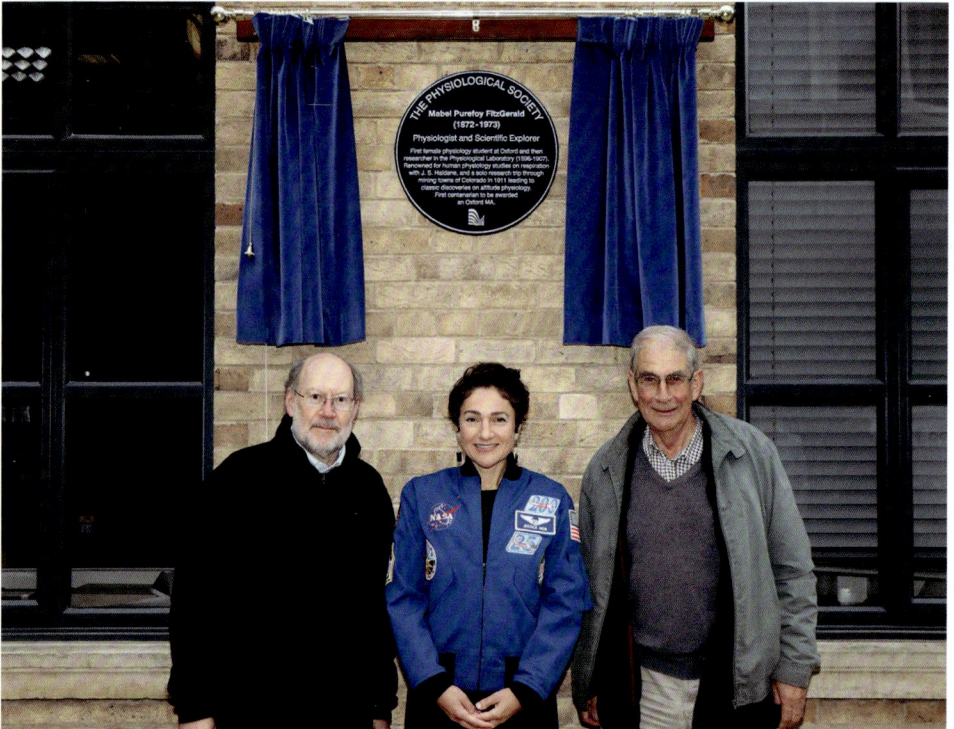

Figure 8. NASA astronaut and physiologist Jessica Meir unveiled a plaque in honour of Mabel FitzGerald on her visit to Oxford to deliver a public lecture on 16 November 2021. Jessica's many achievements include the first all-female spacewalk (on 18 October 2020). The author (left) and his co-investigator Richard Boyd.

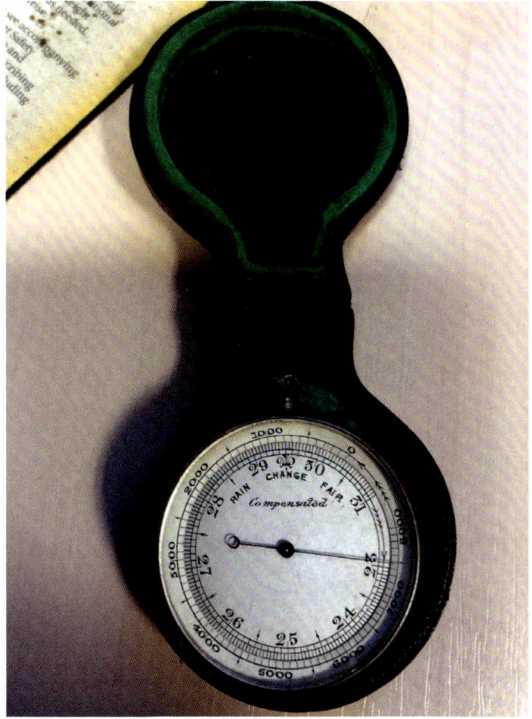

Figure 9. John Scott Haldane's barometer. This instrument was an engraved gift to Haldane in 1891. It is likely that it accompanied Haldane in visits to collieries during investigation of mining disasters. It may also have visited Pike's Peak, Colorado, in 1911. In 2019 it found its way with Nobel laureate Professor Sir Peter Ratcliffe FRS to the Nobel Museum in Stockholm.

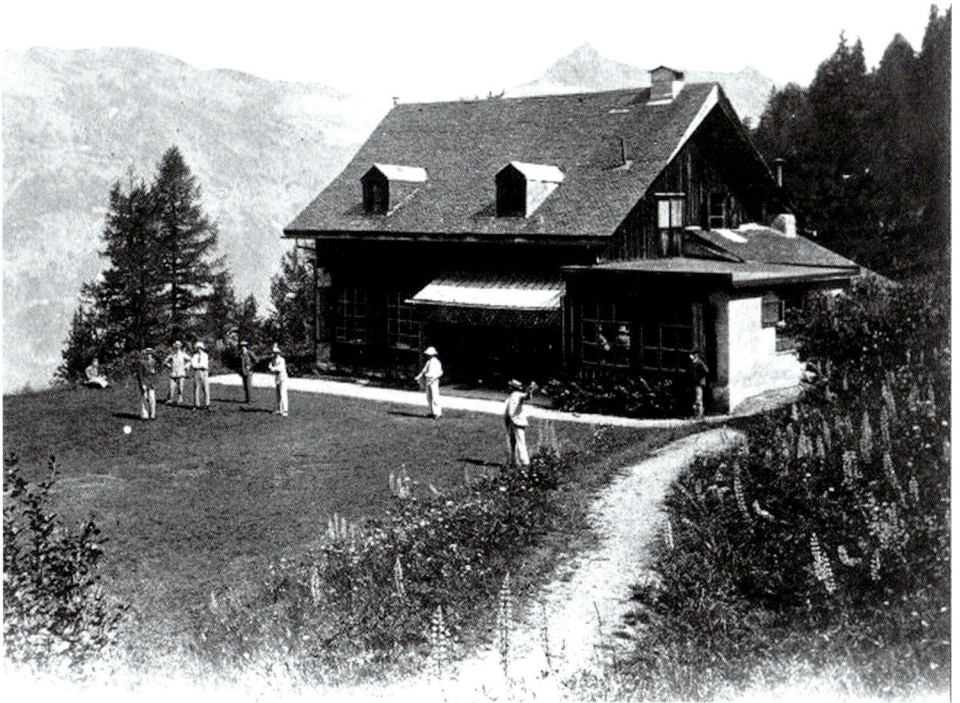

Figure 10. The chalet of David Urquhart built in 1865 on the Mont Blanc massif above the French village of St Gervais-les-Bains. From 1891 it was used by his son 'Sligger' for summer reading parties of students from the University of Oxford. Its successor (after a fire of 1906) is a larger chalet used for student reading parties and known locally as the 'Chalet des Anglais'.

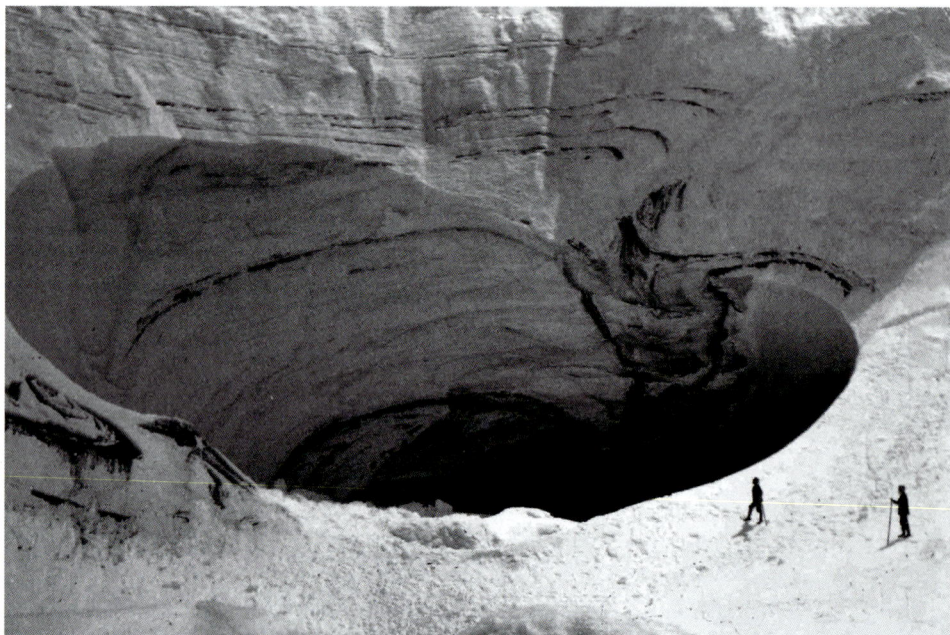

Figure 11. The *Catastrophe of St Gervais* 1892. The hole in the Tête Rousse glacier from which the subglacial lake avalanched down the Bionnay valley of Mont Blanc on the night of 11–12 July.

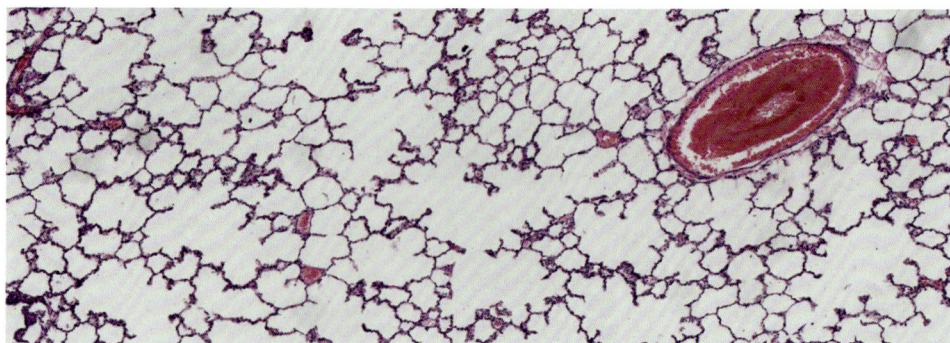

Figure 12. Light microscopic section from human lung (haematoxylin and eosin stain). Polygonal alveoli of diameter about 0.2 mm fill most of the field, many seen collected around the alveolar ducts through which they receive inspired air. One large blood vessel is in view, laden with red blood cells.

Figure 13. Scanning electron micrograph of rabbit lung alveoli showing approximately 20 alveoli of diameter about 0.2 mm. The convolutions made by the capillaries in the alveolar septa (walls) are apparent throughout.

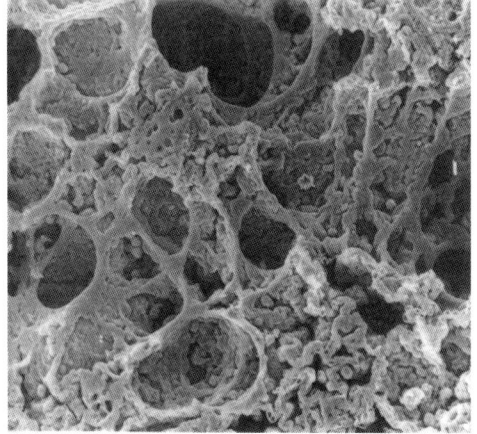

Figure 14. Architecture of interalveolar septa in the lung. (A) Scanning electron micrograph from a human lung shows the capillary network. Doughnut-shaped red cells can be seen at the edges of sectioned capillaries. (B) Transmission electron micrograph showing capillaries containing dark red blood cells. Each capillary has a thin side facing one alveolus and a thicker side facing a neighbouring alveolus. The thicker side contains connective tissue fibres. Scale markers 10 μm.[58]

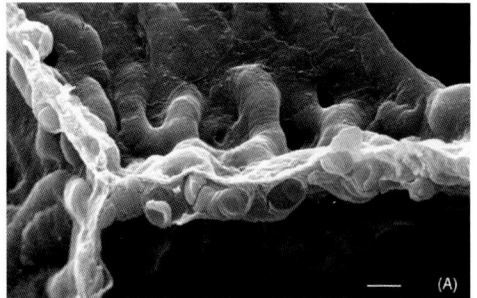

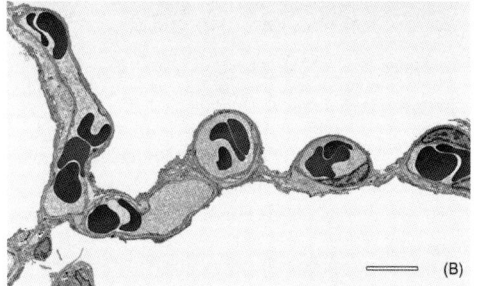

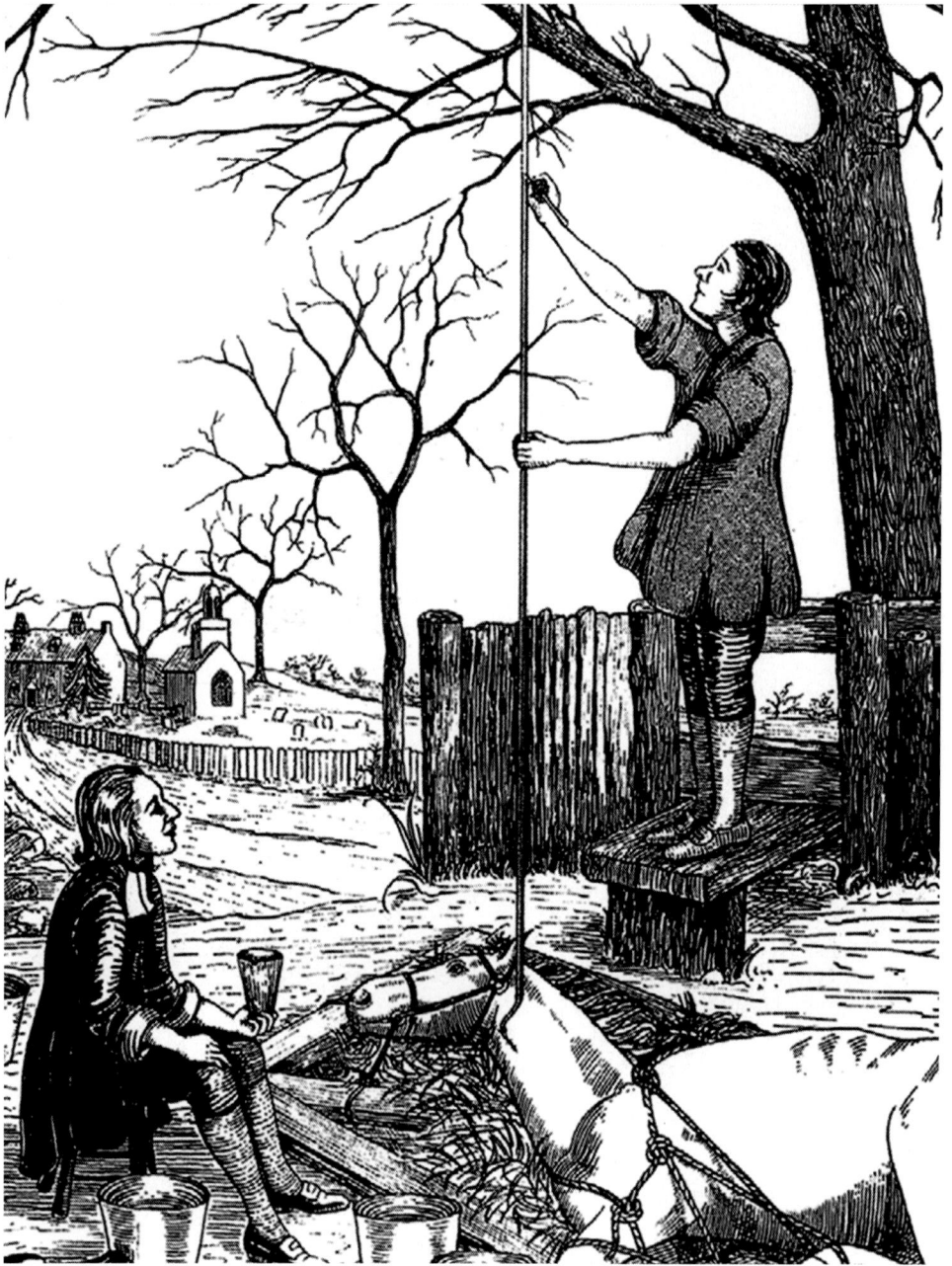

Figure 15. Measurement of the arterial blood pressure of the horse by the Reverend Stephen Hales around the year 1714. A brass cannula in a carotid artery was connected via an excised windpipe of a goose to a glass tube 12¾ feet high. Blood rose in the tube to a height of 9½ feet (290 cm).[17]

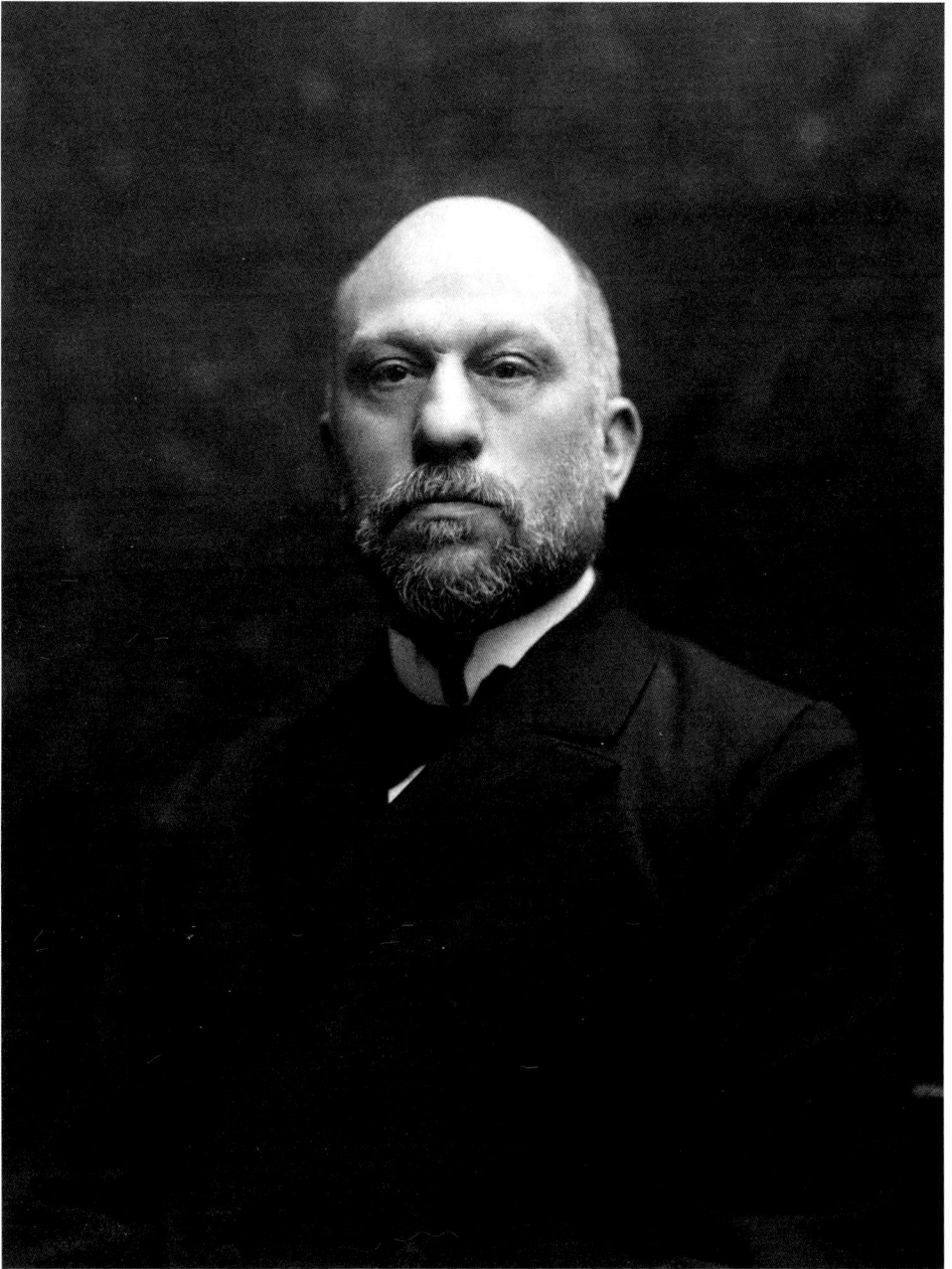

Figure 16. Professor Angelo Mosso, *c*.1910, Italy's renowned researcher into mountain sickness and originator of the Capanna Regina Margherita on the Monte Rosa at 4,559 metres altitude.

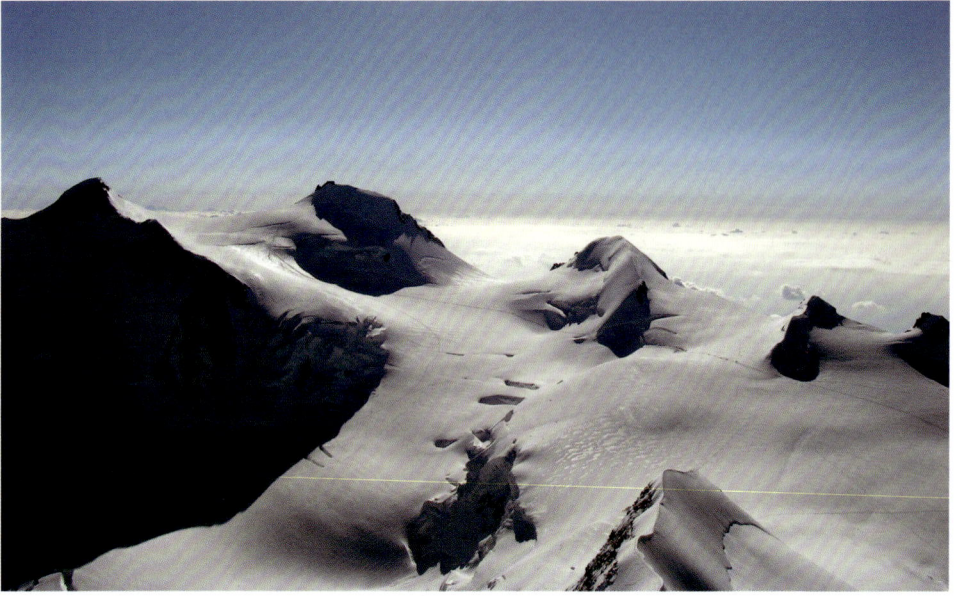

Figure 17. Site of the Capanna Regina Margherita. View from the Lyskamm of the Monte Rosa plateau. The Margherita hut is seen on the summit of the Signalkuppe, second peak from the left, at 4,559 metres.

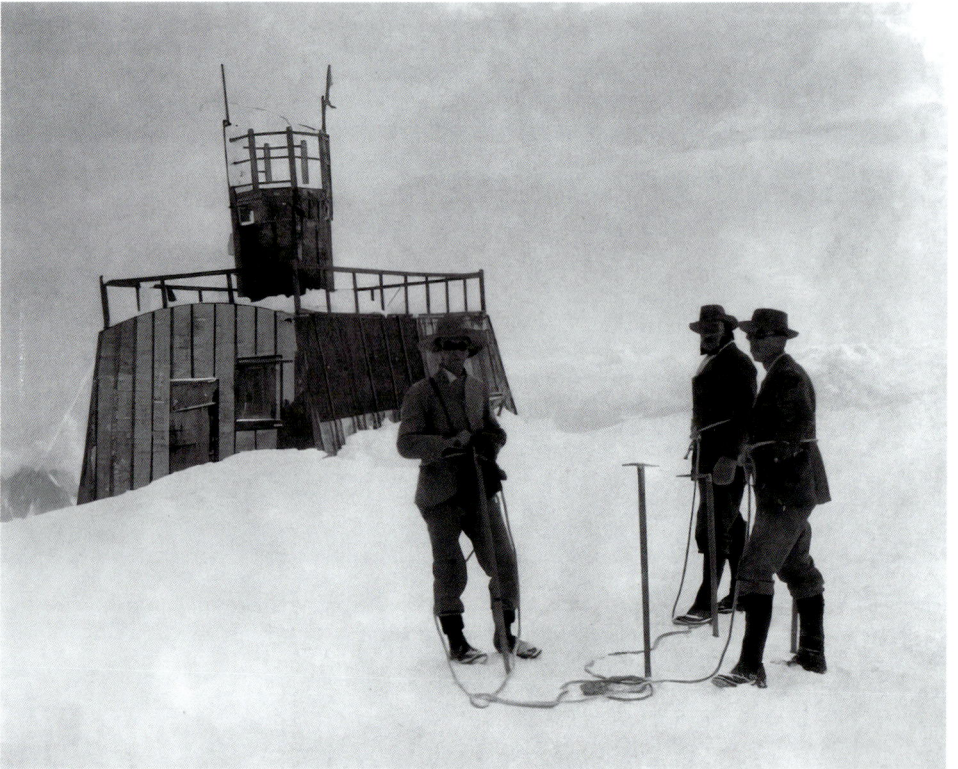

Figure 18. Sligger Urquhart's ascent of Mont Blanc on 20 August 1900. The climbing party of four consisted of Sligger (left), guides Schwarzen and Fuhrer, and Gertrude Bell, who is taking the photograph using Sligger's camera. The Janssen observatory is seen partially sunken in the snow of the summit.

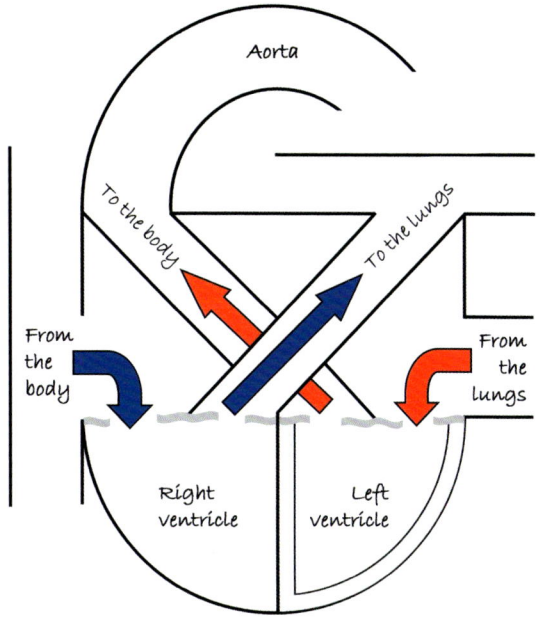

Figure 19. Schematic of the human heart. Venous blood, low in oxygen (blue arrows), arrives from the veins of the 'greater circulation' into the right ventricle, from which it is pumped to the lungs through the 'lesser circulation'. It returns from the lungs oxygenated (red arrows) to the thick-walled left ventricle. From here it is pumped at high pressure via the aorta to the rest of the body. Four valves, shown as grey wavy lines, direct the flow into, and out of, the ventricles.

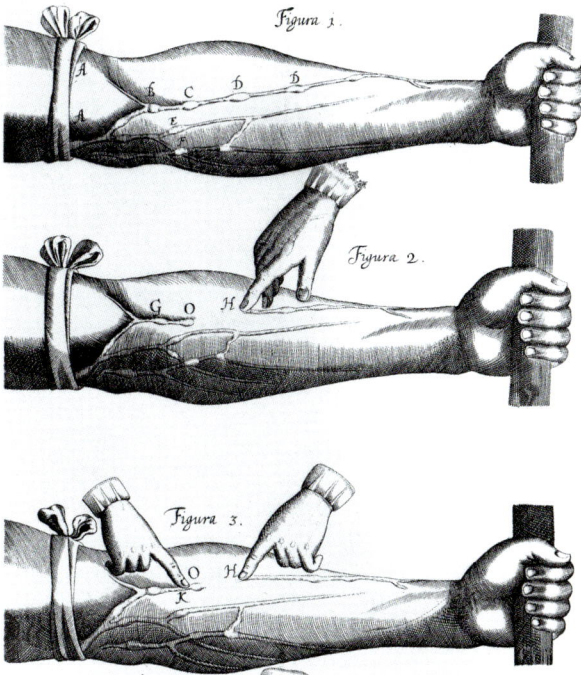

Figure 20. Illustration of human forearm veins from William Harvey's *de Motu Cordis* of 1628.[8] In *Figura 1* we see the forearm with a ligature AA as applied for blood-letting. Locations of the valves in distended veins are shown (B–F). In *Figura 2* occlusion of the vein at H, and emptying of the segment OH by stroking towards the heart, leaves the segment empty because the valve at O prevents backflow towards the periphery. *Figura 3* confirms that the segment remains empty despite a second finger pushing at K towards the periphery.

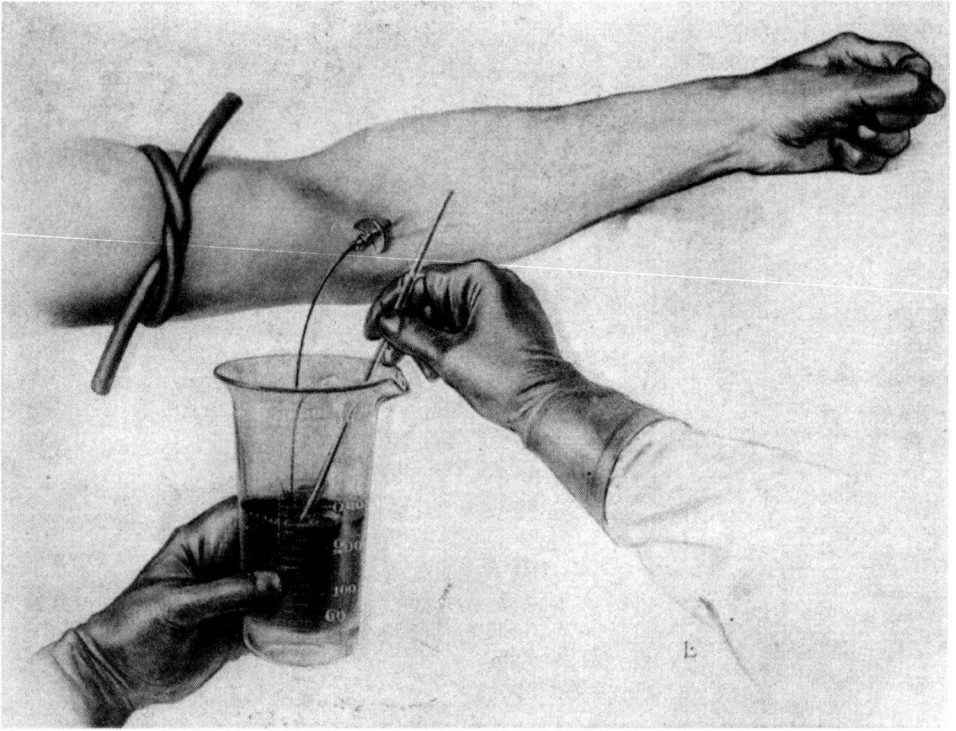

Figure 21. Harvesting blood from the forearm of a donor, as depicted by Lewisohn summarising practice in the period 1914–24.[12] A metal cannula is shown in an antecubital vein pointing towards the hand. Citrate was used to prevent coagulation of blood, with the help of stirring.

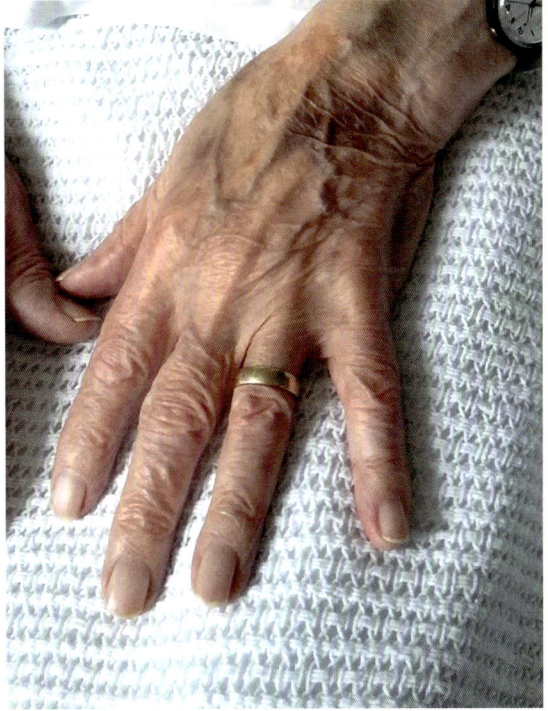

Figure 22a. (*Top*) Bruised hand of an elderly hospitalised patient showing evidence of attempts to sample blood from veins on the dorsum of the wrist and hand. Distress associated with failed phlebotomy is widespread among patients and healthcare staff.

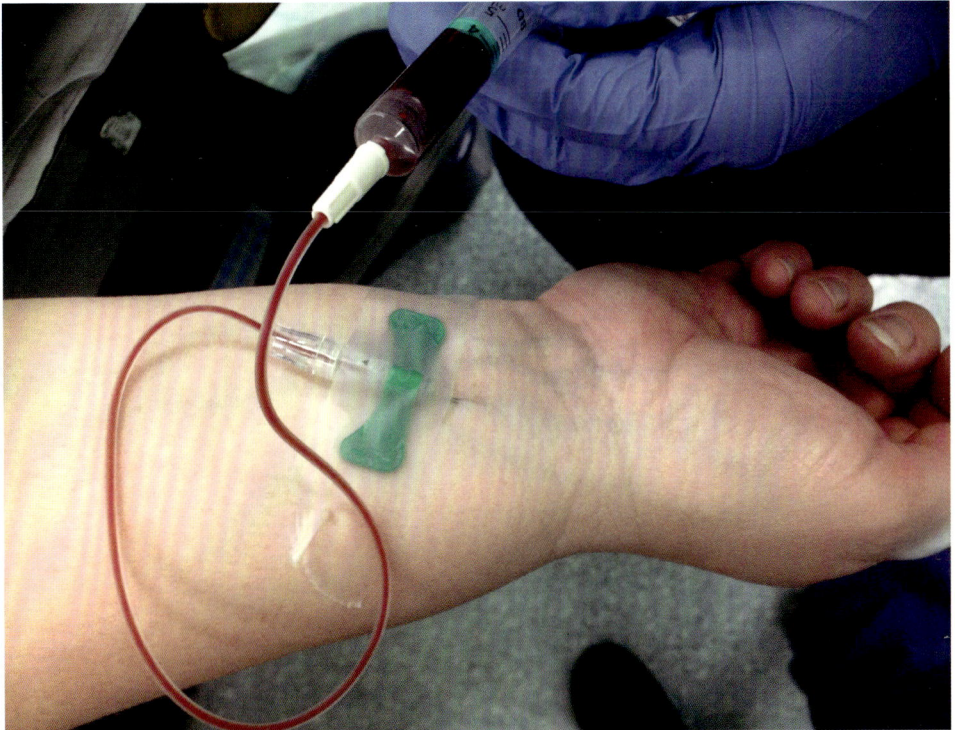

Figure 22b. (*Bottom*) Sampling of blood from a forearm vein of a young patient under anaesthesia via a 'butterfly' needle pointing towards the periphery and therefore facing towards the direction from which the blood is flowing.

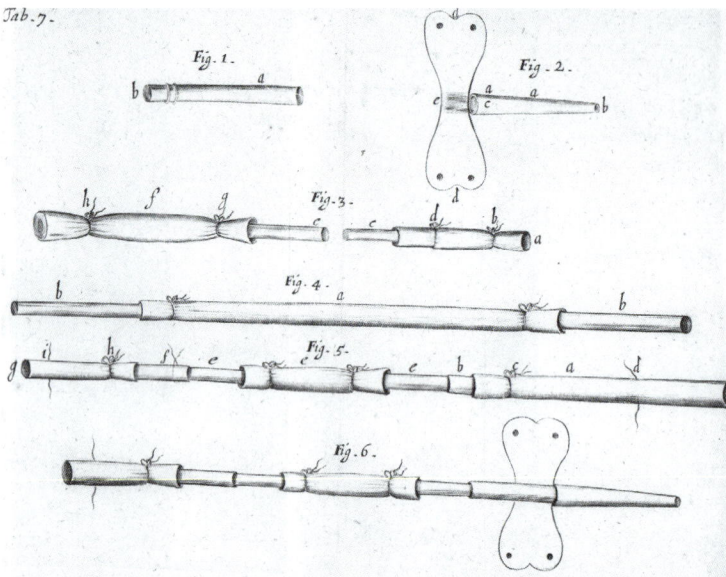

Figure 23. The first 'butterfly' needle. Richard Lower's 1669 assembly of cannulae for vascular access for the purpose of blood transfusion. *Fig. 1* shows a silver tube with two circular raised rings to make tying into a vessel secure. *Fig. 2* is a silver 'butterfly' needle for insertion into a human arm vein, with wings carrying holes "for the passage of the string, which is to bind the plate to the arm". *Figs. 3–5* show the progressive assembly of blood vessels and silver tubes for animal-only transfusion. A length of "cervical artery taken from a horse or an ox" (*a* in *Fig. 4*) is recommended to accommodate movement "when the animals toss and twist around". *Fig. 6* shows "the same apparatus for transfusion of blood from an animal to man".[15]

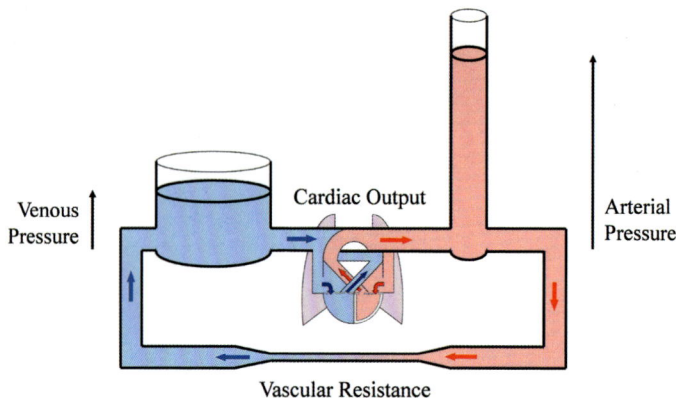

Figure 24. The most basic physiological features of the circulation. The heart and lungs are represented as a single unit which generates a *cardiac output*. This flow of oxygenated (red) blood enters the large arteries which are depicted as a tall thin container open to the atmosphere. The cartoon represents *arterial pressure* by the height of blood in this reservoir. Blood flows from the arteries to the veins through narrow blood vessels represented by a *vascular resistance*. Large veins are depicted as a shallow wide reservoir open to atmosphere. Venous deoxygenated blood is shown as blue. The *venous pressure* is represented by the height of blood in this reservoir.[34] The image illustrates that, in a circulation with a fixed volume of fluid, arterial pressure depends upon cardiac output and vascular resistance.

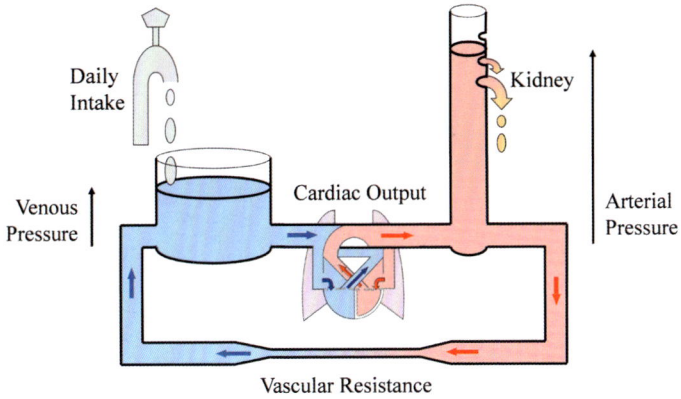

Figure 25. The basic features of the circulation (following Figure 24) with the addition of a daily intake of fluid and a mechanism for its elimination via the kidney. The kidney has an output which depends on many factors. One of these is the arterial pressure. Other factors include its nerve supply, the influence of hormones, and drug medication. This cartoon illustrates that over prolonged periods of time arterial blood pressure depends upon kidney function and daily intake.

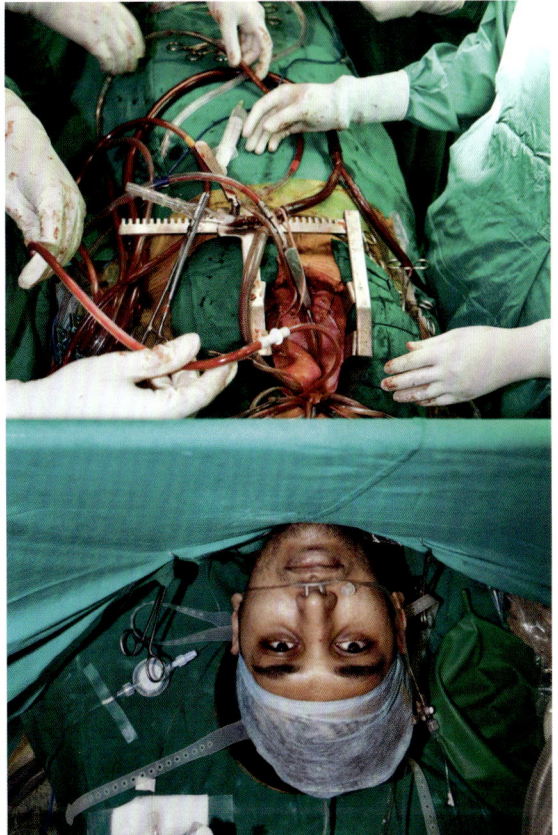

Figure 26. Heart surgery being conducted under epidural anaesthesia on 23-year-old patient Swaroup Anand in Bangalore in or before 2009. The function of the patient's heart is being taken over by a heart–lung machine (out of view).

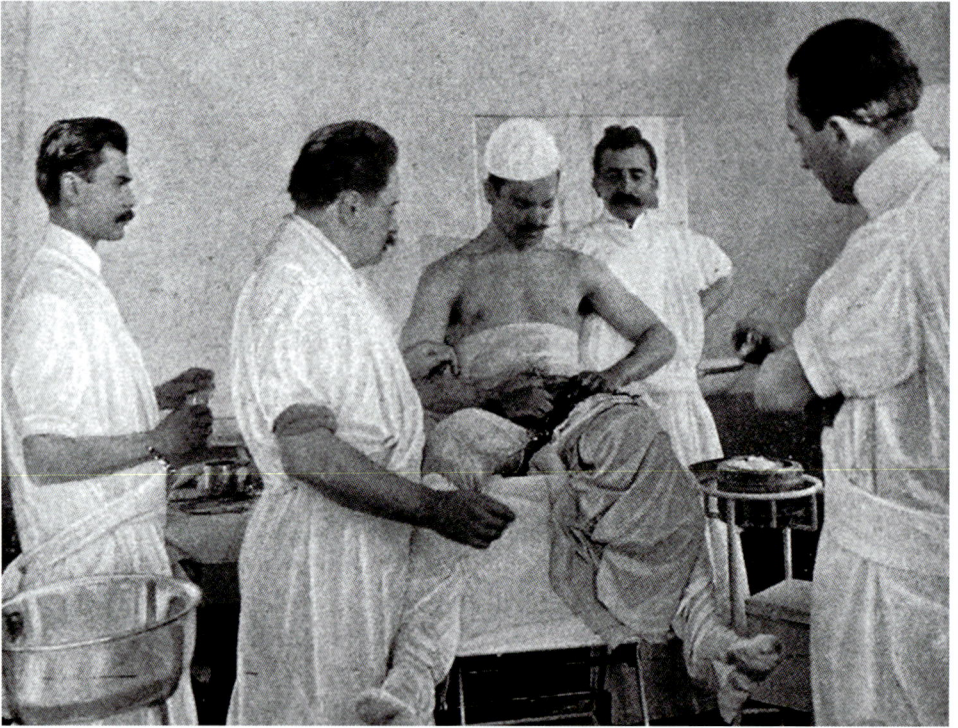

Figure 27. Alexandre Fzaïcou, a 26-year-old Romanian doctor, operating on his own left inguinal hernia under spinal anaesthesia in 1909. The technique was named 'rachi-strychno-stovainisation'. This is the first known occasion on which a surgeon performed a substantial operation on himself.

Figure 28. Depiction of a vertebral bone from the lumbar region of the spine showing a needle passing in the midline from the back through a yellow ligament (*ligamentum flavum*) into the spinal canal which is bordered on all sides by bones and ligaments. The needle then passes across the epidural space and finally crosses the dural membrane (shown in grey). The dural tube is shown here as empty. In fact, in the upper part of the adult spine the dura contains the spinal cord. In the lower (lumbar) part of the adult spine the dura contains nerves passing down from the cord towards their respective points of exit from the lower spinal column. The dural tube contains cerebrospinal fluid, indicated in the image by a drop of liquid at the end of the needle. Note that many structures are not depicted here, including blood vessels and adipose tissue in the epidural space.

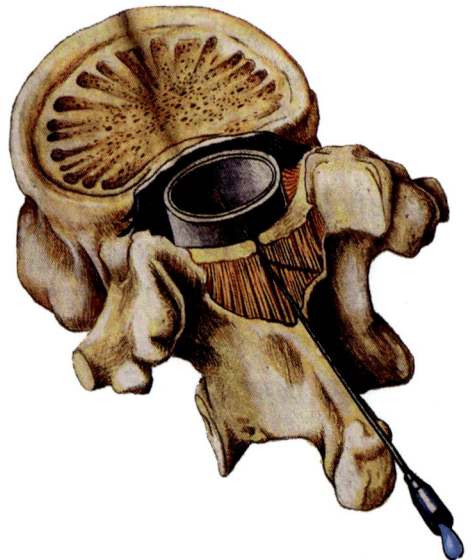

Sligger, Gertrude Bell, Roger Casement, William Tyrrell and another friend, Margaret Stanley, set off from the chalet on 19 August for a climb to the Tête Rousse refuge. They arrived at 4.30 p.m. The plan was for Gertrude to ascend from there with two guides, Schwartzen and Fuhrer. It was at this point that Sligger changed his mind. Gertrude described the events in a letter to her father. "Here Mr Urquhart announced that he would like to stay and do Mont Blanc with me, we all cheered him on, borrowed woollen clothes for him from the *patron*, and the others went down at 5 leaving us two. Mr Tyrrell was much entertained, for Mr U. has hitherto expressed the greatest contempt of all mountaineers and their feats."[55]

Setting off at 2 a.m., the foursome attained the Aiguille de Goûter at 4 a.m. and at 6 a.m. reached the newly constructed observatory of the eccentric Joseph Vallot, with whom they breakfasted for an hour. The summit was reached at 8.30 a.m., a remarkable pace having been set.

> There was no time to lose, the black clouds were hurrying up from the west, we heard thunder and the guides were in a great state of anxiety. I had just had time to photograph the drunken little Janssen observatory, which is gradually sinking into the snow, to cast my eye round a marvellous panorama of peaks rising out of the cloud, and we were enveloped in mist and snow.[55]

The photograph she took with Sligger's camera has pride of place in the chalet diary for that year (Fig. 18). Visitors to Chamonix can visit the top balcony of Janssen's short-lived 'drunken little' summit observatory and the 'Chinese salon' from Vallot's observatory as they are now on display in the town's modern-day Alpine Museum.[56]

This account seems to suggest that we can ascend successfully to high altitude without 'ills of the hills', but the party met with danger during their descent. On returning to Vallot's observatory, "a ridiculous little salon of which he is very proud, fitted up with Oriental hangings and bad Japanese masks", an electric storm broke and the air became charged with electricity. "The steel heads of the axes fizzed and crackled too and one man had his beard singed and blackened." On descending to the refuge on the Grand Mulet rocks, the party experienced a life-threatening slide, held up, according to Gertrude's account, by the "very good man" Schwartzen.[55]

Sligger and George Mallory

You may wonder whether Sligger's ascent of Mont Blanc in 1900 might be the last of his mountaineering associations. A discovery in Sligger's photograph albums by my colleague Stephen Golding has revealed a more lowly association with mountaineering fame; a long-standing friendship has come to light between Sligger and George Mallory, the climber who died on Everest in 1924.[57] Photographs show a rowing party on the Thames at Sandford on May Day 1911 when Mallory, as a history master at Charterhouse, appears to be making what we might now term an 'admissions liaison visit' to Sligger, the history tutor at Balliol. We next see Mallory "in a wistful and camera-conscious mood" beside Sligger's window during a visit to Oxford in 1913, during which Sligger advised him to become a don, like himself. Later photographs show Sligger's visit to Mallory at Charterhouse in 1915 and there is evidence of a continuing correspondence right up to Mallory's three attempts on Everest in the years from 1921.

The last image we have of George Mallory is with young Andrew Irvine, a chemistry undergraduate at Merton College, Oxford, at their camp on the North Col of Everest at an altitude of 7,000 metres. Ascent that far without supplementary oxygen is an early example of remarkable adaptation to altitude. They were setting off on 6 June 1924 with oxygen cylinders on their backs for the attempt on the summit that led to the deaths of both of them. If George Mallory had taken Sligger's career advice he might have avoided this most famous example of the "Ills of the Hills".

CHAPTER FOUR

DECEITS OF THE HEART

Myths and Mysteries of the Circulation

'Newes from the Dead'

Anatomy requires dissection of the dead. How else could early doctors find out which way the pipes and nerves ran around the human body? From 1549 any medical student in Oxford was obliged to view two anatomical dissections and also to perform two. The limited availability of bodies for this purpose was resolved by Charles I in 1636 in a charter that made available the body of any person executed within 21 miles of Oxford.[1]

On 14 December 1650 the housemaid Anne Greene ascended the scaffold, having been condemned of infanticide consequent upon being raped by the grandson of Sir Thomas Read in his house in Duns Tew.[2]

> She was turn'd off the Ladder, hanging by the neck for the space of almost half an hour, some of her friends in the mean time thumping her on the breast, others hanging with all their weight upon her legges; sometimes lifting her up, and then pulling her downe again with a suddaine jerke, thereby the sooner to dispatch her out of her paine.[2]

The coffin was taken to "a private house, where some Physitians had appointed to make a Dissection": Bulkeley Hall, a building off Oxford High Street and the residence of the University Reader in Anatomy, William Petty. On opening the coffin, it came as a surprise to Petty and the physician colleague with him, Thomas Willis, that Anne Greene was still alive.

The detailed account of her resuscitation over the next hours and days is a wonderful catalogue of contemporary therapies, which include potentially helpful measures, such as persuading "a woman to goe into bed to her, and to lye very close to her", and probably unhelpful procedures, including being "bled about five ounces, and that so freely that it could not easily be stopped". "Thus, within the space of a Moneth, was she wholly Recovered." She became a celebrity, her innocence was established, her father collected money from inquisitive visitors, and she went on to marry and have three children. In a strange twist of fate, Sir Thomas Read died within three days of her execution.[2]

The account of this episode, *Newes from the Dead*, was accompanied by over twenty poems "casually written upon that subject", one of which was authored by the young Christopher Wren, then a first-year undergraduate student of Wadham College. His effort is a cryptic hotchpotch of anatomical detail mixed with classical allusions. The legend of Orpheus and Eurydice appears along with "Bowells", "One Breast", "veines", and "Femall Organs".

For Petty and Willis the living body of Anne Greene clearly did nothing to advance their knowledge of "Femall Organs" and yet her resuscitation proved to be a major career boost for Thomas Willis. His medical practice took off, he married the daughter of the Dean of Christ Church, moved to the generous accommodation of Beam Hall in Merton Street, and from 1660 held the university post of Sedleian Professor of Natural Philosophy. Willis is regarded as the founder of neurology, a reputation aided by publications, including remarkably detailed drawings of the brain by Christopher Wren.[3] These famously include the 1664 illustration of the 'Circle of Willis', an oval-shaped loop of arteries at the base of the brain via which the circulation distributes blood to the brain. But who discovered the circulation of the blood in the first place?

William Harvey and Andrea Cesalpino

Across the pebbles of Merton Street, a few yards from Willis' dissection room in Beam Hall, lies Merton College. From 1642 to 1646, during the Civil War, Charles I set up residence in nearby Christ Church and accommodated his queen Henrietta Maria in the warden's lodgings in Merton, the parliamentary warden having made a tactical departure. Henrietta Maria's later move to the West Country for delivery of her baby in 1644 permitted the appointment of Charles' personal physician, William Harvey, to head Merton college for a year from 1645. Although succeeding to this post at the age of sixty-seven, and only briefly, this has enabled Oxford to lay some claim to the man celebrated as the discoverer of the circulation of the blood.

Undergraduate physiology textbooks rarely inform on historical origins but it comes as no surprise that a recent *Introduction to Cardiovascular Physiology* co-authored by a fellow of Merton (my own head of department) maintains Harvey's pre-eminence. "One-way valves in the heart and veins ensure that blood follows the circular pathway … first described by the physician William Harvey. Harvey's originality and ground-breaking introduction of experimentation into physiology and medicine disproved the earlier ebb-and-flow dogma of the previous 1,000 years."[4]

The story, however, is more complicated than this brief summary suggests. John Hemmeter, a professor of physiology in Baltimore, began his essay on the circulation of the blood with a focus on patriotism:

> A very curious impression is made upon the objective investigator to see the scientific judgement obscured by ill-guided patriotism … The Spaniards regard Michael Servetus, born in Villanueva in 1511, as the discoverer of the circulation and have erected a monument in the Museo Anthropologico in Madrid. The Italians have three men to whom the title to this discovery is accredited with more or less historic and scientific correctness, namely: Matheus Realdus Colombus, born in Cremona in 1516; Carl Ruini of Bologna; Andreas Cesalpinus born at Arrago in 1519. Monuments have been erected to Carlo Ruini at Bologna and to Andreas Cesalpinus at Pisa and Rome. William Harvey has been honoured by a monument in London erected by the Sydenham Society, a second at Hempstead, and a third at Folkstone.[5]

Clearly, dissecting this historical record is not for the faint-hearted. It seems that there were several key steps in assembling a concept of the circulation. One early step concerned the heart itself, which has a right ventricle and a left ventricle. Blood is found in both. It had long been thought that blood might get from one side to the other by oozing through the septum lying between the two. Alternatively, blood could leave one ventricle via a blood vessel, and pass through the lungs to find its way to the other ventricle via further vessels. We now appreciate that this 'lesser circulation' does indeed pass through the lungs. The Spaniard Servetus published the resolution of this in 1553 in a largely theological book, which sadly resulted in the author's death at the stake later that year in Geneva. Safe in Catholic Italy on the other side of the border, Columbus of Padua attributed the 'through-the-lungs' solution to himself in a publication of 1559.

It may come as a surprise that anyone could have thought that blood could ooze its way across the thick layer of tissue that constitutes the septum between the ventricles of the heart, but a similar dilemma faced the anatomists about whether blood in tissues elsewhere could pass from arteries to veins through invisible "porosities of the flesh" (to use Harvey's term). The first person to appreciate and publish a clear solution to this problem is now recognised to be Andrea Cesalpino in his *Quaestionum peripateticarum* ('Peripatetic Questions') of 1571. Cesalpino, who writes of the *circulatio* of blood throughout the body from arteries to veins via *vasa in capillamenta resoluta*, a term which suggests that he envisaged collections of tubes or vessels comparable in size to hairs being responsible for providing a pathway through which blood could flow.

Not only is the passage of blood through what we now know to be tissue capillaries clear from Cesalpino's book of 1571, but so too is its passage through the heart. "For two are the vessels of the right ventricle, and two also of the left: of the two, then, one sends in, the other sends out (the blood) by means of membranes properly arranged" – a reference to the valves of the heart, which are indeed 'membranes', albeit of varying shapes and attachments.[6] Cesalpino kept the publications coming, in 1583, 1593 and 1602. These document observations and experimental investigations on animals and on man and constitute a body of teaching that gives the Italian precedence in demonstrating the circulation of the blood, and not just in a quiet backwater, but in Padua where Cesalpino taught and later William Harvey spent formative years in his medical studies; he was to graduate there in 1602.[7]

One of the steps in assembling an understanding of the circulation concerned the valves in the veins. These are small semicircular flaps of tissue, which permit blood in veins to flow in one direction only: towards the heart. We shall meet these again later in this chapter but suffice it to say here that Fabricius of Aquapendente in 1603 in his book *De venarum ostiolis* ('On the Valves of the Veins'), though addressing their anatomy, failed to appreciate their functional significance.[5] Several of the names of the 'discoverers' of the circulation are linked to observations about valves, and we shall see that Harvey modified a diagram from Fabricius for his own publication in 1628.

Harvey's famous book was *Exercitatio anatomica de motu cordis et sanguinis in animalibus* ('An Anatomical Exercise on the Motion of the Heart and Blood in Living Beings'), known as *De motu cordis* for short.[8] Hemmeter describes it as: "without doubt the masterpiece of a man of genius", while at the same time placing it within the progress of the topic, noting that Harvey

> did not discover the lesser circulation. This Servetus discovered in 1546. Harvey did not discover the greater circulation. This Cesalpinus discovered in 1569. Harvey did not discover the venal valves. These Jacob Silvius, Scarpi, and most accurately Aquapendente discovered in 1574. Harvey did not furnish the clear-sighted proofs of the circulation. These were given by Servetus, Colombo, Valverde, Aranzi, Ruini, Rudio, Scarpi, Cesalpinus, and Aquapendente. Harvey never saw the circulation of the blood. Malpigi saw it several years after Harvey's death.[5]

It was by using a microscope that Marcello Malpighi was able to observe blood flowing through the capillaries of a frog's lung in 1661.[5]

A plausible summary of this complexity comes from a Jesuit and enthusiastic citer of assembled Latin texts, George Bishop: "it is impossible to attribute any discovery to Harvey. What Harvey did was to perfect and put in one volume what Cesalpino put in many."[7] Harvey's *De motu cordis* is a mere seventy-two pages long. It succeeded in propagating its message particularly effectively but with limited acknowledgements. One suggestion why Harvey avoided citing two key figures is that "a court physician under such a tyrannical prince, who would have dared to confess himself to Cesalpinus or even to Michael Servetus, would have certainly been executed".[5] This may be reason enough to edit the references in a book when in times of trouble.

Whether this overview of the circulation of the blood leaves us with the exposure of a myth or just a clarification of the progress of anatomical thought, I leave to the reader to decide.

Overview of the plumbing with Harvey's help

Figure 19 shows a schematic diagram of the human heart. In the resting adult, a flow of blood of about 5 litres per minute arrives at the heart from the tissues of the body via the veins. It is dark red, verging on blue, signifying that it is relatively depleted of oxygen. It is pumped from the right ventricle into the lungs via the 'lesser circulation' where it becomes well oxygenated and changes its colour to bright red. This blood then flows into the left side of the heart, from which it is pumped onwards at high pressure into the arterial tree of the 'greater circulation', starting with the aorta. Valves in the heart play an important role in maintaining the forward flow.

Much early debate concerned whether the blood in one ventricle arrived from the other ventricle by seeping through the septum between the two. We have seen that Servetus and Columbus can be credited with establishing the correct route. Another early view was that air from the lungs, either on its own or mixed with blood, made its way into the left ventricle. In his text of 1571, Cesalpino was clear that such bubbling did not occur, but that the air and blood blend only by "touching" (*solo tactu temperat*) each other in the lungs.[6] Then there was the question of whether the blood moved backwards and forwards in any of the arteries or veins. An appreciation of the valves in the heart, Cesalpino's "membranes properly arranged", established that this was a one-way system.

William Harvey's account astonishes the reader with its descriptions of the heart in humans and a wide range of other animals. These include sheep, dogs, oxen, pigs, swans, geese, snakes, frogs, crabs, snails, fish and wasps, some of whom he recognised as having a single ventricle, and some of whom he noted to have no lungs. The translucent living shrimp was particularly revealing. "I have often shown some of my friends the movements of its heart with great clearness. Since the outside of the body did not block our view, we could observe the least tremor of the heart, as through a window."[8]

It is not until we get to Chapter IX of *De motu cordis* that things become quantitative. Harvey's aim was to show that the heart pumps such a large flow of blood that this is inconsistent with the then-popular view that the heart's job was distribution of food to the body. He noted the relaxed human ventricle to contain "two or three ounces" of blood and proposed that perhaps "a half ounce" might be ejected with each beat. Reckoning on more than 1,000 beats in half an hour, he calculated a lower limit of 42 pounds of blood pumped in half an hour (1 pound then equalled 12 ounces), equivalent in current units to about 1 litre per minute in flow. Despite this being only one-fifth of what we now know the cardiac output to be, it made the point that "a greater quantity would eventually be pumped into the arteries and the body than could be furnished by the food consumed, unless by constantly making a circuit and returning".[8]

In Chapter XI the argument moves out to the limbs. Harvey describes the use of "tight" and "middling" ligatures (what we now call tourniquets) around the upper part of a limb. The first of these eliminates the arterial pulse in the peripheral part of the limb beyond the ligature while the second, used for phlebotomy, retains the arterial pulse but causes the veins beyond the ligature to "become swollen". Further, in Chapter XII, phlebotomy, bleeding from a cut vein, gives a further indication of the flow through the heart: "if you figure how many ounces of blood flow through a single arm … in twenty or thirty beats, you will have a basis for estimating how much flows … through all the other arteries and veins of the body".[8]

The discussion moves on in Chapter XIII to the valves in the veins of the arm. It is interesting that Harvey has no depiction of the heart in his book; the only figure is that of the veins of the arm, part of which is reproduced in Figure 20. In Padua, Harvey had been taught by Fabricius, from whose book *De venarum ostiolis* of 1603 Harvey modified a diagram of the forearm for his own explanation of the functions of the valves in veins.[7] This depicts a pleasing experiment, which readers can conduct on themselves or a volunteer with prom-inent veins (Harvey recommends "rustics"). The locations of valves are commonly visible as 'knots or swellings' along the line of veins, or can otherwise be located by finding where a segment of vein (OH in Fig. 20), when emptied by stroking towards the heart, does not fill from the end nearest the heart.

As indicated by these diagrams, some veins lie close to the surface of the limbs. The arteries carrying blood from the heart lie deeper. Harvey noted from dissections that the arteries have no valves. One study of valves in the superficial veins of the human forearm found the veins to be furnished with a valve about every 5 cm.[9] So, what might the function of these valves be? Perhaps it is sufficient here to summarise, as Harvey does, that "the valves are present solely that blood may not move from the larger veins into the smaller ones lest it rupture or varicose them, and that it may not advance from the center of the body into the periphery through them, but rather from the extremities to the center".[8]

Blood-taking and the Great Phlebotomy Myth

To readers who have followed Harvey's line of thought and noted his *Figura 2* (in Fig. 20), it will be obvious that anyone taking blood from a vein in the arm will only be able to withdraw blood that arrives from the direction of the hand. It follows that it would be sensible to insert a needle or cannula to face the hand. There was no doubt about this in the seventeenth century; in his book *Clysmatica nova* of 1667 Johann Elsholtz depicts veno-venous transfusion of blood between humans with a silver cannula in the donor facing towards the hand and the silver cannula in the recipient facing towards the heart.[10] Elsholtz took care to emphasise that "the ends of the tubes, when they are inserted, must be properly directed to pour out and receive blood".[11]

Harvey's and Elsholtz's wisdom continued to be recognised into the twentieth century. Figure 21 depicts a summary of practice during the decade around the First World War. A metal cannula sits in a vein of the tourniqued arm facing towards the hand and provides a generous flow of blood into a beaker.[12] No valves stand in the way of this stream of blood exiting the arm.

It may therefore come as a surprise that the standard practice for modern-day blood-taking is invariably to insert a needle into a vein by pointing the needle *towards the heart*. This is recommended and taught practice but it is frequently beset with problems, as will come as no surprise to readers, be they patients who have been on the pointed end, or medical personnel at the syringe end, of the process.[13] The internet is replete with 'agony' comments about difficulties with the 'blood draw' (to use an Americanism), 'blood test' or 'phlebotomy' (to use UK terms). A common request to an anaesthetist like myself is to take blood from a patient when others have failed, often on multiple occasions, and one of the most frequent sights on the hospital ward is the patient with bruised hands, signifying several attempts at a difficult phlebotomy (Fig. 22a). This challenge of taking blood in difficult cases has caused me to reflect.

Standard practice is to approach a patient's vein in the fold of the arm (the antecubital fossa) with a needle pointing towards the heart. Many patients have a vein accessible here, which lies at a junction of several other veins, and blood usually flows freely into a needle. In those in whom a visible or palpable vein does not exist at this site, in either arm, it is more difficult. For example, if a needle facing the heart enters a vein like those shown in Figure 22a it will tend to obstruct flow from the periphery either by occluding the lumen of the vein or by pressing upon it. Failure often results from attempts in such veins.

The solution is to enter veins in the hand or forearm with the needle pointing towards the hand, taking a lesson from Lewisohn, as in Figure 21. An example is shown in Figure 22b. In this child undergoing surgery the more commonly used antecubital veins were obscured by adipose tissue and a wrist vein presented the obvious site for a sample taken with the needle facing *towards the hand*.

The 'butterfly' type of needle shown here is particularly useful for fine manipulation when access to the limb is difficult because it has 'wings', one or both of which can be held during insertion and then taped to the skin to secure.[14] The butterfly needle rewards further thought; its origins actually lie in seventeenth-century Oxford. In February 1665 Richard Lower, another alumnus of Christ Church and a colleague of Thomas Willis, successfully transfused blood from the neck artery of two large dogs, into the neck vein of a smaller dog. And this was not a trickle. The recipient dog was bled several times and blood from the two others transfused "in such an amount as would equal, I imagine, the weight of its whole body".[15] We read of the recipient that:

> once its jugular vein was sewn up and its binding shackles cast off, it promptly jumped down from the table, and, apparently oblivious of its hurts, soon began to fondle its master, and to roll on the grass to clean itself of blood; exactly as it would have done if it had merely been thrown into a stream, and with no more sign of discomfort or of displeasure.[15]

Figure 23 shows Lower's depiction of the apparatus he recommended for animal-to-animal transfusion plus his device for
animal-to-human transfusion. It is here that we see Lower's silver butterfly cannula for infusion of blood into a forearm vein. In his book
Tractatus de corde we are made aware of a dispute with the French
over precedence in transfusion and read of "the subject of a harmless
form of insanity" in whom Lower "superintended the introduction
into his arm at various times of some ounces of sheep's blood at a
meeting of the Royal Society, and that without any inconvenience to
him".[15] The butterfly needle was put to human use.

The Great Phlebotomy Myth of the modern day is that the only
way to sample venous blood is from a needle pointing in the 'wrong
direction' from the point of view of the valves in the veins, which
prevent the backfilling of the segment of vein in which the needle is
inserted. There is no mention in over 100 pages of the World Health
Organization guidelines on drawing blood of considering alternative
needle directions; the diagrams show needles dutifully pointing heart-
wards.[16] By way of contrast, Lahiru, a doctor from Melbourne, has
recently made a rare elegant short video to show drawing of blood in
an adult from a small hand vein by inserting a fine cannula facing the
fingers; he has some useful advice on how to proceed.[17]

It is interesting to speculate why practice changed about a
hundred years ago.[13] My co-author Matthew Frise and I recently identified three factors: first, the arrival of routine blood tests; second,
the development of relatively fine needles, which could be used to
draw modest quantities of blood without occluding the flow from
the periphery; and third, the dominance of the use of the antecubital
vein. This vein acts as a junction for two or more superficial veins as
well as commonly for a connecting vein coming from deep in the
arm.[13] It is when this most commonly used site for phlebotomy is no
longer available that drawing blood with the now-standard approach
becomes difficult.

A fourth factor, which may be pertinent in accounting for the
standard approach, is the custom of medical staff to face the patient
when they consult or take blood. It is noteworthy, however, that the
use of a butterfly needle enables a phlebotomist to insert a needle
facing away from the heart even when sitting facing the patient. The
wings provide something to hold, whichever way the needle is facing,
as Richard Lower would have appreciated.

The circulation in top gear: the mysteries of exercise

I hope that the reader will permit a sudden change of gear as we move from the circulation in patients at rest to the much-accelerated circulation in healthy exercise. When we lie in bed at rest the flow of blood through the heart, our 'cardiac output', is about 5 litres per minute. A remarkable change occurs when we exert ourselves. At a maximum level of exercise, the cardiac output typically rises about fourfold to around 20 litres per minute. The manner in which the body brings this about has occupied physiologists for over a hundred years and still remains to a large extent a mystery.

Even greater is the increase in breathing that occurs during exercise. During maximal exercise this follows the large increase in oxygen consumption by the body and rises by a huge twelve-fold. One task of physiology has been to try to unravel how the body achieves and regulates a fourfold increase in cardiac output and a twelve-fold increase in breathing. These are remarkable changes.[18]

When physiologists consider how such changes occur they traditionally invoke the engineering jargon of 'control theory'. When I was first studying physiology as a medical student, I recall a lecture by Professor David Whitteridge in which he illustrated control theory by getting us to consider how the gun barrels of a battleship tossing in a rough sea could be made to continue to point in a fixed direction towards a target.

A control system requires a 'sensor', which detects the position or state of whatever is being controlled (in Whitteridge's example, the angle of the gun barrel relative to the horizon). This information is regarded as 'feedback', which can be compared with the desired angle. The difference between these angles (the 'error signal') is then used to move the gun barrel to minimise the error. These engineering concepts are widely applied in physiology, where such *feedback control* is often called a *reflex*. Our eyes have a system analogous to Whitteridge's naval guns that keeps us looking in the same direction if we turn our heads. It is so effective that we take it for granted.

Let us think about how the body might bring about the increase in cardiac output necessary for us to walk up a steep hill. As we make the conscious decision to move, our brain sends out a neural message to the muscles of our limbs to make them contract. These muscles need to increase their blood flow to provide them with enough oxygen. We now know that individual muscles can autonomously

dilate the arteries that supply them in order to satisfy their requirements for oxygen, or at least to some extent. The question arises: how
is the heart made aware that it needs to increase its output to satisfy
this enhanced flow demanded by the muscles? What signal could be
sensed?

Blood pressure in the carotid artery of the neck is one candidate.
If muscles draw more blood from the arteries during exercise, then
arterial blood pressure might be expected to fall and provide a signal
of the need to increase cardiac output to keep the arteries well filled
with blood. The 'baroreceptors' in the carotid sinus we have met in
Chapter Two. These lie in the internal carotid artery in the neck and
measure arterial blood pressure by detecting the extent to which it
stretches the wall of a small outpouching of the artery called the
sinus. The baroreceptors might seem to be just what is needed to
do the job of sensing pressure during exercise, by sending a measure
of blood pressure up to the brain. We envisage this measurement
being compared with an ideal 'target' value stored in the brain. The
difference between the measurement and the target would constitute
the error signal and the brain would then send a message down to
the heart to increase its rate and output. This might seem plausible
but the mystery is that the arterial blood pressure detected by the
carotid baroreceptors may stay virtually unchanged during the transition from rest to exercise despite the presence of a large increase
in cardiac output. The anticipated error signal simply does not exist.

A much-cited demonstration of this was published in 1967 by
Alexander Lind and a colleague, physiologists working for the Coal
Board in Edinburgh. They showed no change in mean arterial pressure
during "an exhausting treadmill-walking test" in a group of men,[19]
from which they were driven to conclude "at present, the mechanisms involved in producing the cardiovascular responses to rhythmic
exercise are unknown".[20] Here, with arterial blood pressure, we have
an example of something we know to be measured and responded
to vigorously by the body when at rest but for which the notion of
feedback control involving an 'error signal' during exercise appears
not to provide an explanation.[21] Traditional control theory seems to
fail to explain how the heart is stimulated during exercise.

To be fair to physiologists, in addition to arterial blood pressure,
many other variables that might contribute to feedback control have
been identified, both before and since 1967. These include pressures

elsewhere in the circulation and neural signals from 'work receptors' in exercising muscles sent to the brain to bring about reflex changes in the heart. The complexity is frankly bewildering and provides scope for much discussion in degree courses in human physiology or sports science.[4]

Florence Buchanan's Oxford discovery of 'feedforward' control

As *feedback* control seems not to provide an answer, physiologists have turned instead to *feedforward* control. Here the notion is that the brain may be able to tell the heart directly and quickly by how much to increase its cardiac output in order to cope with the uphill walk. It is here that we encounter a classic study conducted in Oxford by a pioneering woman physiologist.

Florence Buchanan's education was in zoology at University College London, where she graduated in 1890 having published two papers as an undergraduate. In 1894 she moved to Oxford to work with the Professor of Physiology on electrical responses in muscle. From 1904 she worked more independently in the Oxford Museum of Natural History where the regulation of heart rate in animals and man was of particular interest to her. There, around 1909, she made measurements of the heart rate of volunteers when performing exercise, using an electrocardiogram employing basins of water as electrical contacts. The experiment on a "Mr Moseley of Trinity" involved him "sitting down with one hand and one foot in two basins of salt water, and squeezing, as hard as he could, a dynamometer with the hand of the free arm when he heard the signal".[22] Her discovery was that the heart rate increased *from the very first beat* occurring after the beginning of exercise. This was regarded as too early for any sort of reflex feedback signal from a sensor to go up to the brain and then down to the heart to increase its rate of beating.

In 1913 the future Nobel Prize-winner August Krogh and fellow Danish scientist Lindhard published a paper about "the initial stages of muscular work".[23] They explained that "Miss Buchanan has shown us the very great kindness to take some electrocardiograms on subjects starting work on a stationary tricycle." Her measurements on seven volunteers in their paper (for which today she would certainly deserve to be a co-author) show a rise in heart rate in the first half-second of exercise from 60 to 79 beats per minute. A further rise occurred over six minutes to 121 beats per minute. Krogh and Lindhard wrote that "motor impulses to the muscles irradiate to the centres governing the heart", suggesting that the very early rise in heart rate is a response to a speedy message straight from the brain to the heart, and not a reflex.

The authors not only measured the heart rate but also estimated by how much the cardiac output increased right at the start of exercise. In five volunteers exercising on a treadmill they estimated a fourfold increase in cardiac output within the first twenty seconds of starting the exercise. They used the term 'irradiate' to express the notion that the brain's message to exercising muscles has a parallel connection to the heart. We now prefer the term *feedforward* control to describe the notion that the brain can communicate directly by how much the heart should increase its rate of beating and output to match the requirements of exercise. A mystery was, and remains, how the brain might know *by how much* to stimulate the circulation to match the level of exercise being commenced.

The mystery of breathing during exercise

Just as baffling as the control of the heart in exercise has been the control of breathing. It is in fact a repeat of the same story. It has long been known that the body detects the levels of respiratory gases, oxygen and carbon dioxide, in the arterial blood. In Chapter Two we introduced the reader to the carotid body chemoreceptors, which can do this: tiny organs that lie close to the carotid arteries in the neck. The chemoreceptors send their measurements up to the brain, which uses them to tell us how hard to breathe.

Experiments in resting humans show substantial changes in breathing when stimulating the carotid bodies with low oxygen or high carbon dioxide levels. This initially led physiologists to assume that the large changes in breathing that accompany exercise must be brought about by low oxygen or high carbon dioxide in the arterial blood as the exercising muscles get to work, drawing oxygen from the blood and discharging carbon dioxide into it. But careful measurements showed that the levels of oxygen and carbon dioxide seen by the chemoreceptors commonly change little or not at all during exercise. No 'error signal' can be found to explain the heavy breathing.

Mike Parkes, a physiologist in Birmingham, UK, recently summarised the state of research: "There is still huge controversy over whether carotid chemoreceptors have any importance in controlling breathing during exercise, despite ~80 years of research."[24]

This problem also occupied Krogh and Lindhard in 1913. Half of their paper was devoted to measuring breathing at the onset of exercise.[23] As with the changes in the heart, they were interested to know whether changes in respiration were too fast to be accounted for by feedback from something detected in the blood. In seven volunteers they observed a sixfold increase in breathing within the first few seconds of starting exercise. Perhaps because breathing is something that we can to some extent control voluntarily (unlike our heart rate), they chose to speculate that the "motor cortex" is involved: the part of the brain in which we make conscious decisions to move and breathe: "with regard to the ventilation we think also that the evidence is in favour of an irradiation of impulses from the motor cortex rather than a reflex". One of their reasons for this conclusion was that sometimes volunteers increased their breathing even *before* the exercise was started, i.e. in anticipation.

Learning to ride a bicycle

Let us summarise the problem. We want to understand how the body increases the output of the heart and breathing to match a chosen level of exercise: small changes for light exercise and large changes for heavy exercise. We expect the brain to make use of measurements of blood pressure from the baroreceptors and blood oxygen from the chemoreceptors. We know that the brain receives, and responds to, measures of these at rest, so we expect it to do so during exercise. But the problem is that these measures do not change consistently during exercise, so there is a lack of *feedback* signals informing the brain of changes with exercise. So, we jump to an alternative explanation, the idea of *feedforward* signals: direct messages from the brain to the heart and respiratory muscles for which we have seen evidence going back more than a hundred years. A big mystery surrounding these feedforward messages, if they exist, is how the brain judges how vigorous to make them.

Given these difficulties, we cannot avoid looking to some kind of *learning* to explain what is going on. By this I mean that past experience of exercise on many occasions provides the brain with information that enables it to match its stimulation of the heart and breathing to the level of exercise about to be undertaken. However, the word 'learning' is something we usually associate with activities that have at least some conscious input, such as riding a bicycle. Here we need to extend the concept to apply to the rate and output of the heart, over which we have no conscious control. An engineering term that might be useful to cover this wider sense of learning is *adaptive control*.

Adaptive control uses many experiences over time (presumably since birth) in which *feedback* signals have been available to tell the body how well it is achieving its objectives of matching the circulation and breathing to different levels of exercise. These experiences provide the data from which the brain learns by how much to generate *feedforward* signals to achieve a very targeted outcome. The learning has adapted so well that we no longer see changes in blood pressure or blood oxygen during exercise. The concept has its parallel in cycling. Early attempts to ride a bicycle may lead to wobbling and falls but eventually we learn to cycle in a straight line with only rare deviations and it becomes unconscious or instinctive. We can think of error signals as having served a very useful role over a period in the past, even if they seem to be playing no role in a current bout of exercise.

Learning the control of blood pressure in exercise

My Oxford colleague Peter Robbins conducted an experiment to find evidence for this brain *learning* in controlling blood pressure during exercise. With graduate student Mari Herigstad he devised a cunning laboratory protocol over seven days to deceive the brain into thinking that the measurements of blood pressure it received from the carotid baroreceptors during seventy short bouts of exercise were larger than the actual arterial blood pressure.[25] The aim was to see whether the brain learned to compensate for this fake 'high blood pressure' and showed this by continuing to lower the blood pressure during subsequent bouts of exercise when the deception had been removed.

The deception was achieved by applying a collar to the front of the neck of volunteers, which provided suction (of ~40 mmHg) to the area of the neck in which lie the carotid arteries with their baroreceptors. When suction is applied in this way, the baroreceptor lying in the wall of the carotid artery is fooled into measuring a higher pressure than the actual arterial blood pressure. The reason for this effect is that the baroreceptor measures the pressure difference between the blood inside the carotid artery and the tissue immediately outside the blood vessel wall. When suction is applied outside the neck, the pressure in the tissue outside the blood vessel wall becomes *lower* than normal. The baroreceptor therefore sees a *higher* pressure difference between blood and tissue when the suction is applied, by about 20 mmHg (less than the applied suction and depending upon the thickness of the neck tissues).

Eight volunteers had the suction applied during ten bouts of vigorous cycling exercise, each lasting four minutes, on each of seven successive days, making a total of seventy bouts of exercise. During the period of deception, the brain received a feedback signal from the baroreceptors, which suggested to the brain that there is an error signal: blood pressure was running higher than usual during exercise. The hypothesis behind the study was that the brain would slowly learn over several days to reduce the blood pressure during exercise to reduce this error signal.

The result was that after the seven days the brain had indeed learned to lower the systolic (peak) blood pressure by 7.3 mmHg. Over the following week the brain *re-learned* its normal control of blood pressure and the circulation returned to normal. Control experiments were used to confirm that the result was not an effect of either the neck suction or the exercise alone. The effect of the deception was small, but then the period of learning was short compared with our lifespan, and despite this the whole study took a year to complete. This illustrates how challenging it is to study the role of long-term learning in the regulation of the heart and circulation, and why we know so little about it.

Learning to breathe

Deception of the brain over a period of seven days was also used by Peter Robbins to see whether humans learn how to breathe during exercise. This time the deception was via the chemoreceptors. It was achieved by modifying the gas inspired during exercise so that the chemoreceptors saw *less* oxygen (by a partial pressure in the blood of −8 mmHg) and *more* carbon dioxide (by +8 mmHg). Robbins and graduate student Helen Wood recruited eight volunteers who breathed the modified gas during ten bouts of vigorous exercise, each lasting four minutes, on each of seven successive days, again making a total of seventy bouts of exercise.[26]

During the period of deception, the brain would have received a feedback signal from the chemoreceptors suggesting to it that there were error signals: blood oxygen was running lower than usual and blood carbon dioxide was higher than usual during the exercise. The hypothesis behind the study was that the brain would slowly learn over several days to reduce this error signal by increasing breathing during exercise.

It worked: the result was that, after the seven days, the brain had *learned* to increase breathing during exercise and by about 20 per cent. After stopping the deception, during the following week the brain *re-learned* its normal control and breathing returned to normal. Control experiments were used to confirm that the result was not an effect of either changing the gas breathed or the exercise alone. A year was needed to complete this study too.

This experiment on breathing and the similar one on blood pressure during exercise support the same notion of adaptive control. The chemoreceptors and baroreceptors provide the brain with *feedback* signals, which are used to learn how to calibrate *feedforward* signals. The end result is tight coupling between breathing and cardiac output and the severity of exercise. This tight coupling leads to there commonly being no detectable error signals, just as we learn to ride our bicycle without falling off.

These experiments may point to a solution to the century-old problem of understanding the physiology of exercise. Unfortunately, the findings raise more questions than they answer: how can such learning come about? They are a reminder that we know a lot less than we often convince ourselves we know – a lesson in scientific humility.

How to cheat at Olympic sports

Endurance athletes such as cyclists and runners have hearts that are 30–40 per cent larger than those of untrained people, and their exercise capacity is commonly 60 per cent greater.[27] Performance of this magnitude we know to be associated with years of training. Small additional enhancements make the difference between winning medals and going home disappointed. It might therefore come as a surprise to discover that scientists in California have found a way of speedily increasing the output of the heart and exercise performance by 30 per cent.

Dr Kirk Hammond and his colleagues in San Diego planned an experiment on pigs trained to run on a treadmill while wearing a mask through which their exercise capacity was measured from consumption of oxygen.[28] The intervention studied in this experiment was surgical removal of the sack that surrounds the heart, the pericardium. Normally the maximum volume of the heart is constrained by its enclosure within this sack of tissue. Dr Hammond found that removal of the sack in five animals had little effect on the size of the heart when they were at rest but during exercise increased the volume of the chambers of the heart and the volume of blood ejected by about 30 per cent. Along with this went an increase in cardiac output and maximal exercise capacity.

This removal of the pericardium could not mimic the years of training of an endurance athlete. That training increases the thickness of the heart muscle and not just the volume of the heart. The pericardiectomy mainly allowed the chambers to stretch to a greater volume. Nevertheless, the effect was dramatic.

The researchers were careful to have a control group of five animals in which the full surgery was not performed. These animals had the stress of anaesthesia and surgery to cut open the pericardium, which was then reclosed. The control animals showed a reduction in performance associated with recovery from an operation. Interestingly, when this decline in performance is taken into account, the enhancement of performance in the animals having the pericardium removed amounts to about 50 per cent.[28]

Incision of the pericardium could now be undertaken with keyhole laparoscopic surgery, and conceivably repaired that way too. One is intrigued to debate whether there are unscrupulous practitioners who might use such an operation to enhance performance in competitive sports. In contrast, of interest here is what these experiments may tell us about how the heart is regulated during exercise.

In the preceding discussion about the mysteries of exercise I painted the picture of the exercising muscles drawing whatever blood they need from the arteries to supply themselves with oxygen. Dr Hammond's animal experiments have left us with a further mystery about exercise. Neither we nor the authors of this study have a clear explanation of how surgery on the heart can result in the exercising muscles drawing 30 per cent more blood flow and using 30 per cent more oxygen. They did exclude one possibility; they checked to see whether a rise in arterial blood pressure in the pericardiectomy animals could account for the increased flow to the muscles. It could not. We still require an explanation of this remarkable behaviour of the circulation in exercise but the regulatory authorities for sport might be advised to keep an eye open for its misuse in sporting events. Physiologists have more work on their hands to understand what is going on during exercise. In the next section we shall see how there is much to clarify about the circulation in people at *rest* as well as during exercise.

The great altercation about high blood pressure

In this section I look at a time-honoured debate about the circulation. This is about people at rest and nothing to do with exercise. The topic is high blood pressure; the jargon term is *hypertension*. The topic concerns many people in some way and at some time of their lives, not least because of the need of many to take medications and who then suffer from their adverse effects.

So, what is the problem? Like much in physiology and medicine, the problem is that we continue not to understand the cause of this condition despite efforts extending back at least 150 years.[29] Hypertension is the condition of long-term elevation of the arterial blood pressure. It is associated with diseases that include stroke, heart attacks and kidney failure. Since the 1950s there have been drugs available that can ameliorate high blood pressure and there is emphasis in modern health care on detecting and treating it. It follows that the teaching of medical students about the regulation of arterial blood pressure forms an important part of their education, as does the pathology of when this regulation goes awry.

We are dealing with a dynamic system in which it is difficult to grasp some of the concepts involved. The very concept of 'pressure' itself is foreign to many people. In Chapter Three we noted the reason for often measuring pressure by the height of a column of liquid. We considered the first measurement of arterial blood pressure by the Reverend Stephen Hales from around 1714 using a column of blood. He connected a vertical glass tube to the carotid artery of a reclining horse (see Fig. 15). We recall that in one account of his experiment, in 1733, Hales measured the arterial pressure of a mare as a height of a column of blood of 9½ feet. We noted the convention of stating pressure in terms of the height of a column of liquid mercury as more convenient than using blood. In terms of mercury, the arterial pressure of Hales' horse was about 200 mmHg while the normal value for a human is about 100 mmHg.

The heart generates arterial pressure in a pulsatile manner as each beat ejects blood from the left ventricle into the aorta, which acts as an elastic reservoir, dampening the swing in pressure to some extent. This pulsatile pressure is referred to as having a 'systolic' peak pressure (~120 mmHg) and a 'diastolic' trough pressure (~80 mmHg). The mean pressure of ~100 mmHg drives a flow of blood of ~5 litres per minute through the network of arteries, capillaries and veins that make up the 'peripheral circulation'. In the large veins, and at entry to the right side of the heart, the pressure of blood is usually around 5 mmHg.

Figure 24 represents the physiological characteristics of the circulation in cartoon form. The heart and lungs are shown as a single unit pumping the *cardiac output* into the large arteries. Arterial blood is shown as red to represent it having been oxygenated by its passage through the lungs. The large arteries act as a reservoir at a high pressure. This role can be represented in the cartoon by using a narrow container open to the atmosphere with a depth representing the mean *arterial pressure*, analogous to Hales' vertical glass tube. From these arteries blood enters a meshwork of small vessels as it makes its way through the tissues of the body. These are successively small arteries, capillaries and small veins and are represented by a single narrow tube, having a *vascular resistance*; in this respect, the cartoon is least representative of the actual architecture of the circulation but can represent the resistance of the small vessels.

Within the small vessels, blood gives up oxygen to the tissues and becomes deoxygenated. This is represented using the colour blue. Blood passes from the vascular resistance into the large veins. These act as a large reservoir of blood at a low *venous pressure*. This role can be represented in the cartoon by using a shallow reservoir of wide girth open to the atmosphere. From this reservoir the heart draws blood to complete the cycle of flow.

In a manner analogous to Hales observing the height of a column of arterial blood in his horse, physicians commonly look for the height of a column of blood distending the large veins in the neck of a semi-recumbent patient so as to make a direct measurement of the venous pressure. No glass tube is needed; the height to which the veins of the neck are full can be visualised directly.

The cartoon enables us to see a fundamental relationship. What has to change if arterial pressure is to rise? One or both of two things must occur. An elevated arterial pressure must be associated with a raised cardiac output, a raised vascular resistance, or both. Having noted this relationship, we need to take a trip back to the 1960s to share some astonishment experienced by an American physician.

The professor from Mississippi who proved everyone wrong

It would be nice to lay a local claim to the distinguished physiologist Arthur Guyton, but the Oxford in which he was born in 1919 was the one in Mississippi and not the one in the UK. One may be tempted to associate his unique contribution to our understanding of the circulation with accidents of birth and ill health. His father was a doctor and dean of a medical school, and his mother a teacher of mathematics and physics. As a youngster Arthur built boats and many mechanical and electrical devices. His medical training at Harvard and the Massachusetts General Hospital was interrupted first by Navy service in the Second World War and then by severe poliomyelitis, which ended his hope of becoming a surgeon and left him dependent on a wheelchair. In Oxford, Mississippi, he devoted himself to teaching and research, becoming Chair of the Department of Physiology in 1948. He moved to Jackson, Mississippi, when the medical school moved there in 1955.[30]

In the 1960s Guyton worked with Thomas Coleman, an electrical engineer, with whom he formulated the concept of modelling the behaviour of the circulation using analogue computers. These came before digital computers and represented variables, such as blood pressure, as electrical voltages. The early versions of their model of the circulation, written in computer symbols, were identical to the cartoon model shown in Figure 24, but modified to include the way in which the output of the heart was known to depend upon the venous pressure and with a facility to allow the volume of blood in the circulation to change.[31] They explored making the computer model ever more sophisticated. By 1969 it contained forty-eight 'building blocks', each of which expressed an equation relating one of the variables in the model to one or more other variables. An example would be 'block 44', which related the concentration in the blood of a hormone (angiotensin) to the vascular resistance, the hormone concentration itself being dependent in other blocks of the program on pressures in the circulation.

As the computer model developed, Guyton and Coleman struggled with a key problem. They kept trying to confirm "what without doubt everyone already understood that increased total peripheral (vascular) resistance did indeed cause chronic hypertension".[32] Their computer model persistently showed the opposite: *absolutely no effect of vascular resistance on long-term arterial blood pressure.*[29, 33]

This did not impress some of their 1969 audience. There was talk of the computer model being "revolutionary" and having "startling consequences". The model was seen by one commentator as having so many components that "it can be made to predict anything at all, which means that it can never predict anything"![33] What makes Guyton and Coleman's findings fascinating is that the altercation they put in motion continues to the present day. Nothing has appeared to settle the dispute about whether hypertension is caused by increased vascular resistance or not.

The kidney that would not go away

In a biographical piece Arthur Guyton explained the "ecstatic euphoria" he felt and the "sudden light at the end of a tunnel" when he realised why his computer model predicted the opposite of what everybody thought.[32] This was all to do with building blocks 1 and 2 of his forty-eight-block analogue computer model. He had allowed for his human circulation to have an *intake* of fluid and salt each day and an *output* via the kidney. In other words, the volume of fluid in the circulation could change gradually with time. Crucially, his model reflected the real behaviour of kidneys, namely that the amount of urine they produce depends upon (among many other things) the arterial pressure in the blood vessels perfusing the kidney. These two features of his model are shown in cartoon form in Figure 25.[34] The intake of salt and water is represented by a tap allowing intake to the venous reservoir. The output via the kidney requires a sufficient arterial pressure for the level in the arterial reservoir to be at or above the lowermost hole in the wall of the reservoir.

It may be obvious from inspecting Figure 25 that only one state of affairs is possible if our model has a urine output that matches the daily intake: the arterial pressure will depend only on two things. The first is the behaviour of the kidney; here this is represented by the height and distribution of holes in the arterial reservoir. The second is the amount of daily intake. Changing cardiac output or vascular resistance will not be able to alter arterial pressure for more than a brief period of time.

It is important to note that things are completely different on shorter timescales in which the volume of fluid in the circulation stays unchanged, as depicted in Figure 24. Under this condition, raising the vascular resistance will increase arterial pressure. Similarly, stimulating the heart to have an increase in cardiac output will raise arterial pressure. In this situation, the changes will be maintained indefinitely.

The "revolutionary" conclusion that Guyton was driven to is that, in the long term, the arterial blood pressure cannot be changed by tinkering with the vascular resistance or the cardiac output. The blood pressure *depends only upon kidney function and the daily intake of salt and water.*

Many observations support this conclusion. I shall mention just two.[29] The first is that patients with hypertension who receive a kidney transplant from a healthy donor have their blood pressure normalised. This suggests that it is the kidney that is responsible for setting the blood pressure. The second is that patients who have one or more limbs amputated do not have a change in blood pressure. Loss of a limb involves an increase in vascular resistance because of the reduction in the number of small vessels that can carry blood from the large arteries to the large veins. This shows that changing vascular resistance has no long-term effect on blood pressure.

Despite all this computer modelling and experimental evidence, current teaching about hypertension continues to mislead. A false narrative is widespread and, as we shall see in the next section, it focuses on how hypertension is treated using drugs.

The big myth about treatment of hypertension

The current prevalent dogma about treating long-term high blood pressure with medication can be summarised by citing an educational piece for anaesthetists: "all anti-hypertensive drugs must act by decreasing the cardiac output, the peripheral vascular resistance, or both".[35] This is a statement that can be regarded as completely true and wholly misleading, but it is the approach taken in the most widely consulted pharmacology text for medical students in the UK.[36] This approach has misguided generations of students and medical personnel because it detracts from the key point that the *only mechanism* via which a drug can treat hypertension is by having an action on the kidney. Drug actions that only have effects on the heart or vascular resistance will not work. This is what Guyton and Coleman showed in the 1960s and what all modern computer models of the circulation confirm.[29]

We now recognise that confusion arises because the drugs that are effective in hypertension also have diverse actions on the heart, blood vessels and kidneys. But those actions that do not involve the kidney (or its own blood vessels) have incidental effects, which cannot contribute to lowering blood pressure. It is this complexity of the action of these drugs that has misled so many for so long, often including those who write for education.[37]

Colleagues and I have recently reviewed all publications on drugs used for hypertension since the 1950s. We wished to identify the manner in which they have actions on the kidney. Together with medical student Holly Digne-Malcolm, Matthew Frise and I sought all publications in which patients or healthy human volunteers were administered effective blood-pressure medication *for a minimum of one week*, and in which their kidney function was investigated both when taking the drug and when not taking the drug.[38] This enabled us to see how the drugs were able to allow the kidneys to perform their normal excretion of salt and water while being perfused at a lower arterial pressure. We identified about 130 relevant studies. In many of these, the period for which medication was taken was more than a week, sometimes months or a year.

We found that we could classify all the drugs into having one of two actions on the kidney (or both). Most drugs showed evidence of dilating the blood vessels that lie between the aorta and the glomerular filters in the kidney. In the glomeruli salt and water are first filtered from blood into renal 'tubules' at an average flow of about 125 ml per minute. Further along these tubules, much of the salt and water is reabsorbed back into the blood, leaving the final urine to enter the bladder at a flow of about 1 ml per minute. In this group there were some surprises, such as 'diuretics', drugs which are usually thought of as not affecting blood vessels.[38]

The second mode of action was partial inhibition of the cellular pumping mechanisms that drive the reabsorption of the salt and water back into the blood from the renal tubules. When a drug inhibits this process, a compensation takes place to make sure that the body does not lose an excess of salt and water. This compensation involves a fall in blood pressure. In this group there were also some surprises, such as 'beta blockers', which are usually regarded as drugs acting mainly on the heart.[38] Interestingly, some of the most widely used anti-hypertensive drugs were found to work in *both* of these two ways; these are known as 'ACE inhibitors'.

It is important to reassert that all the families of drugs used to treat hypertension do other things (often many) as well as affecting the kidneys, but these are not relevant to their ability to lower blood pressure. It is worth emphasising also that we do not understand the cause of hypertension. However, extensive research and computer modelling have identified the parameters within which a cause, or multiple causes, must lie and may one day be identified. It is remarkable that some current research literature follows standard teaching in perpetuating a false narrative. An example is a study in 2020 from Yale and Shanghai, which attempts to "have a role in selecting treatment strategies" in hypertension by providing measurements in 34,238 patients of cardiac output and vascular resistance.[39] The thirteen-page paper contains not a single mention of the kidney. This implies that the study cannot inform treatment.

In summary, fifty years of computer modelling and other evidence tells us that the strategy of treating hypertension by reducing cardiac output or reducing vascular resistance is doomed to fail. Drugs widely regarded as achieving these aims also have actions on the kidney and complicate the picture. However, it is these actions on the kidney that lower blood pressure. Teaching of the topic remains deeply flawed throughout the medical profession. Fortunately, the textbook which Arthur Guyton started in 1956 continues to this day in its fourteenth edition and contains a sound account of the physiology of blood-pressure control, and the most recent edition of a favourite UK textbook gives a robustly correct description of both the physiology and pharmacology of hypertension.[4, 40]

As a medical student I accessed my modest savings by visiting the building society then located in Bulkeley Hall, where Anne Greene was brought to be dissected in 1650. I now cycle past it on my way to a coffee or the bank and recall how an understanding of anatomy progressed by dissection of the dead and how, in the short period of my own career, anatomy was advanced in the living by sophisticated imaging techniques, including computer tomography and magnetic resonance. The view I suggest in this chapter is that our understanding of the *function*, or physiology, of the circulation may lag behind our appreciation of its anatomical detail. More work is needed to unravel myths and mysteries of the circulation, and until then the heart will continue to deceive us.

CHAPTER FIVE

A SPOONFUL OF SUGAR

Surgery without Sleep

Open-heart surgery Indian-style

Sometimes an image may be a real shock without being gruesome. In 2010 the *Daily Mail* showed its readers a relaxed-looking twenty-three-year-old patient, Swaroup Anand, staring contentedly into the camera while five surgical hands were operating on his beating heart through an opening in the front of his chest (Fig. 26).[1]

Some details will help to clarify the occasion. Swaroup wears a blue 'J-cloth' hospital paper hat. He has nasal cannulae for trickling oxygen into his nostrils. Hospital staff would recognise the entry port to an 'epidural catheter' parked beside his left ear. Then there is a green surgical drape across the middle of the image, separating Swaroup's relaxed face at the top of the picture from his open chest at the bottom. This drape is sometimes known jokingly as the 'blood–brain barrier' when those on its surgical side are being teased (or perhaps insulted) by the anaesthetic team at the head, or brain, end.

Here the action is definitely on the blood side of the drape. We can see a dense entanglement of plastic tubes, two of which lead into the heart. One contains dark red blood and the second bright red blood. The pumping role of Swaroup's heart is being temporarily taken over by a heart–lung machine (out of view), to which dark deoxygenated blood is being drained, and from which newly oxygenated blood is being pumped to perfuse the tissues of the body.

This is open-heart surgery Indian-style, performed in Bangalore on a conscious and comfortable young man under a form of regional anaesthesia that goes by the name of 'epidural'. The lead surgeon, Dr Vivek Jawali, reported more than 600 operations of this kind by his team since 1999. He explained that patients do not feel afraid during the operation: "We give them headphones so they can listen to their favourite music."

This almost casual surgery inside the heart is a spectacular success of modern medicine. In this account I draw attention to the role of anaesthesia in making possible interventions that would otherwise be unbearable and impossible. In my own time as an anaesthetist particular satisfaction has come from using regional anaesthesia of the spine to enable patients to undergo surgery (or childbirth) while conscious and free of pain. The epidural anaesthetic is one approach. Another is 'spinal' anaesthesia, and a notable event from a hundred years before Swaroup's surgery showed its possibilities when a surgeon decided to operate on himself.

How to repair your own hernia

Alexandre Fzaïcou was a twenty-six-year-old Romanian doctor who was working on a doctoral thesis on spinal anaesthesia. He had enthusiasm for his topic. He also had a hernia in his left groin. In 1911 he published an account of performing a repair of this inguinal hernia on himself after getting a colleague, Professor Juvara, to perform a spinal anaesthetic on him.[2] The name they employed at the time for this version of this procedure hardly slips off the tongue: 'rachi-strychno-stovainisation'. An image in his paper in the French journal *La Presse Médicale* is another stunner (there are several in the paper to choose from), even though the black-and-white photograph does not show the colour of the blood (Fig. 27). It features four impressive moustaches. One is on Mr Fzaïcou, who sits partly covered in drapes, both hands repairing the hernia in his left groin. Three are on his assistants, standing inquisitively close by. "We should be prepared to have ourselves what we would recommend to others in similar circumstances," he wrote, and reassuringly: "I suffered no disagreeable phenomenon, even though I operated on myself, that I had to remain in a sitting position, make the movements necessary to reach the instruments and to wash my hands red with blood, and to make all the other movements necessary to carry out the operation."[3]

The operation took place on 23 September 1909. His minute-by-minute account tells us that the spinal injection took place at 15.47 with a cocktail of the tiny volume of ⅔ ml of 1 mg/ml of strychnine and 70 mg/ml of stovaine (more widely known as amylocaine and

the first synthetically made 'local anaesthetic' drug, first manufactured in France in 1903). The anaesthetic was performed by passing
a needle into the lumbar spine while he sat upright. At 15.50 he had a
ticklish sensation in his lower body, and by 15.52 his feet felt warm. His
perineum was numb at 15.53, and soon he became unable to move his
lower limbs. A change from the sitting to a semi-recumbent position
was found to help spread the area of numbness. At the twenty-minute
point there was discussion because there was still some sensation in
his groin. Fzaïcou turned down Juvara's offer of chloroform and
decided to inject a small volume of the stovaine into the skin of the
groin to enable him to get started.

He took a little over an hour to repair the inguinal hernia. Several
days of discomfort, insomnia, headache and constipation followed,
plus the entry into history as the first surgeon to have performed a
substantial operation on himself. He probably should have used the
full 1 ml of anaesthetic he had prepared rather than just ⅔ ml. Like
baking a cake, this kind of anaesthesia relies for success on attention
to fine detail. By 1911 it had a reputation for killing people and that
was not only because of injecting strychnine, a well-known lethal
poison. And what was that doing in the cocktail anyway?

Strychnine, known for centuries, is a plant poison that kills by
interfering with nerve conduction, producing convulsions and paralysis. Its availability as a rat poison has tempted some to other uses;
Mr William Dove, "an independent gentleman of Leeds", was one
such. We read in the *Lyttelton Times* of August 1856 that "Mr Dove and
his wife had not lived happily together", and that on more than one
occasion he had threatened to "give her a pill that would do for her".[4]
Dove's guilt in having finally done so was confirmed in a manner
regarded at the time as highly scientific: contents of the deceased
wife's stomach were administered to "two rabbits, two mice, and one
guinea pig" and resulted in similar convulsions, twitching and spasms
(and death in four animals) to those seen in the unfortunate Harriet
Dove.

In the later nineteenth century, strychnine found advocates for
its use in small doses as a performance-enhancing drug and recrea-
tional stimulant. In this context it was picked up by Professor Thomas
Jonnesco of Bucharest as an idea for countering some of the depres-
sant effects of stovaine in patients undergoing a spinal anaesthetic for
surgery. But first, some background detail.

The injection of a 'local anaesthetic' drug into the cerebrospinal fluid that bathes the spinal cord was known by the turn of the twentieth century to be a very effective way of numbing part of the body for surgery without the need to put the patient to sleep with a general anaesthetic by vapour such as chloroform or ether. The family of local anaesthetic drugs had been started around 1884 by medical use of naturally occurring cocaine on the front of the eye and was soon continued with the manufacture of amylocaine, procaine and several other 'caines'. When these drugs bathe a nerve, they stop the conduction of nerve impulses, thereby blocking the conduction of sensation and pain.

Pain impulses are among those that travel from the periphery towards the spinal cord, which sits within the canal running through the vertebral bones of the spinal column. Each segment of the body sends its own nerves to an associated vertebral level in the spine spanning from high up in the neck down through the lumbar vertebrae of our lower back and further still to the bones of the pelvis. As these nerves enter the spinal canal they pass across a robust membrane of tissue called the 'dura'. Once inside the dura the nerves find themselves traversing the cerebrospinal fluid that bathes the spinal cord, and then connect with the cord via 'nerve roots'. A local anaesthetic drug injected into the cerebrospinal fluid can block nerve impulses, along with other sensations such as the feeling of touch and of hot or cold, where the nerves are bathed by the fluid (Fig. 28). This is the target site referred to as a 'spinal' injection, which enabled Fzaïcou to operate on himself.

Going in the other direction, from the spinal cord out to the muscles, are other nerves conveying signals telling the muscles to contract. These tend to be carried by thicker nerves than pain signals, and so get blocked more slowly, but nevertheless blocked they are if the drug gets to them. So, Alexandre Fzaïcou would have been unable to move his legs and indeed his assistants may have needed to guard against the possibility of him falling out of his chair during the operation had he become unbalanced while leaning forwards to wash his hands "red with blood", because his muscles would not have responded to attempts to help himself.

The incidental blocking of motor nerves by a drug given specifically for the purpose of blocking sensory nerves is not necessarily an unhelpful adjunct to the injection into the spine. Sometimes it can be really helpful. For example, if a surgeon intends to operate inside the abdomen, relaxing the normally taut muscles of the abdominal wall helps the surgeon to gain access without the patient's intestines inconveniently being squeezed out of the incision (and being hard to squeeze back in). This is what blocking the motor nerves achieves. The loosening of the muscle tension in Fzaïcou's groin will have made it easier for him to repair the hernia.

But there is a problem if the drug blocks the motor nerves to the muscles with which we breathe, and the higher up the spine the injection takes place (or the drug trickles) the more likely this is to happen. In particular, in the neck, the phrenic nerve (which provides the motor signals to the diaphragm, our main respiratory muscle) exits the spinal cord via nerve roots at the levels we label cervical 3, 4 and 5 (Fig. 29). If the local anaesthetic reaches here then breathing may stop and the patient may die. It would seem impossible to use a spinal anaesthetic to remove pain sensation for surgery in the neck, and above it in the head, because the spinal anaesthetic would block the roots of the phrenic nerve and stop breathing. It may come as a surprise, therefore, that one surgeon advocated spinal anaesthesia as the best way to perform *all* surgery *on the head* as well as *all* surgery elsewhere in the body.

Thomas Jonnesco's exorbitant claims

This astonishing claim was made in 1909 in *The British Medical Journal* by Professor Thomas Jonnesco of Bucharest. His alleged pain-free surgery under spinal anaesthesia *on patients' heads* was met with some incredulity.[5] In his paper Jonnesco reports 398 operations performed under his brand of 'general spinal analgesia' (he calls it variably 'analgesia' and 'anaesthesia') in a nine-month period, 103 of which were from injections high in the spine, enabling (often major) operations on the "skull", the "face", the "throat" and the "thorax" in patients as young as two years old. The very notion of these forms of surgery in conscious patients of all ages will find the modern anaesthetist incredulous and wondering whether this paper is 'pulling a fast one' with its claims: "General spinal anaesthesia is absolutely safe; it has never caused death, nor produced any important complications, early or late," and is "infinitely superior to inhalation anaesthesia. Owing to its simplicity, it is within reach of all, and as there is no contraindication it may be employed with any patient." Anaesthetists may further note how redundant they are in Jonnesco's vision of the future of surgery: "As it can be performed by the surgeon himself it does away with the attendance of a person often inexperienced, and never responsible."

We need to think more about Jonnesco's claims and ask whether and how it may have been possible to make this very high spinal anaesthesia work. Was it really possible to block the pain signals in the sensory nerves entering the spinal cord (along with some from the face entering the brain) while not blocking the motor nerves exiting the spinal cord in the neck? How could breathing possibly continue in this situation? Jonnesco claimed that there were two essential components. The first was that the anaesthetic solution had to be injected between the first and second 'dorsal vertebrae'. These are the first two of a stack of twelve 'dorsal' or thoracic vertebrae below the neck, which we now refer to as T1 and T2 (Fig. 29). A photograph in Jonnesco's paper shows a sitting patient leaning forwards so that his chin touches his sternum; a needle is being inserted in the midline of his spine at this level, T1–2. Jonnesco preferred the anaesthetic stovaine but noted other local anaesthetics with which he had less experience.

The second of Jonnesco's requirements was that the solution should contain strychnine as well as the local anaesthetic drug. The strychnine was for "neutralising the depressing action of the stovaine", which he seems to have identified as being an "injurious action on the bulb", i.e. what we now think of as the brain stem, which lies above the spinal cord and connects it to the brain. Indeed, it is striking that Jonnesco does not mention the anatomical origin of the phrenic nerve at C3, 4, 5 and we may conclude that he was unaware of this. His assessment of the complications of his technique was, as we note above, more dismissive than thorough. He lumped together "stoppage of breathing and of the heart" along with "pallor of the face, nausea, or sweating" as "bulbar phenomena – attributable to the excess of stovaine" and admitted to these occurring only when his refined technique was not followed precisely. In other words, he viewed his technique as 100 per cent successful because any failures resulted from a deviation from it.

Further features prove to be important as we follow Jonnesco's description of his technique.[5] A third factor was that the volume of injectate was 1 ml, or thereabouts, with adjustment for the age and condition of the patient. This is small compared with the volume of local anaesthetic used for spinal anaesthetics in current practice. These are now usually administered much lower down the spine to avoid the risk of damaging the spinal cord and a volume of 2–3 ml is commonly used. A clarification of the anatomy will help explain how damage can occur unless spinal injections are limited to the lumbar levels of the spine.

The spinal cord sits within its bathing cerebrospinal fluid, enclosed in the cylindrical tissue membrane, the dura. In adult patients the spinal cord extends all the way from the brainstem and the cranium at the top down to the first of five lumbar vertebrae in the lower back. A needle inserted above this L1 lumbar level, if advanced too far, carries the risk of impaling the spinal cord and producing serious and irreversible damage. Jonnesco characteristically took the view that "the fear of pricking the cord" was "unfounded; even if it happens it is not harmful".

Below the L1 lumbar level the dural tube contains nerves ascending to and descending from their roots within the spinal cord. These nerves are mobile in the cerebrospinal fluid and able to move away from a needle arriving among them. This bundle of nerves is colourfully called the *cauda equina*, from the impression of it as a horse's tail. It is here that it is now common to inject 2–3 ml, i.e. a small teaspoonful and a volume that is enough to produce a complete block of all nerve signals passing up and down in this area. The small volume of Jonnesco's injectate may be of significance in understanding how his technique could sometimes be effective.

A fourth feature of Jonnesco's technique was that the injection had to be performed slowly "so as not to produce an undue impact upon the spinal cord" and the patient was laid flat on their back immediately following the injection. It is this requirement that draws our attention to the way the small volume of fluid might distribute itself within the spinal canal and which aspect of the spinal cord and its nerve roots it might have affected.

The relevant anatomical feature of the spinal canal is that the sensory nerve roots enter the spinal cord on its back (posterior) aspect while the motor nerves exit the spinal cord on its front (anterior) aspect. Herein lies the possibility that a *small* volume of drug injected *slowly* from the rear into the cerebrospinal fluid of a patient laid immediately *supine* might distribute only around the posterior sensory nerves over a limited *span* of the spinal canal and selectively block them, thereby producing anaesthesia for surgery in an area of the head and neck while leaving intact the nerves at the front required for breathing.

A very localised distribution of the anaesthetic drug might also account for Jonnesco's observation that patients could sometimes continue to move their limbs. The anatomy of the spinal cord is arranged such that tracts of nerve cells carrying signals up from, and down to, the lower parts of the body tend to lie quite deep inside the cord. It seems possible that a small volume of drug might fail to penetrate the internal tracts of the spinal cord and leave some of this traffic unaffected. This would mean that sensation and motor function could be retained in the lower part of the body. That this occurred in some cases is apparent from Jonnesco's description of paralysis (paresis) not always being present:

> The immobility of the limbs, the neck, and the head, due to paresis caused by the spinal analgesia, is a great advantage to the surgeon by suppressing movements which might embarrass him. It is true that there may be complete anaesthesia without loss of mobility in the limbs; this rarely happens, but its occurrence ought to be known, as it is not necessary to wait for paresis before beginning to operate.

We might be tempted from these careful considerations to assume that it is possible, by using only 1 ml of drug solution, to keep patients conscious, pain-free and happy during surgery on any part of the body from the head downwards. Perhaps, however, we should first find out what contemporaries thought of Jonnesco's claims before radically revising surgical practice.

A Berlin physician who was particularly exercised by the dangers of anaesthesia was Dr Heinz Wohlgemuth, who wrote a pleading piece in a German medical weekly in 1908 about brutal practices and fatal consequences associated with inexperience and lack of training.[6] He was arguing for advanced training courses in anaesthesia, like one that he had identified in London, and more widely for obligatory training in the subject for all doctors. He noted in anticipation a special thematic session on anaesthesia at the forthcoming 1908 International Surgical Congress to be held in Brussels. Indeed, it fell to Wohlgemuth to write a summary of all the proceedings, surgical as well as anaesthetic, for a Viennese medical weekly.

The report by Wohlgemuth of the anaesthesia session at the international congress that September suggests that quite a commotion blew up when Jonnesco took to the floor to advocate the "absolute safety" of his high spinal anaesthesia. Heated debate involved several supporters but also those delegates who thought spinal anaesthesia should never be used because of damage it might cause to the spinal cord. Jonnesco planned a demonstration, and on a child, would you believe? This took place in the St Jean Hospital and went so badly wrong "that one surely from now on will distance oneself from this kind of anaesthesia", wrote Wohlgemuth.[7] Immediately after the injection the child was beset by "alarming tetanic seizures".

Wohlgemuth reads like the sort of doctor one needs in challenging circumstances, a calm rational voice who in 1901 had himself developed improved safety in general anaesthesia by using oxygen to supplement chloroform. After summarising the rival points of view expressed at the conference about the several kinds of anaesthesia available at the time, he emphasised almost poetically the need for training: "*Die* Narkosenfrage *sei eine Frage des* Narkotiseurs, *nicht des* Narkoticums" ('the *question of anaesthesia* is a question of the *anaesthetist*, not the *anaesthetic*'). His final summary of the conference discussion on anaesthesia was a prediction that remains sound to this day: "There will never be an anaesthetic agent or a mode of anaesthesia that can be both fully effective and completely safe."[7]

The failed demonstration in Brussels of Jonnesco's high spinal anaesthesia was not the only occasion on which he failed to convince an audience. An editorial in 1910 in a US surgical journal recounts events during a demonstration in the Mount Sinai Hospital in New York.[8] Jonnesco injected four patients. Two of them received their injections low in the spine – the sort of lumbar injection that Alexandre Fzaïcou had received before doing his own hernia repair, and the sort of spinal injection that is now a routine method of performing a spinal anaesthetic (although without the strychnine). These two injections by Jonnesco were "quite satisfactory". The other two injections were attempts at his high spinal technique. In the first, more than one attempt was needed and blood was drawn, a bad sign. Moreover, although the operation "involved only superficial tissues on the chest, the patient complained repeatedly of pain and cried out for chloroform". We may get some insight into Jonnesco's bedside manner and distorted assessment of evidence by noting the editorial comment on this failure. "Jonnesco (who, it must be said, does not understand English) explained these complaints as due to nervousness and to the sensations of contact and traction – although both during and after the operation the patient plainly felt pricks on his arms, and noticed numbness only on one shoulder."[8] Jonnesco's second attempt at a high spinal injection shocked the bystanders with its clumsiness and was abandoned, the patient being given a general anaesthetic with ether.

A further indication of Jonnesco's assertiveness and lack of insight into his own limitations comes from the fact that the February 1910 issue of the same journal was persuaded to publish his forceful attempt to rebuff the scepticism of the January editorial.[9] It must have tested the patience of the readers of the day to be told that the surgical patient, a boy, felt no pain but was in a "psychological state" – as well he might have been – and that all of Jonnesco's other 195 high spinal injections had been a success.

The debate about the efficacy and safety of Jonnesco's method of spinal anaesthesia continued apace. In September 1910 a London surgeon, Lawrie McGavin, waded in with detailed case reports of his own.[10] This time *The British Medical Journal* can take credit for a more measured scientific approach than in Jonnesco's 1909 list of 398 operations. McGavin was surgeon at the Seamen's Hospital in Greenwich and had a close acquaintance with Jonnesco, who had injected three patients there during a visit to London. Only one could be regarded as successful.

The Seaman's Hospital had started its life in 1821 as a hospital ship in Deptford and spent long years in two ships named *Dreadnought* until being transferred to land on the Greenwich hospital site in 1870. It took the name Dreadnought Seamen's Hospital and provided care for merchant navy and other seamen. Born in 1868 in Calcutta, Lawrie McGavin was educated at Fettes College, Sandhurst and Guy's Hospital, from which he qualified in 1898. He was appointed surgeon to the hospital in 1902.[11]

McGavin reported eighteen instances of his own use of spinal anaesthetic using Jonnesco's cocktail of strychnine and stovaine. Six were high spinal injections. Interestingly, three of the six resulted in satisfactory analgesia from the top of the head, or forehead, down to the umbilicus or lowermost ribs and provided good operating conditions for surgery on the head, neck and upper arm. A fourth gave patchy numbness, and surgery on the back of the head had to be completed under general anaesthetic. Numbers five and six were failures; they resulted in embarrassed breathing: gasping, a sense of suffocation and "terror". One of the two patients, clearly a seaman, likened the episode to his earlier experience of being "washed overboard and nearly drowned". McGavin concluded that "the unsuccessful cases of high puncture show it to be fraught with danger, and from the humane standpoint unjustifiable". His experiences of the technique had resulted in him being far less enthusiastic than when he reported partial success after Jonnesco's visit to the hospital the year before.[12]

The twelve cases of lower spinal injection in McGavin's series were largely satisfactory, yet he concluded that the addition of strychnine had nothing to offer and "undoubtedly results in a shortening of the period of analgesia usually resulting from the use of stovaine alone". Somewhat modestly, McGavin concluded his paper with remarks which suggest that the Seamen's Hospital may have been a centre for a major advance in spinal anaesthesia out of proportion with its humble origins and facilities. In a remarkable paragraph at the end of his eighteen case reports, McGavin introduces a new factor, writing:

> The above remarks, it must be remembered, apply solely to cases done by the stovaine–strychnine method, the results of which must not be confounded with those of the stovaine–glucose method of Barker. Of these latter cases, considerably over 500 have now been done in the wards of the Seamen's Hospital with perfect satisfaction to the patients, to myself, and to those of my colleagues who have given it a trial.[10]

Arthur Barker's spoonful of sugar

McGavin's report might at first appear to be the kind of inflated claim for success that we have seen from Jonnesco and have come to suspect, but this is from a young surgeon whose case reports are characterised by detail and reflection. Five hundred, indeed! Who is Barker and what has glucose – sugar – to do with it?

Arthur Barker was Professor of Surgery at University College Hospital in London (Fig. 30). He was born in 1850, trained in Dublin and Bonn, and was first appointed surgeon in Dublin in 1876. In 1885 he joined the staff at University College Hospital, becoming professor to the medical school there in 1893.[13] By the time he wrote his momentous first paper on spinal analgesia in 1907, therefore, he had more than thirty years of surgical experience behind him.[14] His paper is a model clinical report: a series of 100 spinal anaesthetics firmly based upon scientific reasoning and laboratory experiments, and delivered with caution and modesty. It includes many useful tips on practical techniques, which anaesthetists may benefit from reading today. His valuable idea was to use a local anaesthetic that was heavier (i.e. denser) than cerebrospinal fluid to allow *gravity* to direct the drug to the nerve roots that needed to be blocked. For this purpose, he added 5 per cent glucose to stovaine to form a cocktail that had a density of 1.030, which was higher than that the 1.007 of cerebrospinal fluid (both relative to water), while not being so dense as to damage the nerves it was aiming to reach.[14]

To exploit gravity, Barker needed a thorough understanding of the curvatures of the spine when patients lie on their backs (the supine position). Patients were asked to lie supine immediately following their spinal injection, which was conducted either with the patient sitting or lying on one side. To aid insight, Barker produced a long glass tube, half an inch in diameter, which matched the spinal curvature of a full-sized section of a female human cadaver frozen in that posture. Using this model spine, he could study and demonstrate how drugs flowed to regions of the spine under gravity.

Readers may find it surprising how curved the healthy spine is. When we lie on our backs, there are two high points in the spine, one in the lumbar region (L2–4) and one high in the neck (Fig. 29). By coincidence the L2–4 level is the one in which it is safe and most convenient to perform a spinal injection: safe because it is below the level at which the spinal cord terminates (L1–2) and so it is in the area where the spinal nerves of the *cauda equina* descending from the cord are unlikely to be damaged by a needle; most convenient because the shape of the vertebral bones in this area makes it easiest to pass a needle into the spinal canal here.

Two low points are present in the supine spine. One is between the high points, around the mid-thoracic area, in the region of vertebrae T5–7 (Fig. 29). The second is low down the spine, below the lumbar region, in the sacrum, a single bone made up from five fused sacral vertebrae at the base of the spinal column. The T5–7 level has a particular significance for clinical practice. It is the level above which spinal anaesthesia can get into difficulties and many saw as best avoided (though clearly Jonnesco was not one of these). Problems include partial paralysis of the subsidiary muscles of breathing, those lying between the ribs (the intercostal muscles), and also the blocking of nerves that regulate heart rate, which may lead to slowing of the heart and fainting. We have already noted that blocking the phrenic nerve roots in the neck stops the vital contribution of the diaphragm to breathing.

Barker inserted a small access portal at the L3 point of his glass models of the spine so that he could inject at that point cocktails of various densities to which the dye methyl violet had been added, enabling him to see how gravity distributed the injectates and with what speed. Before each injection the whole glass tube was filled with fluid with the same density as cerebrospinal fluid so as to mimic the fluid properties of the spinal canal. The conclusion of his experiments was that a dose of the glucose–stovaine mix injected in the lumbar area would flow over a couple of minutes from the site of injection headwards towards T5–7 and feetwards to the sacral area. Some cautious tipping of the operating table head-down could be used to extend the spinal analgesia further headwards if required. He not only tried injectates that were denser than cerebrospinal fluid, but he also visualised the movement (or rather lack of it) of drug that was lighter than cerebrospinal fluid and thereby was able to explain the erratic behaviour some surgeons had reported from injectates that gave unsatisfactory spread of analgesia. In summary: a spoonful of sugar was the way to make 'the medicine go *down*', as it were; with the increased density, gravity could be used to achieve predictable distribution of the analgesia.

Barker's use of glucose and gravity was a brilliant, simple discovery and one that has led to a century of safe, reliable practice in spinal anaesthesia. In my own work as an anaesthetist, I have found particular value in being able to anaesthetise the lower half of a patient for procedures such as removal of the prostate or repair of a vaginal prolapse, while being able to sit beside them at their head and hold a conversation (and sometimes a hand) while the operation is under way.

It is to Barker that we owe a technique of spinal anaesthesia that is safe for everyday use. In 1979 J. Alfred Lee, the great polymath consultant anaesthetist from Southend-on-Sea, made "an attempt to bring to the notice of the readers of *Anaesthesia* some details of ... one of Britain's great pioneers of regional anaesthetic techniques".[15] During my own career among anaesthetists I was not aware of Barker being so little appreciated; having myself been born in a Southend-on-Sea hospital during Lee's time in post there, I would like to think that my mention here of Barker's achievements might extend Alfred Lee's efforts to bring them to the attention of anaesthetists and others.

Barker followed up his 1907 series of 100 spinal anaesthetics with two more reports, each of a further 100 cases. Report number two was characterised by much reticence plus vigorous combat with one Dr Dönitz in Bonn. First, the reticence. In the first sentence of his report Barker states: "With no wish on the one hand to advocate or, on the other hand, to disparage this new procedure, I have hopes that the following study may help to settle its proper value in surgery, whether this will be small or great."[16] Perhaps at this point in his experience this is a little disingenuous; it is difficult not to conclude that he had some intent to 'advocate' what in his view provided remarkably favourable operating conditions.

Second, the combat. Barker politely refers to "Continental *confrères*" laying down "principles of action" that are "diametrically opposed" to his own. In particular Dönitz denied any effect of gravity on the spread of anaesthesia following spinal injection. He attributed the spread to the flow of cerebral spinal fluid with change in posture – a kind of *sloshing* up and down the spinal canal – quite distinct from the flow under gravity that Barker advocated. "It is not a matter of the action of gravity on the analgesic compound at all," wrote the German *confrère*.[17]

In his second report Barker did finally identify two *confrères* who had also concluded that the density of the injected drug was important in influencing its movement. In a paper with a bizarre title referring to "observations during the first one thousand spinal anaesthetics" from the Freiburg women's hospital, Professor Krönig and Dr Gauss reported experiments on corpses in various sitting and lying postures that led them to believe that lighter spinal solutions moved upwards and heavier solutions moved downwards under gravity.[18] A few experiments in patients localised to the upper and lower lumbar segments confirmed this view (but the thousand cases make no appearance). A particularly useful insight came from noticing that the density of stovaine varied with temperature so that it might be heavier than cerebrospinal fluid when injected at room temperature only to become lighter at body temperature. That had the potential to confuse even the most astute observers. A protective Barker discussed their work and noted that his experiments were more conclusive and had precedence.[16]

Dr Len Carrie and the 'Oxford' position

In both his second and third series of 100 cases (totalling 300 eventually), Barker extended his range of surgery, and his success rate, and explored posture, timing and the effects of gravity further.[19] One of his experiments in particular leads us to jump ahead ninety years to what has become known as *the Oxford position* (not a philosophical or erotic one, as the name might suggest) in which to conduct spinal anaesthesia for the surgical delivery of a baby by Caesarean section.

First a description of his experiment: Barker was interested to observe the spread of spinal analgesia in the case of a patient administered the injection in the lumbar region while lying on their side and *remaining in that position*. Following his thinking about the spread under gravity in the curves of the supine spine, he laid his patient on their side with a pillow under the head and another under the pelvis so as to produce a U-shape in the spine with the lowermost point around the lower thoracic vertebrae, T10. The position is nicely illustrated in his photograph in which each palpable spinous process of the vertebrae, from the neck down into the lumbar region, is marked with a pen. He joined up the dots on the vertebral spines with a line that formed a smooth, clear U.[16]

What did he find, and how did it influence the Oxford position many years later? As he anticipated from his experiments with glass tubes, one of which was used to mimic the U-shape of the patient lying on their side, the analgesia spread predictably from the uphill site of lumbar injection, close to the pelvis on the pillow, to the mid thoracic area. In one case this provided good anaesthesia for a below-knee amputation of the left leg of a young man. In another case the conditions allowed surgery on varicose veins of the left thigh and leg.

Note the 'left' here: the injection was performed in both cases with the patient lying with the left side down. In both cases Barker found that the right leg was largely or wholly unaffected; both sensation and the ability to move the limb on that side remained. To Barker this confirmed that his 1 ml of glucose–stovaine cocktail both went downhill under gravity in the U-shape of the spinal curve and also tended to stay in the lowermost half of the dural tube so that nerve roots on the left were affected by the local anaesthetic and those on the right remained largely unaffected.

Those of us who trained in anaesthesia in Oxford in the 1980s had the very good fortune to fall under the tutelage of Dr Len Carrie, the lead specialist in obstetric anaesthesia. A dour Scotsman, he had not only heard of Arthur Barker, but he had also replicated his model, which for Oxford trainees became famous as 'Carrie's glass spine'. A thorough demonstration of the disposition of injectates of different densities in different postures can be enjoyed on a video presented with characteristic authority by Len Carrie himself.[20] Barker makes a brief appearance in the video too: Carrie shows Barker's portrait as he gives him credit (the same portrait I show here in Fig. 30). It is perhaps ironic that the glass spine should be central to Carrie's practice of spinal anaesthesia in women undergoing Caesarean section (i.e. delivery of their babies through an incision in the lower abdomen), and that is because women close to birth cannot safely lie fully supine in a manner that would enable the curves of the spine to be used to distribute the solution. When the mother-to-be lies supine the baby weighs down on the large blood vessels of the abdomen, making the mother feel faint and nauseated. The standard solution to this if the woman does need to lie on her back (for example, for the operation itself to take place) is to put a wedge or pillow under the right hip so that the lower part of the abdomen is slanted at about 15–20 degrees to the horizontal. This displaces the baby sufficiently to prevent compression of the vessels. Unfortunately, this cannot be used in anaesthesia; if this twisted position is adopted immediately after performing the spinal injection, the flow of drug is somewhat unpredictable and may be one-sided.

To the rescue came Len Carrie, inspired by Arthur Barker, using the "Oxford positioning technique" to establish the spinal anaesthetic with a novel inflatable 'wedge' to regulate the degree of tilt during the operation.[21, 22] Carrie's modification of Barker's technique was as follows: for the spinal injection the patient was placed on their left side with three pillows under the head and an air-filled bag under the left shoulder. The left hip also rested on a pillow to encourage the spine to form the U-shape that Barker had shown to be so important. Further, by slightly inclining the couch head downwards by a few degrees the spine was oriented such that the bottom of the U-shape was at thoracic level T4. Taking the analgesia up to this level was regarded as ideal for good analgesia for a Caesarean section.

To prevent the spinal analgesia from being unilateral (as Barker has shown it tended to be), immediately after the spinal injection the patient was turned into the 'right lateral' position, identical to the first U-shape, but with the right side downmost. The patient was left in this position for several minutes before being turned more nearly supine (but with the wedge to prevent compression of the blood vessels) for commencement of the operation.

The wedge that helped in these proceedings had been described by Carrie back in 1982.[23] This was a 3-litre plastic bag for bladder irrigation, emptied of liquid and inflated with air via a small hand pump from the usual device for measuring blood pressure. This primitive but valuable device enabled fine-tuning of the shoulder elevation during the spinal injection and fine-tuning of the wedge under the hip during the operation. Being deflated, it also allowed the patient to be relaxed to the supine position once the baby had been delivered; by improving the position for the surgeon while stitching the wound, this considerate behaviour also helped to maintain an amicable relationship across the blood–brain barrier.

The patient's husband often sat nearby for the delivery and Carrie was a master of defusing any tension in the proceedings (it was not uncommon at the time for husbands to faint.) His subtle good humour can be recognised under 'acknowledgements' in his 1982 paper, which described the inflatable wedge: "I wish to acknowledge the help of Dr Lyn Davies of the Nuffield Department of Anaesthetics Laboratories for a determined but unsuccessful attempt to test the bag to destruction." It would clearly not do to have the wedge bag bursting during the operation.

The 'Oxford position' was perhaps a misappropriation, like 'Carrie's glass spine', when both were so similar to what Arthur Barker described in 1908, but Len Carrie did not hesitate to give Barker precedence. For his spinal injections with patients lying on their side,

Barker had a "padded board" under the hip, a "fourfold blanket" under the shoulder, and a thick pillow under the head to generate a U-shaped spine.[19] Oxford added a little head-down tilt that goes beyond the capability of Barker's couch, plus the flip onto the other side to anaesthetise left and right sides equally. By re-emphasising the importance of position in his teaching and the more recent literature, Carrie has surely saved many of us from embarrassingly inadequate spinal anaesthetics.

The origin (and near end) of spinal anaesthesia

Spinal anaesthesia for the delivery of babies is one of the most valuable applications of a technique that had its origins in a very different setting. Here we take a step back a decade before Jonnesco's exaggerated claims to see how spinal anaesthesia was first used and very nearly ended abruptly.

It was the German surgeon August Bier who led the way by experimenting on himself with "cocainisation of the spine", and also on his assistant and six patients undergoing lower-limb surgery for complications of tuberculosis.[24] Bier demonstrated that a tiny volume of cocaine solution (0.5–1 ml) injected into the spinal canal was capable of rendering up to two-thirds of the body sufficiently free of sensation for major operations to be performed totally free of pain: not a bad contribution to medical science for a few days' work.

In his 1899 report of these events the excitement of the achievement leaps from the page, not least in the way that he and his assistant Hildebrand celebrated the success of their self-experimentation with an evening of cigars, wine and a good meal. Yet what may come as a surprise, despite the evening of celebration, is that this was very nearly the end of spinal anaesthesia. So dreadful were the sequelae in most of their patients and both Bier and Hildebrand that Bier felt "it was no longer justifiable to conduct further experiments on humans".[24] Headaches were debilitating, as was vomiting. These adverse effects seemed to be worse than those after a general anaesthetic by chloroform or ether. Bier spent nine days in bed even after Hildebrand actually failed to inject much cocaine into his spine because of a badly fitting needle but did manage to cause Bier to lose a lot of cerebrospinal fluid. Hildebrand felt unwell, was off his food, and had a headache for several days; he remained weak for three weeks.

We have seen that a major threat to the adoption of spinal anaesthesia subsequently was the irresponsible recommendation of its use
for surgery high in the body by Thomas Jonnesco in Romania. It is
astonishing that, despite announcing in the first sentence of his 1909
publication that Bier publicly repudiated Jonnesco's spinal technique,
the latter was totally dismissive of the concerns raised and was "firmly
convinced that my new method of general spinal analgesia will in a
short time be universally accepted".[5] The passage of time was to be
his judge, and fortunately the critical approach of McGavin and others
brought sense to bear on Jonnesco's claims.[10, 25] It is interesting to read
a laudatory account in 2009 of Jonnesco by two Romanian surgeons
as 'Founder of the Romanian School of Surgery', containing not one
word of criticism of their subject's approach to 'rachianaesthesia',
or indeed any of his other activities.[26] These authors present all of
his demonstrations of spinal anaesthesia round the world as wholly
successful.

Bier had discovered a way of rendering two-thirds of the body
free of pain in conscious people. We will have to account for how
spinal anaesthesia managed to survive despite the appalling after-
effects that persuaded Bier to call a halt in 1898, but first we might
best consider how a small minority of conscious people can have 100
per cent of their body free of pain sensation. These people were born
never to experience pain; their condition gives fresh insight into why
we feel pain.

Zero pain: a mixed blessing

In 2006 a research group in Cambridge led by Professor Geoffrey
Woods and incorporating scientists from Lahore reported six individuals within three Pakistani families who had an inability from birth
to experience pain.[27] All came from the same Qureshi baradari clan
in the north of the country. An 'index case' from a fourth family had
originally drawn attention to the group, but died aged thirteen before
he could be studied thoroughly. Well known to the medical services
for several years, this unfortunate child died after jumping off a house
roof, having previously performed "street theatre", including placing
knives through his arms and walking on burning coals without expe-
riencing pain.

The six who were studied at both clinical and molecular levels were between the ages of four and twelve. None had ever shown evidence of appreciating pain. Thorough examination showed that other modalities of sensation were entirely normal: touch, pressure, warmth, cold, and the ability to sense the position of limbs without looking at them (proprioception). All the children had injuries to their lips and tongues caused by biting themselves, and there were quite a lot of other injuries apparent from bruises, cuts and healed fractures – reminders of how pain serves to protect us from harm even though we usually regard it as undesirable.

Geoffrey Woods and his team set about identifying an inherited abnormality that could account for the inability to sense pain in some members of these three families. The remarkable result of the genetic and molecular hunt was that each family had one or more members with an abnormality in the same molecule: one found in the surfaces of nerve cells and which forms a pore through which sodium atoms can move.

Signals within nerves are conducted by individual nerve cells, called neurones, which have a tubular extension (an axon) that passes all the way from where a signal is generated (such as a painful stimulus in a toe) to the point where the signal is passed on to another cell (such as in the spinal cord). Axons may be extraordinarily long: the length of some running from the foot to the lower spinal cord. In contrast to this enormous length, the diameter of a neurone is only about 1–10 micrometres (millionths of a metre). Given that a human hair is typically about 100 micrometres in breadth, we can imagine between 10 and 100 axons bundled together within the breadth of a hair.

Going down further in size we identify the molecular structures that Woods' team found to be disrupted in their patients. These can be envisaged as doughnut-shaped protein molecules with a diameter of about 0.01 micrometres, which surround a pore in the wall of the axons.[28] These molecules are known as 'sodium channels' and have been given the name $Na_v1.7$. Their pores provide a route for charged sodium atoms to move rapidly across the cell wall from outside the cell to inside the cell as an electrical signal goes past from one end of the neurone to the other. They are one of the main elements that make the passage of such signals (called action potentials) possible.

As an action potential passes along the axon the sodium channel opens, revealing a pore just big enough for sodium atoms to pass through (about 0.0001 micrometres in width, or one-hundredth of the size of the molecule itself). We now understand that when Bier administered cocaine to his patients and his assistant, the cocaine molecules blocked *all* the sodium channels in *all* the types of nerve to which they had access via the cerebrospinal fluid. Cocaine, and its later relatives such as stovaine and modern-day lidocaine and bupivacaine, indiscriminately act like temporary plugs in all types of sodium channel in all types of nerve, whether sensory or motor.

Woods and his colleagues identified abnormalities in their patients in one type of sodium channel. These were mutations that completely stopped the pore opening and therefore prevented sodium from being able to pass through. As an example of how powerful our knowledge of molecular biology has become, Woods' paper provides a good illustration. Not only were the three individual mutations identified in the sodium channel for the three families down to the smallest building blocks of the $Na_v1.7$ molecule, but artificial sodium channels with these changes were manufactured with molecular tools, like miniature faulty buttonholes, and inserted into some human kidney tumour cells, in which the electrical properties of the sodium channels could be studied and compared with normal ones; it was confirmed that they stayed shut. This is a classic example of engineering at the molecular level, which enables components of living cells to be assembled and studied in cells in which they are not normally to be found.

Two mysteries remained. The first was that the molecular abnormalities differed in the three families. One might expect that clan members from the same area in Pakistan might have inherited *identical* molecular abnormalities in the building blocks of the sodium-channel protein from an ancestor in whom a single mutation occurred. Indeed, another study of patients with congenital indifference to pain published later by Goldberg and colleagues identified ten different mutations in $Na_v1.7$ in nine families of seven different nationalities.[29] One might well expect families from different geographical locations to have acquired different mutations; why the Pakistani families had different mutations seems not to have been explained.[27]

Second, why were only pain signals affected and no other types of sensation? Up to this point it had not been suspected that pain signals in nerves could depend upon one particular type of sodium channel that other modalities of sensation appear not to use (though interestingly Goldberg and colleagues identified loss of smell in patients they reported).[29] Attempts are now under way to exploit this apparent selectivity by identifying molecules that might be used to block pain sensation by inhibiting the function of $Na_v1.7$ in the way that the mutations inhibit it.[30]

We have seen how around 1909 Thomas Jonnesco envisaged simplifying surgery by using only his version of strychno–stovaine analgesia instead of general anaesthesia. That turned out to be a pipe dream but the findings in patients with congenital insensitivity to pain open up the possibility of pain-free surgery in conscious patients by using a temporary blocker of $Na_v1.7$. That really would be an exciting and powerful development.

Caesarean section under spinal anaesthesia

To return to a previous clinical example, the possibility of being operated on while being awake raises the interesting question of whether patients are willing to be treated in that way even if they experience no pain. Most are knowledgeable about general anaesthesia and my own practice tells me that many patients are fearful of having surgery while they are conscious and express a preference to be asleep. However, the investigation of the Oxford position in preparation for a Caesarean section actually arose in part because expectations and practice for this operation were changing from general anaesthesia to spinal anaesthesia; mothers-to-be, often accompanied by a partner or relative, wanted to be awake during the delivery and able to hold their baby as soon as they were born. Furthermore, evidence was accumulating to suggest that *regional* anaesthesia (as in spinal anaesthesia) avoided some of the risks of general anaesthesia, even though it carried its own risks.

It is fascinating to see how rapidly the increase in regional anaesthesia for Caesarean section occurred worldwide. A flurry of surveys recorded this historic change. In one area of the UK between 1992 and 2002 the rate of regional anaesthesia for elective Caesarean section rose from 69 per cent to 95 per cent.[31] Even for emergency procedures, for which establishing good regional anaesthesia can take longer than a general anaesthetic, the rate increased from 49 per cent in 1992 to 87 per cent in 2002. German doctors observed similar dramatic changes: between 1996 and 2002 the use of regional anaesthesia for elective Caesarean section throughout Germany rose from 39 per cent of cases to 73 per cent.[32] Over an even shorter time period, from 2003 to 2006, a survey in Nigeria found an increase in the use of regional anaesthesia in Caesarean section from 18 per cent to 71 per cent; these data comprised around half elective and half emergency operations.[33] We have gone, therefore, from Bier concluding in 1899 that no further spinal anaesthetics in humans could be justified because of dire after-effects to an expanding use in obstetrics and other areas of surgery.

We can now return to thinking about why Bier spent nine days in bed and his colleague Hildebrand was almost as seriously debilitated after giving each other a spinal anaesthetic. We now suspect that the loss of cerebrospinal fluid through the hole in the dural membrane through which a needle has passed to inject the local anaesthetic commonly causes headache. This may be because the fluid normally provides some buoyancy to the spinal cord and the brain, and loss of fluid leads to a distortion of the anatomy inside the skull, and pain. The bigger the hole produced by the needle, the more of this fluid can drain from the dural tube, the longer it is likely to do so, and the worse and more persistent the headache seems likely to be. Bier's account draws attention to something that has become well known: "that I felt completely healthy while lying down, and that the disturbances only made themselves apparent when I made myself upright".[24] We now suspect that sitting or standing up increases the pressure in the cerebrospinal fluid and therefore increases the leakage of the fluid through the hole in the dura. We now encourage patients with this kind of headache to lie down to give the hole time to close without much flow of fluid. In some persistent cases, we can inject some of the patient's own blood around the hole in the dura to stop the leakage with a blood clot, a so-called 'blood-patch'.

This problem of headache has been diminished over the years by using finer needles for spinal injection, with tips designed to be less traumatic to the dural membrane. In 1990 Len Carrie was able to report an incidence of 'spinal headache' in obstetric patients of 3–6 per cent with a 26-gauge spinal needle. These have an outer diameter of a little less than 0.5 mm. He also used a needle with a bevel, which has a cutting action, and recommended the practice that the bevel should be in line with the long axis of the spine so as to avoid cross-cutting the tissue fibres of the dural membrane. This was thought the best way to minimise the tendency for the hole to remain patent to fluid.

A development then came along that reduced the incidence of headache still further. In 2017 Dr Xu and colleagues surveyed twenty-five well-conducted studies that compared a bevelled needle with a 'pencil-point' designed to push gently through the tissue strands of the dural membrane without cutting them at all.[34] In this kind of needle the presence of the solid point at the end prevented there being a hole in that position so a hole was placed on the side of the needle, through which the local anaesthetic was injected into the spinal canal. Analysis of the twenty-five studies showed a clear benefit to the pencil-point: the rate of spinal headache was reduced to a third. Further progress has been made with even finer needles; in 1990 Carrie reported an Oxford study of 100 patients in whom a 29-gauge needle was used.[22] This needle has a diameter of a little over 0.3 mm and no headaches occurred at all in his group. But there is a catch with these needles: they are so fine and flexible that they are difficult to insert into the patient through the strong tissues around the spine and so their success rate can be impaired. This problem has a solution, which we shall consider a little later. For the present, it will be clear to the reader that since 1899 multiple and often small steps in technical development have been able to turn spinal anaesthesia from a liability into a superb means of preparing patients for surgery.

There could be other reasons why Bier and Hildebrand got into difficulties, and one especially needs to be mentioned: they may well have suffered a degree of meningitis from the introduction of infection into the cerebrospinal fluid. They made no mention of preparing the skin for the injection (and skin harbours bacteria) and it is unclear whether attempts were made to sterilise the needles and the cocaine solution. Bare fingers were used over the end of the spinal needles to control the loss of fluid. Today, access to the cerebrospinal fluid requires the most vigorous sterile practice, usually involving 'scrubbing up', with gowns, gloves and masks – equipment that Arthur Barker advocated with enthusiasm.

August Bier and the German helmet

There is one iconic object for which the surgeon August Bier might be much better known than his spinal anaesthesia if the world at large knew about his association with either. Junior doctors questioned on this might well reply "Bier's block", the widely known method of anaesthetising a whole limb by filling its veins with local anaesthetic after making sure that the limb is isolated from the rest of the body with a tourniquet. And very useful this has proved, for example for reducing wrist fractures in patients.[35]

No, it was not Bier's block, important though it is, that I want to consider. I am thinking of something both cuboid and round, metal and leather: something designed to protect the back of the head from shrapnel blasts but also with a slight peak at the front to keep the rain from the face. Bier designed the *Stahlhelm* that we now recognise as the symbol of the German military from 1916 to 1945. It replaced that icon of Prussian militarism, the *Pickelhelm*, the leather helmet with a spike protruding from the top that seemed more likely to cause injury to its wearer than the wearer's foe. Bier's design was found to be highly effective at reducing injuries, although his initial versions were so deep that they impaired the wearer's hearing. The influence of the *Stahlhelm* on contemporary military and police headgear can be seen today; the current US Army helmet, though made of Kevlar, bears a striking resemblance and many countries use something similar. I have been known to wear a *Stahlhelm* for a few minutes when lecturing about Bier's contributions to medicine, to keep my audience attentive.

When sugar is not needed: epidural anaesthesia

Developments in anaesthesia and surgery have often come from the military, and no better example is there than that of the Spanish surgeon Fidel Pagés Miravé who in 1921 devised a valuable modification to spinal anaesthesia. Pagés qualified in medicine in Zaragoza in 1908 at the age of twenty-two, moving the same year to train in surgery at the Spanish Military Academy in Madrid. From 1909 to 1911, when Spain was at war with the Berbers in North Africa, he served treating war wounds and then attended many military medical locations in Spain, Menorca and Vienna. In 1919 he was co-founder of the Spanish surgical journal *Revista Española de Cirugia*.[36] In November 1920, while he was in Madrid conducting a spinal anaesthetic, he had an innovative idea. He decided to stop advancing his spinal needle just before it passed through the dural membrane into the cerebrospinal fluid, so that he could inject local anaesthetic outside the dura to block the nerve roots as they entered the dural tube. He realised that the volume of drug required to do this would be much larger than the 1 ml or so used for spinal injection, and made up a volume of 25 ml by dissolving some tablets of novocaine in serum. After twenty minutes he had achieved a 'band' of numbness around the lower abdomen and the outsides of the legs, and was able to repair an inguinal hernia without the least discomfort to the patient.

This, which we now call 'epidural' anaesthesia, refers to it being an injection *outside* the dural membrane into what is termed the epidural space (Fig. 28); it is a 'potential space' in that it is a region containing blood vessels and adipose tissue – loose tissues into which liquid can be injected – but it is not a space in the sense of being an empty compartment. Pagés gave his technique a name that emphasised the *segmental* nature of the band of anaesthesia around the body that resulted from the injection: *anestesia metamérica*.[37, 38] Unlike an injection into the cerebrospinal fluid of the lumbar dural tube, which can reach all the nerves passing up and down in the *cauda equina*, epidural injection bathes only those nerves close to the site of injection. In Pagés' description of his first case he noted that the perineum, scrotum and parts of the legs and feet remained unaffected, consistent with this 'segmental' blocking of nerves around part of the lower body but sparing the lowermost nerves that leave the spine via the sacrum. A translation of his Spanish account into English (albeit missing Pagés' fine diagrams) is available in the anaesthesiology literature.[39]

We now estimate needing a volume of about 2 ml of drug to fill up each vertebral segment of the epidural space. This means that Pagés' 25 ml would have extended up and down by a total of about twelve vertebral levels, i.e. from above the umbilicus down to the back of the lower limb, ideal for repair of an inguinal hernia.

Three factors seem to have inhibited wide appreciation of Pagés' epidural technique. First, he was immediately embroiled in the worsening war in the Spanish enclave of Melilla in North Africa. Second, he published his results in two Spanish journals only. Third, he tragically died in a road accident in 1923 at the age of thirty-seven. Rapid dissemination of this technique did not occur until Professor Achile Dogliotti of Turin independently described his "new" method of "segmental peridural spinal anaesthesia" in both Italian and German in 1931, and again in 1933 in the *American Journal of Surgery*, with the assistance of X-ray images to show the spread of injectate in the "dead and the living".[40] It must have come as a blow to Dogliotti's self-esteem to find out eventually that he had been beaten to the discovery by ten years, but he can take credit for disseminating epidural anaesthesia. He became a surgical celebrity, dying at the age of sixty-eight, a more satisfactory age than the unfortunate Pagés.

You might well ask where this leaves the spoonful of sugar and the Oxford position. Well, no glucose is needed for an epidural anaesthetic. The injection is made into the epidural space, a narrow compartment that surrounds the dural membrane and approximates in shape the bony spinal canal that runs through the vertebral bones (Fig. 28). This canal is distinctly triangular in section, similar in outer profile to the Swiss Toblerone chocolate bar, and so the epidural space approximates to a triangular cylinder.[40] The thickness of the epidural space in the lumbar region is variably between about 2 mm and 6 mm and gravity is still important in determining the spread of the drug, even in the epidural space.[41] Dogliotti included a sketch of a patient on his side in preparation for a lumbar epidural injection, head on pillow: "I attach great importance to the position of the patient. It is necessary that he should lie on that side on which the deeper degree of anaesthesia is desired."[40] We, the subsequent users, have learned that the degree of head-up or head-down tilt is also important in determining the spread of the analgesia.

Then there is the question of headache. The epidural needle does not puncture the dural membrane so headache is out of the question unless the needle inadvertently advances too far. Unfortunately, if it does, and since an epidural needle is thicker than a spinal needle, it often leads to a postural headache of the sort that August Bier described so well. Thicker needles are in fact usually used so that a fine plastic catheter (tube) can be passed into, and left in, the epidural space for continued use over hours or sometimes days, the needle being slid back over the catheter and discarded.

The epidural needle also leads to a further twist in the headache saga. If it successfully reaches the epidural space, it can be used as a guide for a super-thin 29-gauge spinal needle, which has a very low risk of leaving a leak and a headache. The spinal needle can then be withdrawn, an epidural catheter passed, and we achieve a combination of the two approaches.

Oxford's study of combined spinal–epidural

A combination of a spinal and an epidural anaesthetic offers the possibility of benefiting from the advantages of both. The spinal anaesthetic has a rapid onset over minutes while having a duration of only about an hour. The epidural anaesthetic has slower onset but can last for several hours, or indefinitely if a catheter is used for top-ups. The epidural needle can act as a guide for a very fine spinal needle through the tissues of the back.

Oxford in the person of Len Carrie can claim credit for the first series of forty-one cases of this 'combined spinal–epidural' in obstetric anaesthesia for Caesarean section back in 1984.[42] He used the then relatively new drug bupivacaine. It is interesting to see how that study of 1984 was a step in the evolution of Carrie's thinking. It was a study without glucose and without his Oxford position, and all did not go smoothly: "unpredictably extensive spread of analgesia" occurred and there was a "high incidence of hypotension". When more attention to the sugar and the position was given, the results improved. My Oxford colleagues have continued trying to perfect this 'combined spinal–epidural' anaesthesia for Caesarean section, with and without the Oxford position.[43]

Back to Bangalore

This is not the place to discuss all the twists and turns, refinements and controversies, that have been generated by the types of regional anaesthesia of the spine that I have visited in this chapter. The literature on spinal and epidural anaesthesia for Caesarean section (let alone normal childbirth) is vast, and always fascinating. We have seen that Jonnesco's advocacy of surgery in the head, neck and chest under his strychno–stovaine anaesthesia was over-ambitious and frankly dangerous because of the risk of damage to the spinal cord or death from asphyxia.

What may come as a surprise to some readers (including anaesthetists) is that a hundred years after Jonnesco's *British Medical Journal* paper of 1909 a fresh bout of enthusiasm has appeared for performing surgery using 'thoracic spinal anaesthesia' despite the risks associated with passing a needle into the cerebrospinal fluid close to the spinal cord in the chest area. Much of the enthusiasm emanates from a centre in Brazil though several doctors armed with modern imaging techniques to help guide their needles are reporting a variety of operations in the chest and abdomen conducted in this way.[44]

It is time for me to draw a halt by returning to brave Mr Swaroup Anand with whom we started: having open-heart surgery while lying awake in Bangalore with his life supported by a heart–lung machine next to the operating couch. It was Fidel Pagés' discovery that made Swaroup's operation possible. A needle that is not advanced far enough to cross the dural membrane into the cerebrospinal fluid is a needle that cannot damage the spinal cord. If judiciously inserted into the epidural space high in the thoracic vertebrae, it is possible, with attention to dose and posture, for the anaesthesia to go high enough to catch nerves to the area around the heart. With such a 'thoracic epidural' the heart can be operated on in conscious patients without excessively compromising breathing.

The first published experience of awake heart surgery under epidural anaesthesia from Bangalore was a study in 2003 of fifteen patients having 'off-pump' heart surgery, i.e. not requiring a heart–lung machine.[45] These operations were repairs to the arteries on the outside of the wall of the heart that supply the heart itself with blood. The heart can be left beating as this type of operation is performed. In 2005 came a report from Bangalore of eleven patients having 'on-pump' heart surgery in which the heart is stopped, for repair of a hole in the heart or replacement of a valve.[46] You may ask at what position the epidural needle is inserted for this sort of operation. The answer is just where Jonnesco advocated his high spinal analgesia (or the vertebra one level *above* that). There is a slight irony here about the risks of stopping breathing. In ten of the eleven patients reported by the Bangalore team, breathing spontaneously stopped when the heart–lung machine was being used ('on-pump'): of course, the patient doesn't need to breathe if the bypass machine is doing their breathing for them, as we have seen in Chapter One. Had Jonnesco known about this possibility he might have advocated even wilder things, with or without a spoonful of sugar.

Chapter Six

GASES, VAPOURS AND INJECTIONS

Anaesthesia's Ingenious World

Three visits to the dentist

Pulling teeth has long been an opportunity to test whether pain can be abolished. In 1844 Horace Wells, a dentist in Connecticut, in his bid to eliminate pain delivered nitrous oxide gas contained in an animal bladder via a wooden tube. He was systematic in his approach; he first had the gas administered to himself by a chemist colleague for a dental extraction "which was one without any painful sensations". The trial was then extended to his patients: "I then performed the same operation for twelve or fifteen others, with the like results."[1]

Wells had come to the idea of using nitrous oxide by linking two observations. First, its inhalation had a reputation for producing 'nervous excitement'; many know it as 'laughing gas'. Second, "that an individual, when much excited from ordinary causes, may receive severe wounds without manifesting the least pain". He liked to imagine the possibility of losing a limb in combat with no pain "at the time", and that similar insensitivity to pain could result from the excitement of "passion" and being "intoxicated by liquor". He convinced himself that his method worked "with one or two exceptions". Unfortunately for history, one of these exceptions occurred when Wells demonstrated his technique in a hospital setting in January 1845. This account is my first of three notable visits to the dentist.

Wells' event, a demonstration to students of the use of nitrous oxide in a patient undergoing an amputation, was arranged at Harvard Medical School by surgeon John Collins Warren. This plan had to change when the patient refused to go through with the operation. Wells lectured to the class and asked whether any of the students needed a tooth extraction; one volunteered. Also present was dentist

William Morton, later to achieve fame for using ether by inhalation in a surgical operation. It appears to have been an evening with a large attendance and one senses that the students may have been in a flippant mood, perhaps stoked by having inhaled nitrous oxide themselves. However, the operation did not go according to plan. The account by medical student Antony Taft goes as follows:

> Dr. Wells was introduced to our class by Dr. John C. Warren, then Professor of Anatomy at the University. Dr. Wells then made a statement of his discovery, spoke of its importance, and his hopes of introducing it, the anaesthetic agent, into general use in surgical operations. On the same or the following evening, Dr. Wells proceeded to administer the nitrous oxyd gas to several of the students and spectators present. At this time Dr. Wells extracted a tooth for some one under the influence of the gas. The patient holloed somewhat during the operation, but, on his return to consciousness, said he felt no pain whatever.[2]

The extent to which the patient suffered pain is unclear. Wells himself wrote: "Unfortunately for the experiment, the gas bag was by mistake withdrawn much too soon, and he was but partially under its influence when the tooth was extracted. He testified that he experienced some pain, but not as much as usually attends the operation."[3] Spectators were said to have "laughed and hissed" and "several expressed their opinion that it was a humbug affair".[3, 4] Wells headed for home the next morning a dejected man and suffered a breakdown, which ended his professional career.

My second and third notable visits to the dentist are also distressing. We move on to the year 1897. The patient in this case was Oxford cycle and motor mechanic William Morris, then around twenty years of age. His teeth had been neglected and toothache forced him to the dentist, who administered nitrous oxide and proceeded to carry out multiple extractions on two occasions.[5] Morris found the experiences terrifying and described them as nightmares of prolonged suffocation. He retained a vivid memory of these two visits to the dentist throughout the rest of his life.

Baron Nuffield and the golf club

Step forward to the 1930s. Morris was by then a wealthy manufacturer of motor vehicles and also an enthusiastic golfer at the club at Huntercombe near Oxford, where he and Mrs Morris made their home (and also bought the club). Here at weekends he came into contact with visiting staff from Guy's Hospital in London. One of these was Robert Macintosh, from whom we have a personal account of having administered to Morris a general anaesthetic for a "small operation" in London, of which he recounted: "I am not being immodest when I say that this had an inordinate affect (*sic*) on the patient."[5] Macintosh had at his disposal a new anaesthetic in the form of a barbiturate, which could be administered intravenously, avoiding the suffocating experience of his patient having to breathe from a facemask. Morris awoke from the anaesthetic, "looked at his watch and enquired why the operation had been postponed"! Henceforth, conversation at the golf club acquired a new topic. "Later, at Huntercombe, he frequently referred to what he described as the magic of this experience."

Changing anaesthesia from inhalation via a mask to injection via a needle might not have had much effect on the development of the field were it not for the fact that William Morris became one of the most generous benefactors to medicine and was personally dogmatic about its priorities. In the summer of 1936 Morris, who had become Baron Nuffield two years earlier, was engaged in dinner conversation at the Huntercombe club. Talk turned to a request from the University of Oxford for money; at the meeting of the British Medical Association in Oxford a few days previously the Regius Professor of Medicine, Sir Farquhar Buzzard, had advocated the establishment of a postgraduate medical school. He followed this up with an appeal to Nuffield for a million pounds to support professorships in medicine, surgery and obstetrics. Over the dinner Macintosh remarked, "I see they have forgotten anaesthetics again," a comment that seeded itself with Nuffield.[5]

The pomposity of the university is amusingly revealed by the course of events over the next few weeks. Nuffield announced himself favourably disposed to fund a postgraduate medical school and increased the sum offered to include a fourth professorship, the first in anaesthetics in the UK. Support for a speciality with such a lowly status caused embarrassment in the upper echelons of the university and Buzzard informed Nuffield that acceptance of his offer of

a chair in anaesthesia would "expose both the University and Nuffield to ridicule". It took a couple of weeks for the Regius Professor
to realise that Nuffield's offer was an all-or-none proposal, that a
lower-grade employee in anaesthesia was not acceptable to the ben-
efactor, and that Nuffield wanted Macintosh to be the first professor
in the field. The Nuffield Chair of Anaesthetics was finalised before
the final generous donation of £2 million was announced publicly.
Historian Jennifer Beinart summarised the events as the "bitter pill
had been swallowed before the sugar coating was added".[6]

As we shall see, the poorly planned and executed attempt to
relieve the pain of dental extraction at Harvard in 1845 only set back
inhalational anaesthesia by a year or so, though it did lead to personal
tragic outcomes for both Wells and Morton, whose claims to be orig-
inators were not recognised in their lifetimes. By way of contrast,
we should be grateful for the distress experienced by William Morris
while visiting the dentist. Without his experiences in the dentist's
chair we might never have had the establishment of anaesthesia as
an academic discipline deserving of efforts to improve its accepta-
bility and safety. The Nuffield Department of Anaesthetics was to
make major contributions to anaesthesia, both in equipment and
techniques.

This was the department in which I was privileged to begin my
anaesthetic training as a senior house officer in 1984. I was required to
train full time for three months before availing myself of two years
of part-time work in the scheme of Rosemary Rue, which I describe
in Chapter Eight. A similar pattern of some full-time work and then
two years of part-time work followed when I was appointed a registrar in 1986, my formal years of training as a 'junior doctor' being
complete in 1989.

In this chapter I hope to engage the reader in some of the excitement of the evolution and practice of anaesthesia. One theme will
trace the rivalries between different agents (we may call them 'drugs'
in the widest sense), be they gases, vapours, or liquids for injection.
Another theme will be the gadgetry involved in delivering these
agents. It is striking how seemingly modest modifications to masks,
tubes and needles have made great strides in the ease and safety with
which patients can be anaesthetised. A third theme will be the very
recent pressure the profession is coming under to stop it contribut-
ing to global climate problems. First though we must return to the

1840s to look at the early rivalry between nitrous oxide gas and ether vapour.

Rivals: nitrous oxide gas and ether vapour

Today it is difficult to imagine that an operation such as amputation of a leg or excision of a bladder stone once had to be accompanied by appalling agony, as was the case up to the 1840s. From about 1842 a jumble of accounts exists of success using nitrous oxide or ether in patients undergoing dental surgery or relatively minor operations. We have seen Horace Wells' advocacy of nitrous oxide. The trigger that most effectively sparked the international use of inhalational anaesthesia was a demonstration in Boston on 16 October 1846 by Wells' former pupil William Morton of the use of ether in a man having a tumour excised from his neck. The wrangling that followed these events for recognition of priority and possible financial gain is not a topic for this chapter but it is notable that Wells took his own life at the age of thirty-three and Morton died at forty-eight, a 'disappointed man' and still in debt.[7]

However, the use of ether took off rapidly after Morton's demonstration in Boston. Morton's technique was to soak a sponge with liquid ether in a glass globe with a wooden mouthpiece on one side and a hole open to the air on the other. It took a few minutes of breathing through this 'vaporiser' for the patient to reach a sufficient state of 'etherisation' to tolerate incision in the skin. Interestingly, of all the anaesthetic vapours that have appeared since the 1840s, ether is from two points of view the most unsuitable for getting from the bottle to the patient's brain, where it has its action. First, vaporising it from its liquid state requires so much heat that as it vaporises it tends to freeze the apparatus from which it is being delivered. Second, it is so highly soluble in blood and body tissues that it takes a very long time to get from the lungs to the brain.

To understand these problems better, it may be helpful to take a moment to consider two points. The first is the difference between a *gas* and a *vapour*. Ether arrives in the hospital as a liquid in a bottle. It remains a stable liquid under normal atmospheric conditions of pressure and temperature. If allowed to take in heat from its surroundings, however, the liquid slowly evaporates to give off ether vapour. It is in the form of vapour that it is inhaled for its anaesthetic effect. So much heat is needed to convert the liquid ether to its vapour that it tends to freeze nearby equipment. By way of contrast, nitrous oxide cannot form a liquid in normal environmental conditions of pressure and temperature, so we call it a gas. It can be converted to a liquid form either by cooling it down to about minus 90°C or by restraining it in a metal cylinder under a pressure equivalent to about 140 times atmospheric pressure. The distinction between gas and vapour is thus simply a matter of the form in which the anaesthetic agent exists at normal environmental conditions of room temperature and pressure.

The second point of note is how we measure the *potency* of an anaesthetic gas or vapour. This is done by noting the average percentage of atmospheric pressure that needs to be occupied by the agent in the lungs (and consequently in the brain) of a patient to allow them to tolerate a skin incision. I shall define more carefully what we mean by 'tolerate' later in this chapter. For ether, the anaesthetic dose is about 2 per cent – that is, if 2 per cent of the gas in the lungs (which normally consists of about 75 per cent nitrogen, 15 per cent oxygen, 5 per cent carbon dioxide and 5 per cent water vapour) is ether vapour, then the patient is likely to be adequately anaesthetised for surgery.

But there is a big qualification to be made about the last point, and this is that it may take a *very long time* for the level of ether in the brain (strictly its 'pressure' in the brain) to become the same as the level in the lungs. If the anaesthetist were to give the patient 2 per cent ether vapour to breathe, it would take hours for this anaesthetic level to be reached in the brain. This is because the blood and body tissues act as a thirsty reservoir for the ether as it makes its way from the lungs to the brain, i.e. the ether goes into solution in the blood and tissues. The way out of this is to give about 20 per cent in the inspired gas to 'overpressure' the blood with enough ether to bring the brain to the required level within a few minutes. After that, the inspired concentration needs to be eased back to prevent the hazards of excess.[8, 9] In this sense we can think of ether as the *slowest* of anaesthetics.

Nitrous oxide has neither of these two disadvantages but it took a lot longer to become established. It was produced as a gas and initially carried in bags. This obviated the problem with ether of converting liquid into vapour. In contrast to ether, nitrous oxide turned out to be the *fastest* inhalational anaesthetic. This is because it is so *insoluble* in blood and body tissues that the brain quickly reaches the level of gas in the lungs. Whereas with ether it might take hours for the brain to catch up with the lungs, nitrous oxide needs only about ten minutes.[8] However, there is a drawback, and that relates to the potency of nitrous oxide. In contrast to ether's anaesthetic level in the brain of 2 per cent, the anaesthetic level for nitrous oxide in the brain is about 100 per cent. This means that giving enough nitrous oxide to induce anaesthesia excludes all the oxygen and the patient will die if without oxygen for a few minutes.

Joseph Clover exploited the advantages of nitrous oxide in the face of its hazards, and advocated its use at a meeting of the British Medical Association in Oxford in August 1868.[10] Bags, tubing and mask, all made from 'India-rubber', with stopcocks and a valve were assembled for the reliable inhalation of the gas. In a summary of experience published six years later Clover gives us the flavour of the applicability of nitrous oxide:

> I had the pleasure of showing the use of it at the Oxford meeting. Since that time, I have given it in 6,960 cases ... It is by far the best anaesthetic for many short operations, such as the extraction of teeth, opening abscesses or boils ... It is well suited for examining hysterical cases, wrenching stiff joints, and reducing luxations of recent date ... I do not think it suitable for cases where it is necessary to keep the patient quiet more than three or four minutes ... I have never kept a patient unconscious for more than between six and seven minutes.[11]

In 1846 Clover had been a student at University College, London, and recounted seeing "Liston perform the first capital operation under ether that was done in this country"; this was an amputation through the thigh on 21 December 1846.[11] Clover's early preoccupation was with urological surgery and we do not know precisely what motivated his transition to anaesthesia but one speculation is that the unexpected and early death of the famous anaesthetist-cum-epidemiologist John Snow in 1858 increased demand for Clover's expertise.[12] Despite success with nearly 2,000 cases of other anaesthetics by 1868, Clover became attracted by the effectiveness and safety of nitrous oxide when delivered by his personalised gadgetry.

Oxford's first surgery with anaesthesia

We have noted that Clover witnessed the first arrival from the United States of ether anaesthesia in London in December 1846. As a resident of Oxford, I naturally wanted to know how long it took ether to make the journey from London to Oxford. I was delighted to discover that the anaesthetist who first interested me in taking up the profession, Dr Mike Ward, had explored the hospital archives to answer this question.

Anaesthesia with ether took two months to cross the Atlantic from Boston to London but little more than another two months to make its way to Oxford. An entry for 4 March 1847 in the register of operations at the Radcliffe Infirmary tells of a patient who experienced major surgery with and without anaesthesia:

> Case 117 Charlotte Launton of Yarnton; at 16, this girl was admitted under Mr Parker in February 1845 with necrosis of the right tibia ... A large part of the shaft of the tibia was removed, without anaesthesia ... the girl remained in the Infirmary for 19 months. On 10th February 1847 she returned and the leg was removed above the knee without anaesthesia ... On 4th March the operation was the Double Flap & ether was used with complete success ... Discharged June 16th 1847.[13]

Further examination of the register reveals an interesting transition occurring within months. Twelve operations used anaesthesia within its first twenty months of use but only four of those involved ether. The other eight involved a rival, chloroform, which was first used in Oxford on 24 April 1848. It was chloroform that was most acutely to raise concerns about anaesthesia-related deaths.

Anaesthesia-related deaths

A few years into my career as an anaesthetist in Oxford I reported a case of cardiac arrest associated with a then relatively new anaesthetic drug given by injection, propofol.[14] A healthy twenty-five-year-old male was scheduled for reduction of a fractured nose. During the intravenous injection of propofol the patient's pupils dilated, he went white, and the electrocardiograph (ECG) monitor confirmed that his heart had stopped. He was resuscitated and lived but his surgery was postponed. A decade later, a review of many trials and reports found that the heart stopped in one in 660 propofol anaesthetics but that the risk of death from these cardiac arrests was very low at 1.4 in 100,000 cases.[15] The authors of this review estimated that these deaths constituted approximately one-fifth of all anaesthesia-related deaths. Propofol has gone on to establish itself as the most popular anaesthetic in modern practice.

Joseph Clover had a succinct summary on this subject: "The fact that death may be produced, if signs of danger are disregarded, applies to all anaesthetics."[16] His emphasis on observing signs in his patients is seen in a famous image of Clover demonstrating how to administer chloroform with an early version of his apparatus in 1862 (Fig. 31). He is shown posing with his father as a substitute patient, one hand holding the mask and the other hand feeling the pulse. When I started administering anaesthetics in 1984, ECG monitors were not always available where anaesthesia was induced; a finger on the pulse was as important then as in Clover's experience.

Chloroform was introduced into clinical practice in 1847 in Edinburgh where obstetrician James Simpson popularised its use for pain relief during childbirth. It becomes our focus as we think about early deaths from anaesthesia. Chloroform liquid yields a pungent vapour, which produces anaesthesia at a level in the brain of 0.5 per cent and has a solubility in the blood that makes transmission from lungs to brain faster than for ether. Part of its attraction was that it was more appealing to patients than ether because it put them to sleep faster. As the evidence from the Oxford register of 1847 suggests, within months it rivalled ether as an anaesthetic. Added to its favourable properties are unfortunately some that rendered it too frequently lethal; the most immediate of these was that it could stop the heart suddenly, within minutes of first being inhaled.

There is a parallel here with my report of propofol stopping the heart during injection in a healthy young man, for it was found that chloroform could produce sudden cardiac arrest in the early stages of administration. The first report was that of a fifteen-year-old girl, Hannah Greener, scheduled for removal of a toenail on 28 January 1848. It is a sad irony that she had successfully undergone an anaesthetic with ether several months before the fatal chloroform. The coroner investigated, his account including "a struggle or jerk" as the operation was started, attributed to "the chloroform not having taken sufficient effect", and that "the time would not have been more than 3 min from her first inhaling the chloroform till her death".[17]

It is interesting to note that two reports of fatalities attributed to ether anaesthesia preceded the death of Hannah Greener. The first was from Colchester in February 1847 in a fifty-two-year-old man having a bladder stone removed by surgeon Roger Nunn.[18] The account of his death two days after surgery suggests to us now that it was unrelated to ether but it illustrates the belief among surgeons that the pain and stress of surgery (without anaesthesia) helped the patient to survive surgery. Nunn wrote:

> Pain is doubtless our great safeguard under ordinary circum-stances; but for it we should be hourly falling into danger; and I am inclined to believe that pain should be considered as a healthy indication, and an *essential* concomitant with surgical operations, and that it is amply compensated by the effects it produces on the system as the natural incentive to reparative action.

The second claim of an early death attributable to ether came from Grantham. The patient was described as "a respectable woman of the name of Anne Parkinson aged twenty-one years" and her problem was a tumour growing on the back of her thigh.[19] Her death was also two days after surgery and would similarly now not be associated with the ether she received, but her story contains a little detail that I find both touching and amusing. Mrs Parkinson seemed determined to have the tumour removed whether or not ether was administered. Her surgeon, Mr Robbs, had been asked "what he thought of the application of ether, and he said he had no faith in it". Apparently for the assurance of both patient and surgeon two trial anaesthetics were administered three days and one day before the operation itself, so that the 'fatal' anaesthetic for the surgery itself was the third. At the inquest Mr Robbs announced that he "had no doubt whatever that the ether alone was the cause of death, and it was a duty he owed to the public to say so", though his opinion is now difficult to support.[19]

The sudden death of patients in the early stages of inhalation of chloroform became widespread partly because chloroform was favourably regarded and easier to use than ether or nitrous oxide. The mode of these deaths from anaesthesia was hotly debated for seventy years. Suggestions for the mode of death included cessation of breathing, aspiration of stomach contents (or of the brandy used in attempts to revive the patient), and "cardiac paralysis", these possibilities variously being regarded as attributable either to "overdosage" or the patient being too "light".[17] It was work by Goodman Levy presented at the Royal Society of Medicine in 1914 which seems finally to have established the cause of "sudden death under light chloroform anaesthesia".[20] Combining experiments on cats with observations on patients, Levy concluded that the combination of adrenaline and chloroform in the blood triggered fibrillation in the ventricles of the heart. Fibrillation is a fast, chaotic uncoordinated contraction of areas of heart muscle, which renders the heart ineffective as a pump. It rapidly leads to the death of the patient. The adrenaline was important because even on its own it is elevated in the blood in moments of fear and strongly stimulates the heart. The fatal events in patients were indeed commonly associated with a state of anxiety in the early stages of receiving a high dose of chloroform to try to settle them.

Chloroform finally fell from favour in the interwar years after decades of being the most common anaesthetic. Hans Killian, a leading figure in German anaesthesia, in his textbook of 1934 reported statistics of deaths, where he estimated that fatal complications of ether occurred in about 1:15,000 cases, whereas with chloroform the chances were 1:2670 when it was delivered in a similar manner.[21] His figure for nitrous oxide deaths was in the range 1:40,000–1:50,000. We noted earlier an incidence of death for propofol that is more favourable than all these.

It is interesting to make a comparison of the way these drugs stop the heart. The gases and vapours tend to produce the chaotic electrical activity of fibrillation, whereas propofol tends to produce a sudden ceasing of electrical activity, which we call 'asystole'. An important feature of ventricular fibrillation is that it rarely spontaneously reverts to a normal rhythm or responds to medication. In modern practice an electrical shock is the most effective means to 'defibrillate' the heart. This was not known or available in the peak years of chloroform usage. Had electrical defibrillators been available, along with monitoring, which could confirm a diagnosis of fibrillation in the first place, it may be that chloroform could have lasted longer.

In contrast to fibrillation, asystole is more commonly spontaneously followed by a normal rhythm. Indeed, the common faint is a brief period of asystole and from this we are aware that a cessation of electrical activity is often temporary. This is likely to explain why death from propofol anaesthesia is much less frequent than cardiac arrest.

From hasty to prolonged anaesthetics

Prolonged and intricate surgeries were not possible in patients writhing in terrible pain in the pre-anaesthetic era. Even after the introduction of anaesthesia, keeping surgery brief remained advisable. I have already noted Clover's comment about nitrous oxide only being suitable for operations lasting three or four minutes. In the case of nitrous oxide, the practice was to administer it as a pure gas despite risking asphyxia from absence of oxygen. Indeed, for some time it remained unclear whether it was nitrous oxide itself that rendered patients comatose or the lack of oxygen getting to the brain. Edmund Andrews, Professor of Surgery in Chicago, explained the need for hasty anaesthesia with nitrous oxide in his paper of 1868: "If any attempt is made to continue its action, the patient becomes purple in the face, showing all the signs of asphyxia; *subsultus tendinum* [twitching of tendons] then supervenes, and shortly after he almost ceases to breathe, and, if allowed nothing but pure nitrous oxide, would doubtless die in a few minutes."[22]

Andrews advocated using a mixture of 80 per cent nitrous oxide and 20 per cent oxygen to "enable us to anaesthetize a patient for the longest as well as for the shortest surgical operations" but long operations raised the problem of the mixture's "great bulk". He noted that a "gasometer" could be used in hospitals, but home visits would require him to carry a "large rubber bag". This was for his wealthy recipients. "In city practice, among the higher classes … the bag can always be taken in a carriage, without attracting observation."[22]

As we have noted earlier, another problem with reducing the dose of nitrous oxide (so as to include oxygen in the mixture) is that the average anaesthetic level for nitrous oxide of around 100 per cent would not be reached. The need to keep the dose high, combined with the fact that dental extractions are commonly speedy procedures, helps to explain persistence into the modern era of the use of 100 per cent nitrous oxide in dental anaesthesia.[23] Indeed, I have a haunting memory of a black mask in a childhood visit to the dentist where I am likely to have received the asphyxic gas. But this eventually had to end; following a small number of newsworthy deaths in children, dentists in the UK were no longer permitted to administer general anaesthesia in their surgeries after 2001.[24] This step represented professionalisation of anaesthesia in the UK to a practice largely led by physicians with training in anaesthesia.

The duration of surgery under ether or chloroform was not limited in the same way as with nitrous oxide, as long as the patient's access to air, and ventilation of the lungs with that air, was maintained. We have seen that ether and chloroform are delivered as liquids and require conversion to vapour before they can be inhaled. Their administered concentrations in air, up to about 20 per cent for ether and 4 per cent for chloroform, only minimally reduce the concentration of oxygen from the normal value of about 21 per cent in dry room air. A challenge with both these agents was getting the patient calmly off to sleep given the vapours' slow uptake and pungent characteristics. They tend to induce coughing, salivation and a phase of irrational excitement. Joseph Clover had found his own solution to this challenge during induction of anaesthesia. "The most pleasant way is to give nitrous oxide till consciousness is lost, and then administer the ether of moderate strength."[11] By 1876 he was able to describe apparatus combining a pressurised cylinder of nitrous oxide (no more bulky bags in carriages) with an ether vaporiser for "administering nitrous oxide gas and ether, singly or combined".[16]

Two things became necessary for the safe prolongation of surgery and anaesthesia. First was astute observation and monitoring of the patient; the finger on the pulse was at least a start. The second was equipment that could provide a steady-state supply of a measured concentration of anaesthetic gas or vapour, together with oxygen to maintain life. Andrews' proposal of a gas–oxygen mixture carried in bags and Clover's apparatus for adding ether to nitrous oxide were approaches that laid the groundwork for the conduct of anaesthesia well into the twentieth century and also into my own career as an anaesthetist: a judicious mix of oxygen with nitrous oxide and an anaesthetic vapour has been widely used for *maintaining* anaesthesia during prolonged surgery. What changed in the 1930s was the way most patients were initially 'put off to sleep': intravenous drugs became the routine way to *induce* anaesthesia in the manner that Lord Nuffield found so agreeable.

Another cause of death: the hearty meal

In considering the risk of death under anaesthesia we have so far thought of cardiac arrest and the hazard of 100 per cent nitrous oxide. I now turn to the need to maintain the pathway for breathing. Uptake of oxygen and anaesthetics by the lungs requires a clear airway all the way from the mouth or nose down to the lung alveoli. Figure 32 depicts the upper airway and shows how the pharynx is a site where the normal pathway for food and drink is in competition with the inhalation of air. Food is a potential obstruction and the most likely place it can come from in the patient undergoing anaesthesia is the stomach.

John Snow kept detailed notes of some 4,000 anaesthetics delivered by him in the ten years up to his death in 1858. On 18 November 1848 he administered chloroform to "Mrs Evans ... a lady about 50, whilst Mr. Ashton Key applied actual cautery to the *os uteri* for malignant excrescence".[25] Problems with food soon set in:

> The patient had eaten a hearty dinner 2 hours before which, by the result, did not seem at all digested. She began to vomit before she was insensible, and the inhalation was left off for a short time and then resumed, and she vomited again two or three times during the preparatory examination with specula and hooks and during the operation, to which she was totally insensible. On recovering her consciousness, however, she did not feel any sickness.

Many of Snow's entries include related comments: "no sickness"; "vomiting"; "vomiting of a copious meal taken half an hour before". None of these patients had their pharynx blocked but today's anaesthetist would be horrified at the thought of conducting hundreds of procedures in patients in whom little or no effort was made to ensure an empty stomach because of the risk to the patient's life from the remnants of regurgitated food obstructing the airway.

Anaesthesia not only obtunds the normal responses to pain but also reduces or eliminates the protective reflex of coughing, which helps to clear the airway if obstructed. If Mrs Evans was "totally insensible" to the hooks in her vagina, she is likely to have lost her ability to protect her airway. It is remarkable that Snow experienced only three deaths associated with anaesthesia during his ten years of records. Interestingly, the account of one of these deaths, in a thirty-three-year-old "healthy-looking, well made man" on 7 April 1857, records that "he had drunk a pint of bottled ale a quarter of an hour before operation" but at post-mortem the "stomach contained only mucus".[25] There is the possibility that the ale found its way into the lungs and that in effect he drowned.

This death was only one week before Snow "administered chloroform to her Majesty the Queen in her ninth confinement", Prince Albert having administered chloroform "on a handkerchief" before Snow arrived! It is pleasing to read that "the Queen's recovery was very favourable". Two of Snow's three fatalities were actually associated with administration of the vapour amylene, including the one shortly before he attended Queen Victoria. The second was in July 1857. These events seem to have contributed to amylene being abandoned.[26] Ellis cites correspondence suggesting of Snow that "these deaths affected him very seriously, and his sudden and early demise may, in some measure, be attributed to their effects on him".[25]

Clover's opinion by 1876 was that "with respect to vomiting, I think it most important that the patient should have an empty stomach, and prefer that neither food nor drink of any kind should be taken for from four to six hours beforehand. I see least sickness after operations done before breakfast."[16]. This did not preclude the benefits of a little pre-medication to relax the patient. "I like to give a teaspoonful of brandy, without water, a few minutes beforehand … If wine be given, or if the patient must have some water with the brandy, then they should be given half-an-hour before inhaling, to allow time for their absorption."[11]

In 1946 a study from the United States became a classic on the topic of food getting into the airways and the name of the author led to the use of the term 'Mendelson syndrome'.[27] It reported sixty-six cases of aspiration of stomach contents into the lungs out of 44,016 patients having anaesthesia with a mixture of both nitrous oxide and ether for delivery of babies. Of these sixty-six patients, six were found to have breathed in large lumps of food and two of these patients died as a consequence. A point of particular note is that the two patients who died had been starved for six and eight hours from eating a full meal to the time of surgery; even Clover's four to six hours would not have prevented these fatalities. The syndrome name itself became attached to the damage to the lungs that develops after surgery when acid from the stomach is aspirated into the lungs, even if solid food is not involved. In 1956 a study from the UK in a general surgical population found that 110 (18 per cent) of 598 anaesthesia-related deaths were associated with either regurgitation of food or vomiting.[28]

It is unfortunate that for decades the practice of starvation before surgery swung to an extreme that served no useful purpose. A practice of 'nil by mouth after midnight' became the default for patients having surgery at any time of the following day and was widely applied as rigorously to liquid as to solid food. For many patients the misery of prolonged denial of food and drink may be worse than the operation itself. Surveys have repeatedly shown that patients have been starved for far too long, commonly over twice the recommended length of time for both food (six hours) and drink (two hours).[29] We have seen that even an eight-hour fast following a meal cannot ensure an empty stomach,[27] and it is clear that no patient is protected from the risk of aspiration of stomach contents, however long they are starved.[29] Conversely, the healthy stomach can fully absorb into the blood 500 ml of water within about thirty minutes.[30] Perhaps most encouragingly for UK patients, many of whom are wedded to a cup of tea first thing in the morning, is the finding that, whether or not tea contains milk (which is often denied to patients), a cup of tea is absorbed from the stomach in about thirty minutes.[31] As the years grew busier, in my own hospital I found myself increasingly making tea for patients as part of my pre-operative visit. Nobody else seemed to have the time or job description to do so.

A study from Berlin illustrates well how hard-wired into the hospital culture long starvation times can be. In 2018 anaesthetists at the Charité hospital set about trying to introduce a practice for most surgical patients of encouraging them to drink water, tea or coffee (with some milk) *up to the moment they were transported from the ward to the operating theatre.*[32] Initial efforts failed to reduce average fasting time for drinks below eleven hours. A renewed effort in 2021 involved a 'fasting card' for each patient plus further staff education. Over four weeks of trying hard the fasting time was progressively reduced, but only to about six hours. A third cycle of innovation, involving a blast of posters in the wards, lectures to the ward staff, and revision of flyers and webpages, finally led over four months to a mean fasting time of around three hours. I sense that the challenge of achieving better fasting times for surgical patients illustrates wider problems in reforming health care in large and complex organisations.

From handkerchief to vaporiser

I have noted the need to turn liquid anaesthetic to vapour. The gadgetry needed to achieve this has occupied many for over a century and a half. One cannot minimise the equipment to less than a handkerchief. For his obstetric administration James Simpson used a folded handkerchief over the patient's face, judiciously supplied with drops of chloroform. Over decades various wire frames were devised to support a cloth or gauze for this type of 'open-drop' administration, the most famous of which is the Schimmelbusch mask. Earlier wire masks tended to travel with the gauze from one patient to another and in his 1893 textbook on aseptic wound care, Berlin surgeon Curt Schimmelbusch was particularly concerned that gauze held over a patient's face should not be a route of transmission for bacterial diseases such as erysipelas or diphtheria. Schimmelbusch's metal mask provided a clip for easily mounting fresh gauze each time the mask was used, the metal being sterilised between cases.[33] A modification (dating from 1904) by New York surgeon Sidney Yankauer is shown in Figure 33.[34] The extensive wire mesh provided good support to the gauze and, together with a trough around the mask, helped to prevent liquid anaesthetic from getting onto the patient's skin or into the eyes.

My student introduction to ether anaesthesia came in 1982 when I travelled to India to gain experience as a medical student. In St Luke's Hospital in Hiranpur I watched the hospital porter use one of these masks to administer open-drop ether while I assisted Dr Bryan Thomson to operate. These masks continued to be used widely in the 1950s and still find use in developing countries.

In 1934 in his assessment of the risk of fatality with different agents, Killian formed the opinion that open-drop ether carried twice the risk (~1:15,000) compared with techniques using *"Dosierung mit Apparaten"* or some kind of measured vaporiser.[21] His figure for the risk of fatality with chloroform of 1:2,670 was for the open-drop method. The question of why chloroform remained the most popular anaesthetic for so long, despite accumulating evidence for its tendency to put the heart into fibrillation, has been a topic of intense historical interest.[35] Several factors have been identified. First, given that the mortality from early surgery was so high, the relatively low mortality attributable solely to the anaesthetic tended to be hidden. In the mid nineteenth century, mortality in UK hospitals from amputation stood around 40 per cent with or without chloroform anaesthesia.[35] Second, induction of anaesthesia tended to be faster and smoother with chloroform than ether for reasons I have already noted.

A third reason for continued use of chloroform has a uniquely Oxford connection. Because it was less flammable than ether its use was advocated in the Second World War by airborne regiments, transport of flammable liquids and pressurised nitrous-oxide cylinders by aircraft being avoided. The founding of the Nuffield Department of Anaesthetics under Robert Macintosh's leadership in 1937 was timely in leading to development of equipment that supported the war effort, one aspect of which was devising reliable and accurate anaesthetic inhalers. A special design was that of the Epstein–Suffolk–Oxford (ESO) chloroform inhaler of 1942 (Fig. 34). It had to be relatively lightweight and robust enough to withstand a heavy landing. The first twenty ESO inhalers were ready a week before D-Day in June 1944 and many more were subsequently supplied. The chloroform concentration (right-hand dial, Fig. 34) could be set up to 4 per cent and the temperature (left-hand dial) compensated for.[36] The predecessor in my university post, Dr Dan Cunningham, will have been familiar with this unique device; he parachuted into France on the morning of D-Day as a member of the Royal Army Medical Corps and spent many weeks attending to casualties.

The combination of ingenious equipment design and the production facilities of Nuffield's factories led to much wartime production in Oxford. An 'Oxford vaporiser' for ether, based upon Macintosh's experiences during the Spanish Civil War in 1937, became available in 1941, some 2,000 being rapidly manufactured and distributed throughout the world. Macintosh described them as "foolproof" and explained that "during some of the worst fighting in North Africa and in Europe, anaesthetists working single-handed were able to supervise four operating-tables at the same time and keep the surgeons supplied with a constant stream of anaesthetised patients".[37] Having at times had difficulty keeping the surgeon operating on one patient satisfied, I find the notion of keeping four happy concurrently unimaginable!

The reader may have wondered why the terms *inhaler* and *vaporiser* have both appeared. Historically these have been somewhat interchangeable in popular use but allude to devices with different properties. All early devices, handkerchief included, had to provide a pathway of low resistance from which a spontaneously breathing patient could *inhale* an anaesthetic mixture. In most devices, the inhaled mixture is formed by some air passing through a chamber containing the anaesthetic liquid, therefore becoming highly saturated with vapour, and mixing this with some unmodified air which bypasses this chamber. The concentration of vapour in the inhaled mixture is altered by changing the proportion of air passing through the vaporising chamber. In order for the patient to be able to 'draw' the air 'over' the liquid anaesthetic it was important that the pathway for the air was not too narrow or tortuous. Given that no inhaler could avoid all resistance, increasingly devices incorporated a means by which the anaesthetist could assist the patient's breathing. An example is the bellows seen on the top of the ESO inhaler in Figure 34.

The term *inhaler* was limited to *vaporisers* from which a patient could breathe for at least some of the time without having to be assisted. The term *draw-over vaporiser* became a modern name for such a device. In contrast to these vaporisers, devices became increasingly common in which air (or a gas mixture) at a high pressure is needed to overcome the resistance of the pathways through the vaporiser. These are designed for hospital environments in which air, oxygen, nitrous oxide and other gases are supplied from high-pressure sources, including cylinders. The resistance they offer to the flow of gas may be a hundred times greater than those suitable for draw-over anaesthesia but this presents no problem if pressurised gases are available.[9]

A cultural divide has arisen between two types of medical environment. One is the modern hospital with 'on tap' high-pressure gases. The second is the environment commonly found in developing countries in which anaesthesia has to rely on room air, using a draw-over vaporiser with or without some supplementary oxygen. Such settings may also lack a reliable electricity supply. These limitations have famously included battlefield anaesthesia such as in the Falklands campaign. Since 1981 my colleague Dr Mike Dobson has run an annual Oxford course on Anaesthesia for Developing Countries, with daughter courses throughout the world. The approach to anaesthesia in eighty low- and middle-income countries contrasts strikingly with what is taught in the more developed world; Dobson's guide is appropriately entitled *The Right Stuff* and an Oxford ether vaporiser continues to feature prominently in this manual.[38]

Another key development had occurred in 1956, when the drug halothane was introduced into clinical practice. At the Royal Infirmary in Manchester, Michael Johnstone used the high-pressure apparatus of the day (a Boyle's machine) to deliver halothane in a 50:50 mixture of oxygen and nitrous oxide to 500 patients undergoing surgery.[39] Most of his patients were initially put to sleep with an intravenous barbiturate drug called thiopentone. In Oxford that same year Roger Bryce-Smith and a colleague studied halothane as a sole anaesthetic for both induction and maintenance in most of their series of 310 patients.[40] In some they used the open-drop method with the halothane administered using a wire facemask; in others they used an Oxford ether 'draw-over' vaporiser modified for halothane and supplied with air.

No anaesthesia-related death was reported in either study. It is clear that the 'halothane in air' approach in Oxford led to more difficulties than the Manchester protocol. The high concentrations of halothane (up to 3 per cent) needed in the Oxford study led to "depression of respiration which occurs not infrequently and may be sufficient to cause cyanosis … In our opinion, this disadvantage is great enough to warrant limiting the use of the agent to all but skilled anaesthetists until more is known about its properties."[40] In Manchester, the method of putting patients off to sleep with an injection of thiopentone and maintaining the anaesthesia with about 1 per cent halothane added to a mixture of oxygen and nitrous oxide was especially successful and set the standard drug cocktail for the following thirty years. Some took the view that finally a 'safe chloroform' had been discovered. However, as the 1956 Oxford study showed, halothane delivered in air using the open-drop method or using a draw-over vaporiser is not an easy drug to use. To this day, ether remains in favour in many less well-resourced settings.[38]

Tubes, bags and bellows

The plumbing associated with anaesthesia may not appear to be the profession's most exciting aspect but it has occupied much thought and ingenuity since the days of Horace Wells' animal bladder and wooden tube. Anaesthetic has to get to the patient's lungs. Unless 'open drops' are being dripped, the anaesthetic arrives via an *inspiratory tube*. Modern anaesthetic machines are designed to deliver a steady flow of gas (and vapour). If a patient is to breathe spontaneously from such a flow there needs to be a flexible *bag* or *bellows* somewhere in the system to allow the in-and-out excursions of breathing to connect to the steady flow of gas. The final ingredient of a 'breathing system' has to be a means for making sure that gas flows in the right direction: a *valve* is needed, and sometimes more than one.

In Joseph Clover's equipment (Fig. 31) we note a tube over his shoulder linking his reservoir bag of chloroform in air to a facemask which contains a valve sitting just above Clover's thumb. The valve ensures that the patient breathes in gas from the bag and expires to the room air. Similarly, with the ESO chloroform inhaler (Fig. 34) we see a tube leading to a mask with a valve. This 'draw-over' inhaler permits the intermittent flow of the patient's inhalations to draw air through the device with each breath. The presence of the bellows allows for the anaesthetist to assist breathing manually. Two further valves hidden inside the inhaler ensure that air moves in only one direction.[36]

A final ingredient of some breathing systems is an *expiratory tube* carrying gas away from the patient back to the anaesthetic machine. This may serve to take the gas straight to a scavenging system and then to the open air, or may direct the gas to return to the patient after being refreshed.

By 1954 there were so many different ways of connecting tubes, bag and valve that a physicist working in the Cardiff anaesthetic department, William Mapleson, set to work categorising them and clarifying how they worked.[41] His classification of the five main permutations became widely known as Mapleson's A to E (an F was later added). This is not the place to assault the reader with an extensive account but one key point is important: a breathing system needs enough gas; sufficient flow of gas out is needed to allow the patient to flush out carbon dioxide gas from the lungs.

An example of a breathing system much used in the UK is shown in Figure 35. It was described by the Canadian anaesthetist James Bain and a colleague in 1972.[42] By using a single co-axial tube, it had the great convenience of merging inspiratory and expiratory tubing. The valve by which gas could leave the system and the flexible bag (or bellows) were located well away from the patient. Some early accidents were attributed to the inner tube becoming broken while invisible in the opaque outer tube. Newer versions, like that shown in Figure 35 from my own hospital, have a transparent outer tube. In Mapleson's classification this system is labelled 'D'. It has been a workhorse for me over several decades.

An anaesthetic colleague in Oxford's John Radcliffe Hospital, Dr John Lehane, shared my exasperation that in 1987 the flow requirements of these various Mapleson systems still remained to be solved.[7] Long surgical cases permit anaesthetists working together to discuss and think, as John and I did. We were looking for a general solution applicable to any patient. John favoured using a diagram to represent any patient's pattern of breathing and on it to depict solutions to these gas-flow requirements. He thought that this would be more appealing than writing down equations. This diagram we duly published, finding that the five Mapleson systems fell into three categories.[43] We also put to rest a widespread myth that the commonly used system D (including the Bain version in Fig. 35) required different flows during spontaneous and assisted ventilation.[44] Mapleson, reflecting on the fiftieth anniversary of his classic paper, kindly referred to our "extremely elegant graphical analysis".[45] The fame that John and I hoped our solutions would bring never arrived. In part this was because they consisted more of academic nit-picking than of practical significance but also because by this time the Mapleson systems were falling out of favour as the cost of anaesthetic vapours had become very substantial and global warming had raised its head. This was because these systems require a high flow of gas and are wasteful of resources as well as being highly polluting of the atmosphere.

As the 1980s progressed into the 1990s, halothane was gradually replaced in developed countries by much more expensive anaesthetic vapours, including isoflurane and sevoflurane. The breathing system commonly used in the UK, shown in Figure 35, had a greedy requirement for a fresh flow of anaesthetic gas and vapour to keep the tubing well flushed. It needed two to three times the volume of gas being breathed each minute, amounting to about 10 litres per minute.

The solution to this excessive requirement of these Mapleson systems came to the UK around the year 2000. It followed an earlier tradition in the United States: the 'circle system' became widely used, in which the patient's expired gas was returned to them after being refreshed. This meant that the expired gas was passed through a canister of soda lime, which absorbs carbon dioxide; it was then joined by a low flow of fresh anaesthetic gas and vapour (around 1 litre per minute) before returning in the inspiratory tube to the patient. The Bain and other wasteful systems are reserved for short periods of time, such as first putting the patient off to sleep; in the UK this is traditionally done in a separate 'anaesthetic room' – the domain of the anaesthetic team alone – before transferring the patient into the operating *theatre* (as we still, surprisingly, call it).

Then along came global warming. Alarming results have been widely claimed from analysis of the environmental impact of inhalational anaesthetics. A unit of an 'anaesthetic hour' has become popular to compare these agents with the environmental effect of miles driven in a petrol-fuelled car.[46] This unit is based upon using a standard low flow of 1 litre per minute in a circle system for one hour. The anaesthetic vapours isoflurane and sevoflurane respectively are said to be equivalent to 8 and 4 miles of driving. Adding 60 per cent nitrous oxide gas to a mixture (a widely used percentage) adds 60 miles. A once-popular modern vapour, desflurane, yields such an astonishing 190 miles that many hospitals have now withdrawn it. I once thought that my cycle ride to work was a useful contribution to avoiding the effects of a car journey. Now I am being told that my normal day 'in theatre' might easily have been equivalent to driving between 500 and 1,000 miles.

But here we bump into controversy. The anaesthetists seem to have been using a measure of the 'global warming potential' (GWP) of anaesthetic gases and vapours, which the climate scientists argue is misleading.[47] GWP is a theoretical metric that was designed for multigas climate policies (such as the Kyoto Protocol), where emissions of different compounds need to be placed on a common scale to aid international negotiations. It is defined as the ratio of the *cumulative* radiative forcing (based on a concept called 'radiative efficiency') over a time horizon (usually 100 years) from the instantaneous release of 1 kg of a trace substance relative to that of 1 kg of carbon dioxide. But it tells us nothing about how the climate system will respond and what the impacts of anaesthetic gases might be.

Speaking to an anaesthesia research meeting in 2022, Dame Julia Slingo FRS, former chief scientist at the UK Meteorological Office, told her audience that "GWP and, by implication carbon-dioxide-equivalent, are fundamentally unsound measures of potential climate

impacts of anaesthetic gases." According to this view volatile anaesthetics as a whole make a minute contribution to greenhouse gas
radiative forcing, only 0.01–0.02 per cent of the effect that results from
the carbon dioxide associated with human activity, and that lifetimes
are so short and their concentrations so low that "their contribution
to radiative forcing will be lost in the complexity and 'noise' of the
climate system".[48]

Despite these differences of opinion, a cultural move is under-
way towards promoting regional anaesthesia (for more on which see
Chapter Five) or total intravenous anaesthesia in place of inhalational
anaesthesia.[49] Later in this chapter I shall explore intravenous anaesthesia but not before dealing with a few especially useful gadgets:
ways to secure the airway. This has to be done whatever kind of
general anaesthesia is being administered; all patients have to breathe.

'Tubing' the patient

A patient who is unconscious under anaesthesia cannot be relied
upon to maintain a clear airway through which to breathe. Snoring
indicates a poor airway during normal sleep; even worse obstruction
may occur in the unconscious due to collapse of the upper parts of
the airway or displacement of the tongue. In addition, the anaesthetic or other drugs administered may slow or stop breathing even
if the airway remains clear. I look now at the challenge of maintaining the airway and breathing, and some of the solutions offered. We
have already encountered one means of achieving this: the mask. A
custom of requiring one or both of the anaesthetist's hands to secure
a facemask, and apply traction to the lower jaw when needed, has
endured from the earliest days of anaesthesia (Fig. 31) well into the
modern era, and the ability to ventilate an unconscious patient via a
mask remains a key skill for any doctor.

The passage of a tube into the airway through the mouth or nose
offers an excellent way of maintaining it unobstructed yet it was only
relatively late in the development of anaesthesia that passage of a
tube into the patient's trachea became practically feasible. Figure 32
shows how indirect is the route from the mouth or nose into the
trachea, there being an acute curve at entry to the trachea from the
pharynx. The route into the oesophagus is more direct and so one of
the risks of attempting tracheal intubation is that the tube is passed

into the oesophagus by error, with potentially fatal consequenses because the lungs are then denied ventilation.

A major incentive to the advance of intubation of the trachea was plastic surgery on the faces of soldiers injured in the First World War. In most cases there was a need to keep a mask well out of the way of the surgeons while they operated. Sometimes the injuries were so severe that no mask could be used anyway. In 1921 anaesthetist Ivan Magill reported 3,000 anaesthetics administered to patients in Sidcup with facial injuries.[50] In many he used a gently curved rubber tube introduced through the nose and manipulated with forceps in the mouth into the trachea. Tubes of the 'Magill' shape and Magill's forceps remain a useful part of the anaesthetic tool kit.

In 1955 Aubrey F. Alsop from the Nuffield Department of Anaes-thetics described a tube designed for passage through the mouth and having an L-shape to prevent kinking if the head was flexed for-wards.[51] Figure 36 shows a version that includes an inflatable cuff to provide a complete seal in the airway. These rubber items were reus-able after sterilisation and are a notable contrast to the more modern devices shown in the figure, all of which are discarded after one use and contribute to the heavy burden of plastic waste. The items shown include a plastic Portex tube for either oral or nasal use, which has the shape of the early Magill tubes. Like the Oxford tube shown, this version incorporates a cuff that is inflated with air after insertion (and in the image), providing an airtight seal.

A unique event in which the reliability of the cuff in sealing the airway was of especial importance was Macintosh's experiments in 1943 on the effectiveness of life jackets for airmen landing in the sea. The aim was to ensure that an unconscious victim would be buoyant face-up. The means of obtaining an unconscious volunteer was to administer anaesthesia through a tracheal tube to Squadron Leader Pask from Farnborough and throw him into a swimming pool to observe the result. Macintosh described the experiments in 1945:

> E.A.P. was anaesthetised on three separate occasions for several hours each. Wearing various jackets, he was placed in good and unfavourable positions in smooth and rough deep water. The self-righting properties of the jackets were then assessed. Without a jacket he sank to the bottom of the bath. Ciné films

recorded these experiments, and a study of the films has resulted
in modifications to more than one jacket.[37]

In this unusual application, the cuffs on Pask's tracheal tube not only
prevented a leak of gas out of the lungs but also prevented water
from the swimming pool getting into his lungs. The cuffs had been
filled to water to help ensure a seal at whatever depth he sank to.
He was surely deserving of the award he received of an OBE in the
Honours List of January 1944.[6]

As referred to above, a problem with tracheal tubes is getting the
tube there in the first place. It is not possible to look through the
nose or mouth of a patient and see into the trachea; the route is
too tortuous. An instrument called a 'laryngoscope' can be used to
force a view of the larynx and vocal cords leading into the trachea.
Traditionally, these were long, straight metal tubes with a U-shaped
cross-section and were pushed with difficulty into the mouth and
pharynx, a manoeuvre which, according to Macintosh, "jeopardises
the patient's upper teeth or takes a minor divot out of the posterior
pharyngeal wall" (a *divot* being like a chuck of turf turned up by a
golf club – a reminder of his love of the game).[52] We can see from
Figure 32 that the route from the lips to the trachea passes teeth, the
tongue and a flap of cartilage behind the tongue called the epiglottis,
which dutifully covers the entrance to the trachea to prevent food
from entering the trachea when we swallow. Magill had modified an
earlier design of laryngoscope to have a slightly tilted end to offer "an
advantage in elevating and controlling the epiglottis".[53]

In 1943 Macintosh came up with a brilliant simple improvement
for which all anaesthetists have subsequently been grateful. He
devised a laryngoscope with a curved blade designed to follow the
curvature of the tongue and tug gently at the back of the tongue in
order to pull the epiglottis out of the line of sight without touching it
directly.[52] The device had a blade with a Z-shaped cross-section to dis-
place the tongue to one side rather than try to flatten it and was also
well lit by its own internal bulb. It remains the gold-standard means
of tracheal intubation. That is not to say that the manoeuvre is easy.
In some patients a direct view cannot be achieved and it remains difficult to intubate the trachea. Various gadgets such as optic fibres or
a camera are increasingly available to help look along a curved path.

With most devices there remains a risk of levering on the upper teeth and thereby causing dental damage. I have observed that this risk seemed more of a hazard when anaesthetists stood above the head of the supine patient, as they usually do, from which position the upper teeth are not always easily visible. This led me to develop a practice of standing beside the patient with Macintosh's laryngoscope to instrument the airway from a position in which the teeth (if present) were more readily visible.

Of the several airway devices that have proved immensely useful in anaesthesia, two more are included in Figure 36. Anesthesiologist Arthur Guedel of Beverly Hills, California, was concerned about the damage to lips and teeth of metal tubes used as oropharyngeal airways. Such devices prevent the patient biting shut the mouth and help to keep the tongue from obstructing the airway. His original design of 1933 was a rubber outer tube reinforced at the outermost section, where biting occurs, with an inner metal tube.[54] Modern disposable designs, like that shown in Figure 36, are made from plastic. Many of us have found ourselves using a Guedel airway in almost every patient for whom we wish to ventilate the lungs via a facemask.

Finally, Figure 36 includes a device that should have been invented long before Archie Brain actually thought of it. Brain's laryngeal mask is a brilliant gadget, which has revolutionised anaesthesia and wider medical care within my professional lifetime.[55] Brain had a flair for invention but was discouraged by his school teachers from studying science. He won a scholarship to Worcester College, Oxford, to read modern languages. Despite family pressure to enter the diplomatic service, he followed his French and Spanish degree by studying medicine in Oxford and London. Then as a lecturer in anaesthetics he became fascinated by the anatomy of the upper airway. As an alternative to inflating a cuff around a tube within the trachea, he explored whether an airtight seal could be achieved at the back of the pharynx in a device that remained outside the trachea and would therefore be easier to introduce. In 1983 he "noted that an airtight seal could be effected against the perimeter of the larynx posteriorly by an elliptical cuff inflated in the hypopharynx. This observation led to the concept of the Laryngeal Mask."[55] Figure 36 includes a modern disposable version.

Brain's laryngeal mask can be inserted into the airway without instrumentation and used more widely than by anaesthetic staff. It is used in half or more of general anaesthetics, freeing up busy hands

that might otherwise be occupied holding a facemask.[56] The extent
to which it can be safely used in place of a tracheal tube remains a
matter of debate. If we are looking for anaesthetic gadgets of historic
gravity, Macintosh's laryngoscope and Brain's laryngeal mask are in
competition for first prize.

The alternative to gases and vapours: intravenous anaesthesia

For Lord Nuffield, having an intravenous (IV) anaesthetic administered by Robert Macintosh was a form of "magic" compared with the
experience via a mask that he had previously endured. It is now taken
for granted that an injection is likely to be the route to being anaesthetised for most patients. Since the 1930s the custom has been for the
intravenous anaesthetic to be a brief means of 'inducing' anaesthesia
while the following 'maintenance' is achieved mainly using a vapour,
with or without nitrous oxide gas. For nearly a century most anaesthetics administered in hospital have been hybrids: IVs followed by
gases and vapours.

Oxford can arguably lay claim to being the site of the first intravenous anaesthetic.[57] Around March 1656 the aristocratic chemist
Robert Boyle, who had recently set up residence in Oxford, assembled a team to administer an infusion of opium in fortified wine to a
large dog. Christopher Wren, then twenty-four years of age, crossed
the High Street from All Souls College to Boyle's laboratory in Deep
Hall to provide the surgical expertise for access to a leg vein using
the "Pipe of a Syringe". They were assisted by "some eminent Physitians, and other learned Men" who may well have included the young
Robert Hooke.

We shall meet the site of this event in Chapter Seven, in the
context of exploring Hooke's law. At the time, Deep Hall belonged to
Christ Church and immediately neighboured University College, to
which it now belongs. Boyle showed support for the then-struggling
Univ by donating a generous £81 to help with the completion of its
dining hall, which pleasingly to this day has the completion date 1656
inscribed on one of the roof beams. In later years, after University
College purchased the site of Deep Hall, the dining hall was extended
into what was once its garden area. Staff of the college like myself
now sit for dinner precisely over the spot where Boyle encouraged

speedy "recovery" of his anaesthetised dog, which was "whipp'd up and down the Neighboring Garden, whereby being kept awake, and in motion, after some time he began to come to himself again". The dog made a long-term recovery and became something of a celebrity.[57]

It took from 1656 to the early 1930s for intravenous anaesthetic drugs to become well investigated and used. Intravenous alcohol had its advocates but the most widespread application came with barbiturate drugs. An early study by Magill in 1931 illustrates the diversity of approaches. He administered pentobarbitone intravenously to 180 patients but also gave it orally or rectally to another 82 patients.[58] In some cases he also administered nitrous oxide and ether. Of the intravenous route, Magill noted that patients "are unanimous in their appreciation of this method of induction" but he emphasised "that a drug of such potency should only be in the hands of experienced persons fully conversant with all the principles of general anaesthesia".

For the first decade of my own career, thiopentone was the induction agent of almost universal use. This short-acting barbiturate had become popular in the later 1930s. It could produce profound depression of the heart, circulation and breathing: the ratio between the dose that could be fatal and the therapeutic dose for anaesthesia was about 3.9 but lower in compromised patients.[59] It has been held responsible for causing many deaths when used in injured personnel at Pearl Harbor in 1941 but when data eventually came to light the risk was shown to have been wildly exaggerated.[60] It was necessary to avoid important adverse effects in its use but it served very well for half a century.

The arrival in the 1980s of a non-barbiturate drug, propofol, extended the use of intravenous anaesthesia from the first few minutes getting the patient off to sleep to maintaining anaesthesia throughout an operation. Prolonged infusion of barbiturates was not suitable for maintaining anaesthesia over many minutes or hours, because of their accumulation in the body, which led to slow recovery of consciousness. Although propofol carries a similar ratio to thiopentone of fatal to therapeutic dose (about 3.4) and a similar profile of hazards, recovery of consciousness after propofol is faster than with thiopentone, especially after prolonged infusion.[59] Its use is also less likely to be dogged by sickness and vomiting. Propofol has become the standard anaesthetic agent and prolonged use by infusion has heralded a new name: total intravenous anaesthesia, TIVA.

TIVA offers the possibility of avoiding environmental damage that may be associated with nitrous oxide gas and anaesthetic vapours. The increasing availability of infusion pumps has allowed programs to be developed in which the rate of infusion into a vein is rapid initially and then decreases in an attempt to maintain an appropriate level of drug in the blood (and brain), keeping the patient anaesthetised over however long is required for the surgery. However, a major difficulty arises with this technique. Anaesthetists have no immediate measure of the concentration of propofol in the blood and therefore no direct measure of whether it is sufficient to keep the patient asleep. I shall address a particular aspect of this problem in the next section.

Those other drugs used by anaesthetists

A property of all anaesthetic agents, whether gases, vapours or intravenous drugs, is that the dose needed to prevent the patient's movement in response to a painful stimulus is higher than the dose required to simply produce unconsciousness, usually by about 50 per cent. When it was discovered that the South American arrow poison curare and other 'neuromuscular blockers' prevent movement by paralysing the activation of muscles by motor nerves, the possibility was raised of giving lower doses of anaesthetics to maintain unconsciousness while still preventing the inconvenience of movement during surgery; curare was introduced into anaesthetic practice in the 1940s. The benefits of neuromuscular blockers exceed simply stopping movement: muscles maintain a tone (tension), which itself can make access to the abdomen and other parts of the body difficult for surgeons if the muscles are tight. These drugs remove the tone completely, greatly easing many types of surgery. However, they also stop breathing and make it necessary to take over ventilation of the lungs entirely: bag or bellows.

A serious problem is that if a patient were to be paralysed with a neuromuscular blocker while at the same time remaining conscious then the patient would be *unable to move at all* and consequently unable to signal distress. In pre-operative visits to patients I have met several who recounted periods of being awake during previous surgery, some having suffered extreme pain. One of the most common fears expressed by patients during such pre-operative visits is that of 'not being properly asleep'. The term 'accidental awareness during anaesthesia' became attached to this experience, degrees of which extend from merely overhearing some conversation between medical staff to the agony of being operated on without pain relief. I myself as a patient have had a fairly inconsequential experience of this kind, waking up after an operation and finding myself unable to breathe.

Studies of awareness have been revealing. My colleague Jaideep Pandit led a UK National Audit Project over twelve months in 2012–13 with the aim of assessing the incidence of and risk factors for accidental awareness.[61] The survey covered ~2.8 million general anaesthetics. The overall incidence of awareness was 1:19,600 but with great variability. For example, during Caesarean section the incidence was 1:670. A major finding was that most cases of awareness were in patients paralysed with neuromuscular blockers and that, of all anaesthetic techniques, TIVA combined with such blockers conferred the greatest risk (almost fourfold) of accidental awareness. What might be the reason for TIVA creating a particular risk?

The reason is a fundamental difference between inhalational and intravenous anaesthetics. The percentage of a modern anaesthetic vapour such as isoflurane in the brain *equilibrates* over a period of minutes with the percentage in the lungs, the primary route via which it arrives in the body and leaves the body. By measuring that percentage in expired breaths at the mouth the modern-day anaesthetist has a window into the level in the brain. In settings where such breath-by-breath monitoring is unavailable, the percentage in the lungs can be judged from the percentage inspired, and that is known from the dial on the vaporiser from which it is being administered.

Contrast the use of propofol: the anaesthetist can set a rate of infusion into the blood on a pump driving a syringe. However, the level reached in the blood and the brain depends upon *both* the rate of infusion *and* how fast the propofol is being eliminated from the blood, mainly by metabolism in the liver.[59] Since this speed of elimination can vary between individuals threefold, the concentration of propofol in the blood and brain achieved by a single rate of infusion can also vary threefold. With this uncertainty goes the risk that the concentration in the brain may be inadequate to prevent accidental awareness.

This problem could be addressed if monitoring of propofol concentration in the blood could be achieved in real time. Some have

looked at measuring propofol in expired breaths but found this not
to be possible. Another approach is to use monitors of brain electrical activity, which show promise in discriminating consciousness
from unconsciousness. A summary by my former anaesthetic tutor
John Sear in 2011 remains pertinent: "because of wide variability in
therapeutic drug concentration window (related to age and type of
surgery) and inter-subject kinetics, propofol dosing is best titrated to
effect".[59] The problem remains that this 'effect' is difficult to judge
when a patient has been paralysed with a neuromuscular blocker.
When Pandit's survey was conducted, 5.8 per cent of surgical cases
received TIVA. The percentage has increased markedly in recent
years and may have now reached 50 per cent in the UK. This way of
doing things may offer benefits for the environment but brings its
own challenges.

   The anaesthetic drug cupboard contains much else besides bottles
of anaesthetic, ampoules of propofol and neuromuscular blockers.
The family of morphine-like analgesics plays a ubiquitous supplementary role to the sleep drugs, both during and after surgery. There
are anti-sickness drugs; drugs to raise the blood pressure and drugs
to lower it; drugs to help prevent bleeding. We have drugs to help
patients wake up and start moving again. The early pioneers would
be astounded to see the pharmacopoeia that is now available. Dr John
Snow has left us a wonderful record of his prescriptions for digitalis,
gentian, hemlock, opium and rhubarb.[25] It would be so fascinating to
be able to show and discuss with him our present repertoire.

The brain after surgery

The aim of general anaesthesia is to change the brain but only temporarily for the duration of the operation. It has long been recognised
that the immediate post-operative course of some patients may
include a brief period of confusion or delirium, often associated with
drugs, electrolyte disturbances in the blood, derangement of sleep
and sometimes infection. More recently, concerns have arisen over
possible long-term effects of anaesthesia and surgery on cognitive
function, and even the possibility that these may increase the risk of
developing dementia.

   This is not the place to review what is becoming a major topic of
interest and now reaching a wide audience in the national press, but

two major points seem pertinent to this chapter.[62] The first is that it remains unclear whether anaesthetic agents themselves might be playing a role in accelerating cognitive decline, or whether the stress of surgery itself may be a main factor. Thus, for example, one study found that overall cognitive decline associated with spinal and general anaesthesia was similar, though there was a suggestion that memory might be worsened more by general anaesthesia.[63] This points the finger at the trauma of surgery itself rather than drugs acting on the brain.

The second point bears on our observation of the increasing use of TIVA. There is a suggestion that the anaesthetic vapours such as isoflurane may have a more deleterious effect on cognitive impairment than intravenous drugs such as propofol; I have had patients asking for TIVA because they were aware of this possibility. A large study of twenty-eight trials comparing the different techniques in the elderly found that it could pool data from seven of these, incorporating 869 patients, to draw the conclusion that there was "low-certainty evidence that TIVA may reduce post-operative cognitive dysfunction".[64]

Locally a unique opportunity presented itself for us to assess cognitive decline after surgery in a group of elderly volunteers recruited from 1988 onwards in the Oxford Project to Investigate Memory and Ageing (OPTIMA).[65] This long-term study involved participants with varying levels of cognitive impairment ranging from none at all to full dementia. It followed them with an annual assessment called the Cambridge Cognitive Examination. From a twenty-four-year period, we identified 394 volunteers out of a database of about a thousand, who had at least two assessments and participated for between three and twenty-three years. We interrogated the database to find episodes of moderate or major surgery, and statistician Dan Lunn helped us explore whether surgery was related to the subsequent rate of cognitive decline. The main finding of the study was that cognitive decline was accelerated after surgery in these elderly patients (average age seventy-three years) but that this occurred only in those who already displayed some degree of cognitive impairment before their surgery.

A group in Wisconsin, in the United States, noted our findings and set about exploring in their registry whether cognitive decline might occur after surgery in younger volunteers with a mean age of fifty-four years when examined over a single four-year period.[66] They found a small degree of memory loss associated with surgery.

These and other studies allow benefits of a proposed operation to be weighed against possible adverse effects on the brain but clearly we need to know more about these effects.

The surgical team

My emphasis on gases, vapours, other drugs and gadgets has perhaps detracted from the more human aspects of working in a team. Senior anaesthetists in the UK tend to work individually but with a nurse or practitioner assistant providing minute-by-minute support. My assistants have been the salt of the earth in the daily toil, and exceptional in moments of crisis. A more junior doctor colleague in training is sometimes also to hand to assist with the increasingly complex tasks and to learn as an apprentice. On occasion I have been privileged to work with a doctor whom I admitted from school to university to study pre-clinical medicine with me some six years earlier.

Then there is the surgeon to get on with. The anaesthetist Gordon Ostlere made his fame with his series of *Doctor in the House* novels, and their film and stage adaptations. He also wrote a student guide to anaesthesia, which included advice on how to manage one's surgical colleague:

> Always keep an eye on what the surgeon is up to, unobtrusively, however. Nothing annoys a surgeon more than seeing his anaesthetist flying around the theatre like a septic poltergeist. A good anaesthetist should have the character of a Jeeves: he should exercise a strict but subtle control over the surgeon, anticipate his wants, cool his unwise enthusiasms, and encourage him in despair – but from the background. The anaesthetist should make himself the centre of the theatre only when the surgeon is in difficulties before an audience of his distinguished contemporaries.[67]

That a surgeon I have worked with for twenty years recently took me out for a celebratory dinner, I take to be evidence that I may have conducted myself at least partly appropriately.

I return finally to that precursor of TIVA in seventeenth-century Oxford. For that first intravenous anaesthetic, on the dog in 1656, we have seen that there was a team of "some eminent Physitians, and other learned Men". Christopher Wren was the surgeon who made "a small and opportune Incision over that part of the hind leg where the larger Vessels that carry the Blood, are most easie to be taken hold of".[68] A "Ligature" was applied and a "Plate of Brass ... almost the shape and bigness of the Nail of a Mans Thumb" used to prevent the vein from "starting aside" when "exposed to the Lancet". I picture Robert Boyle standing ready to pass over the "Syringe" with its "slender pipe" for Wren to slide into the vein for the injection of the "warm solution of *Opium* in Sack".

The purpose was to conduct a scientific experiment. Boyle wanted to know whether intravenous administration of "poysons" would have the same effect as giving them orally. He wished to explore whether "being carried by the circulated Blood to the Heart and Head, it may be found whether their strength be that way more unfringed, and their operation more speedy (or otherwise differing) then [*sic*] if they were taken in at the mouth".[57]

It is a tragedy that the team's success in "stupefying" what became Boyle's "carefully tended" and "admired" pet was not applied further, when it could have allowed nearly 200 years of pain-free surgery in humans before Horace Wells took up his animal bladder full of nitrous oxide in 1844. As intravenous anaesthesia increasingly takes over from the gases and vapours, one wonders whether more effort in the laboratory of Deep Hall might have enabled the gases and vapours that filled a century of anaesthetic practice to be bypassed entirely, leaving intravenous anaesthesia alone in the intervening 400 years.

CHAPTER SEVEN

THE PADDYWHACK

Body Tissue Anomalies

Those scary laws of thermodynamics

We have visited many parts of the body. Now let us look at some properties of the body's tissues themselves, including arteries, ligaments and skin. On the one hand they may seem just to be the passive conduits or the stretchy bits that hold the more vital parts of our body together; on the other, any deficiencies in them can lead to us 'coming undone' in most unpleasant ways.

On close inspection body tissues have some perplexing and interesting behaviours. Unfortunately, there is a big catch to understanding these behaviours: we need the laws of thermodynamics to do so, but most people prefer lighter reading. A particular hurdle is what these tissues have to tell us about 'entropy', something we need to define and grasp. To many, the word has a ghostly air: pertaining to something inscrutable, material for physicists, perhaps, trying to understand the origins of the universe. But we need entropy to understand the behaviour of the long string-like molecules inside the elastic fibres of the tissues. Let's make a light-hearted start with the laws of thermodynamics in song.

Michael Flanders and Donald Swann were a British comedy duo internationally renowned in the years of their public performing between 1956 and 1967. In 'The First and Second Law' they not only wrote a song that guaranteed vigorous laughter in any audience but produced the most succinct summary ever of two laws of nature: the laws of thermodynamics.[1] The song, accessible online, is a delight:

The first law of thermodynamics:
Heat is work and work is heat.
Very good. The second law of thermodynamics:

Heat cannot of itself pass from one body to a hotter body.
Heat won't pass from a cooler to a hotter.
You can try it if you like but you far better not-er!
'Cause the cold in the cooler will get hotter as a rule-r,
Because the hotter body's heat will pass to the cooler
Heat is work, and work's a curse
And all the heat in the universe
Is gonna cool down
'Cause it can't increase
Then there'll be no more work
And there'll be perfect peace
Really?
Yeah, that's entropy, man!

You may wonder whether Flanders and Swann were appropriate authorities to guide us in the laws of thermodynamics. Arguably not. They had met at Westminster School where they put on a revue in 1940. Both went up to Christ Church, Oxford, a connection I am pleased to claim because that was the college I myself attended while studying for a doctorate on the main topic of this chapter: the paddywhack. Flanders read history and Swann read modern Greek and Russian, neither particularly associated with thermodynamics. Their education was disrupted by the war and for Flanders was cut short in a manner of which our shared college may not be so proud. In 1943 in the Navy he contracted poliomyelitis, which resulted in him being in a wheelchair for the rest of his life; his disability appears to have been the reason why Christ Church rejected his request to return to his studies. Fortunately for both Flanders and Swann, talent won through and their duo became one of the most popular stage events of the era.[2, 3] They were a seated duo. Flanders performed in his wheelchair alongside Swann seated at the piano. We shall meet further wisdom from the pair later in the chapter.

This chapter contains, inter alia, an event which took me to the store-room of an art gallery in Copenhagen. First, however, we join the distinguished physiologist Charles Roy in applying the laws of thermodynamics to stretchy body tissues to shed a little light on *five anomalies* of their behaviour: five ways in which these body materials differ from inanimate materials we meet in everyday life. A historical detour into the seventeenth century will be needed to get to the bottom of one of these anomalies. An increase in pace will take us to a whole world of 'rubber-like' or 'entropy' elasticity and then on to a grand finale of the 'sluggishness-of-the-stretchiness' of body tissues, which physicists call 'viscoelasticity'; this is about tissues needing time (often lots of time) to change shape. The need for time to change shape is itself a manifestation of a strange phenomenon called 'glass transition', in which a tissue can be transformed from being stretchy, like rubber, to being rigid like glass when it is cooled or dried out. We'll finish up with something useful to doctors: the skin-turgor sign of dehydration, for which we will have an explanation. It sounds complicated, and is, but bear with me.

My own battle with the laws of thermodynamics started while studying at Hertford College in Oxford in the first year of my course in Engineering Science. The first law didn't seem too difficult to grasp once I realised that the convention of measuring heat in units of *calories* and work in *joules* was not a good idea if they were, in some sense at least, the same 'stuff': two forms of *energy*. At that time (in 1971) the United Kingdom was struggling with units of measurement. Two years previously, the government had set up the Metrication Board to try to drag us away from imperial units such as feet, inches, pounds, pennies, pints, fathoms and furlongs, to metric units based upon multiples of ten favoured by the countries of mainland Europe. Some steps in this process became mandatory in the late 1970s and were accelerated by the UK's entry into the European Economic Community in 1983.

My school and university years were spent in the turmoil of this stumbling transition, which continues today as we purchase our beer in pints and our petrol in litres. To add to the confusion, calories were strictly neither imperial nor metric units, but just something to add another level of complexity, like the *millimetres of mercury* for measuring pressure that as students we struggled to understand. Mercifully, however, we usually now measure both heat and work in the SI (*Système International*) unit of joules. With the climate crisis upon us thermodynamics has shot to the top of the public agenda, which is all about heat waves and heat pumps.

The first law of thermodynamics helps us think of heat and work as being two manifestations of energy: things that can be entered on a balance sheet and summed or subtracted at the bottom to give us the net gain or loss of energy from a 'body' (as engineers like to call

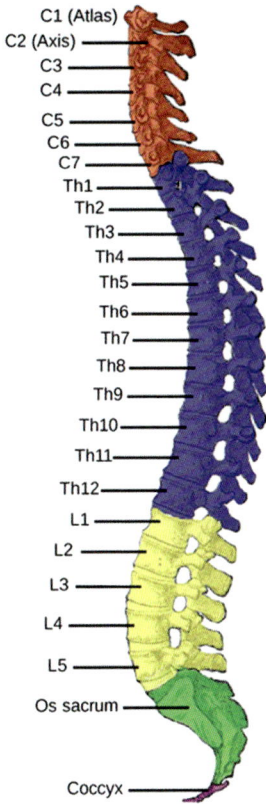

Figure 29. The bones of the human vertebral column seen from a side view: 7 cervical, 12 thoracic, 5 lumbar, 5 (fused) sacral and the coccyx. In this view, the vertebral bodies form a curved column which faces the front of the body and lies to the left; the spinal canal lies between the vertebral bodies and the vertebral spines which lie close to the skin of the back facing the right in this view. A patient who lies on their back (supine) will have lowermost points around T5–7 and in the sacrum. The uppermost points will be around L2–4 and in the cervical region.

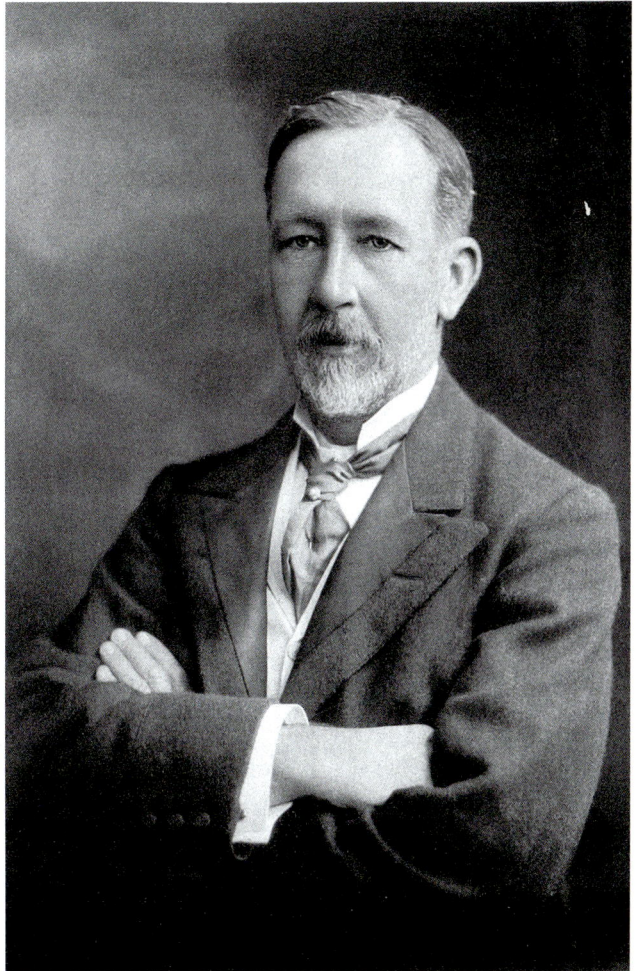

Figure 30. Portrait of Arthur E. Barker c.1915 by Anton Mansch. As Professor of Surgery at University College, London, Barker introduced and thoroughly assessed the use of glucose (sugar) to increase the density of spinal local anaesthetic injectate so that gravity could be used to produce predictable safe spread of anaesthesia when the mixture was injected into the less dense cerebrospinal fluid.

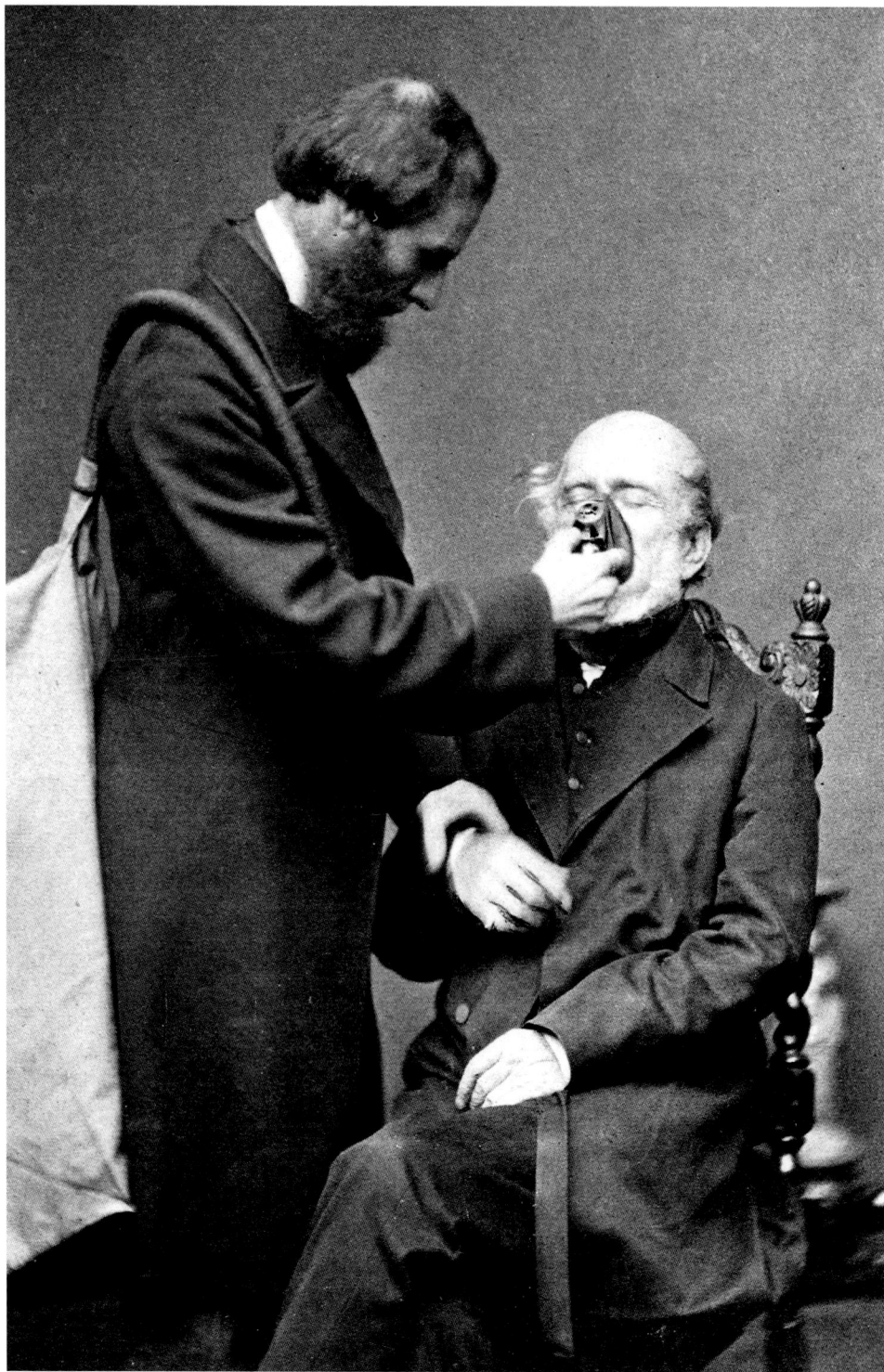

Figure 31. Joseph Clover posing with his father to illustrate the administration of chloroform in 1862. Chloroform liquid was added to a measured volume of air in the bag seen behind Clover to achieve a concentration of ~2–4 per cent. Note the finger on the pulse.

Figure 32. Anatomy of the airway sketched as a midline section through the face and neck. The oropharynx is where inhaled gas from the nasal cavity or the mouth shares the pathway for food and drink crossing from the mouth into the oesophagus. Our vigorous reflexes normally prevent food, drink or stomach contents from passing into the trachea and lungs. Anaesthesia obtunds these reflexes.

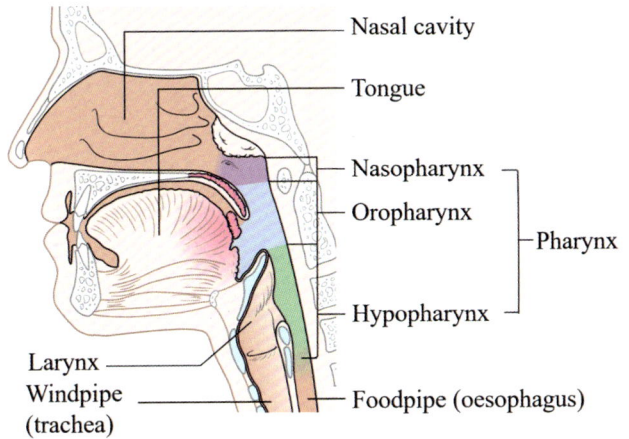

Nasal cavity
Tongue
Nasopharynx
Oropharynx
Pharynx
Hypopharynx
Larynx
Windpipe (trachea)
Foodpipe (oesophagus)

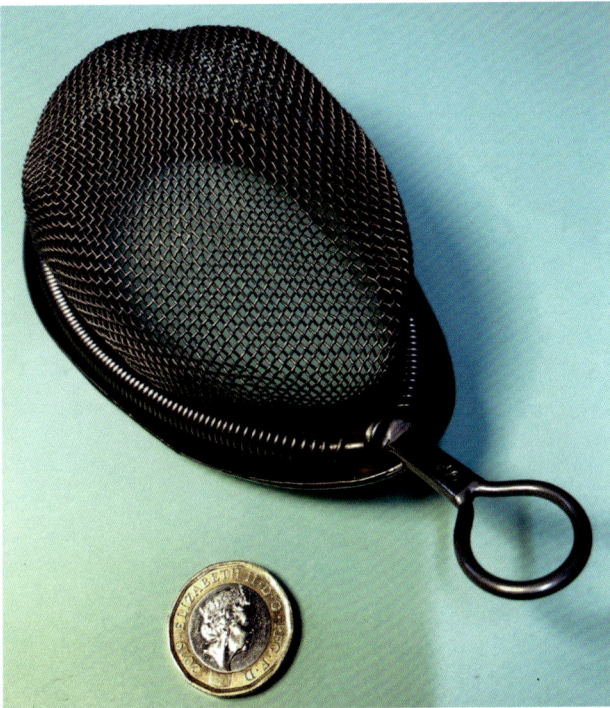

Figure 33. Wire facemask for the administration of open-drop chloroform or ether anaesthesia. Commonly known as the *Schimmelbusch mask* following an original design by Curt Schimmelbusch in 1893, the mask was combined with layers of gauze held in place by the sprung loop with finger-ring. This version was designed by New York surgeon Sidney Yankauer in 1904. It was widely used into the 1950s and still finds use in developing countries

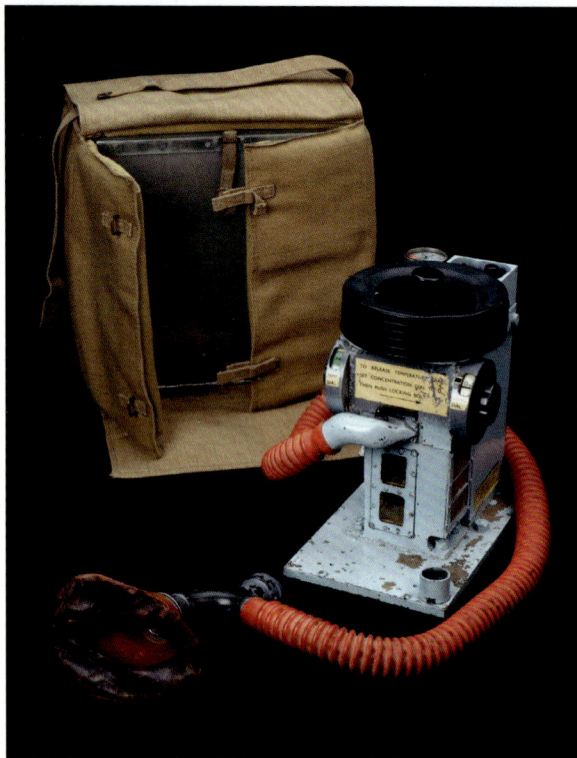

Figure 34. The Epstein–Suffolk–Oxford chloroform inhaler of 1945 designed in Oxford for military use by airborne troops. The advantages in the military setting of using non-flammable chloroform in air were seen to outweigh its known drawbacks. The 'frontpack' was designed to be held on a parachutist's chest.

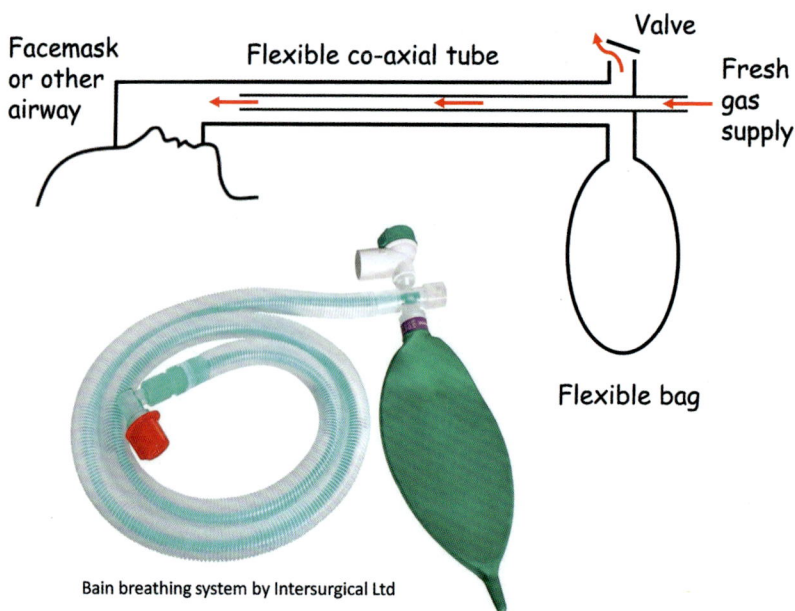

Bain breathing system by Intersurgical Ltd

Figure 35. Bain anaesthesia breathing system supplied with a steady flow of gas from an anaesthetic machine. Gas flows down a narrow central pipe of a flexible co-axial tube to the patient. The outer tubing provides a route for expired gas to pass to both a flexible bag and an escape valve. The bag can be squeezed by hand or replaced by a ventilator bellows if breathing needs to be assisted. The Intersurgical Ltd version is shown with a red cap sealing where a mask or other airway is attached.

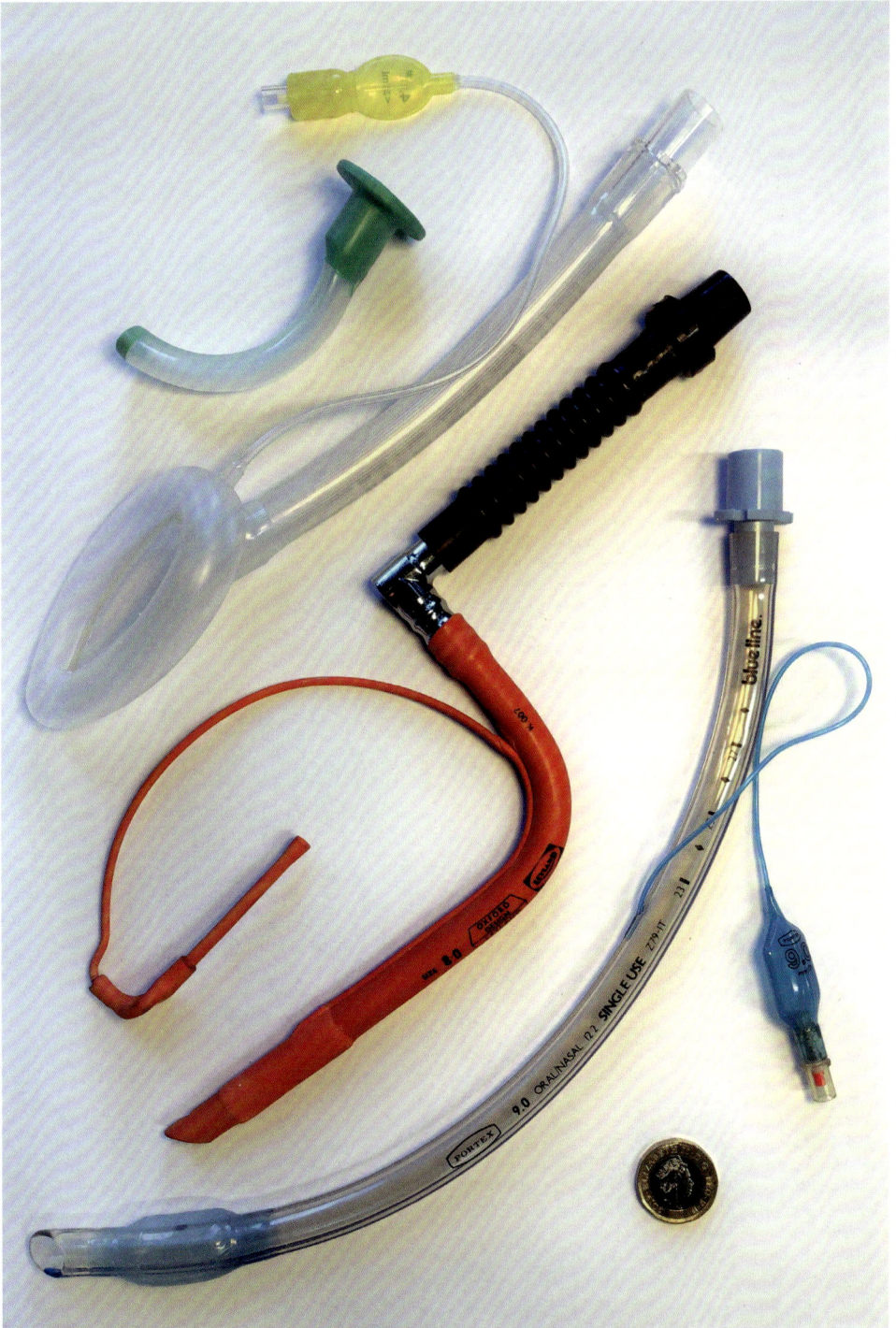

Figure 36. Gadgets for maintaining a patient's airway. From top left: Guedel's oropharyngeal airway, Brain's laryngeal mask, Oxford oral tube, Portex endotracheal oral/nasal tube.

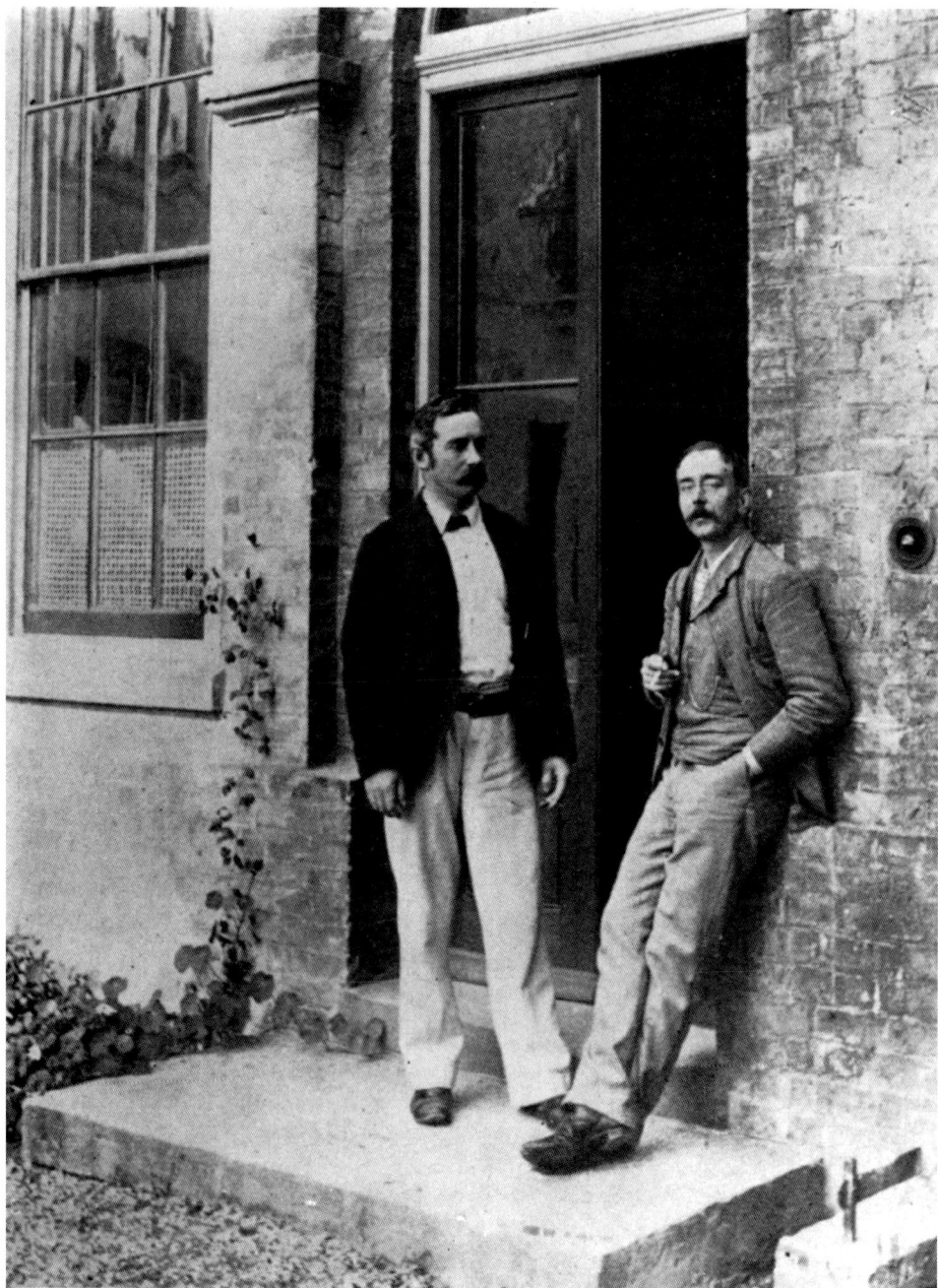

Figure 37. Charles S. Roy (left) and Charles S. Sherrington at the door of the Old Pathological Laboratory, Cambridge, 1893.

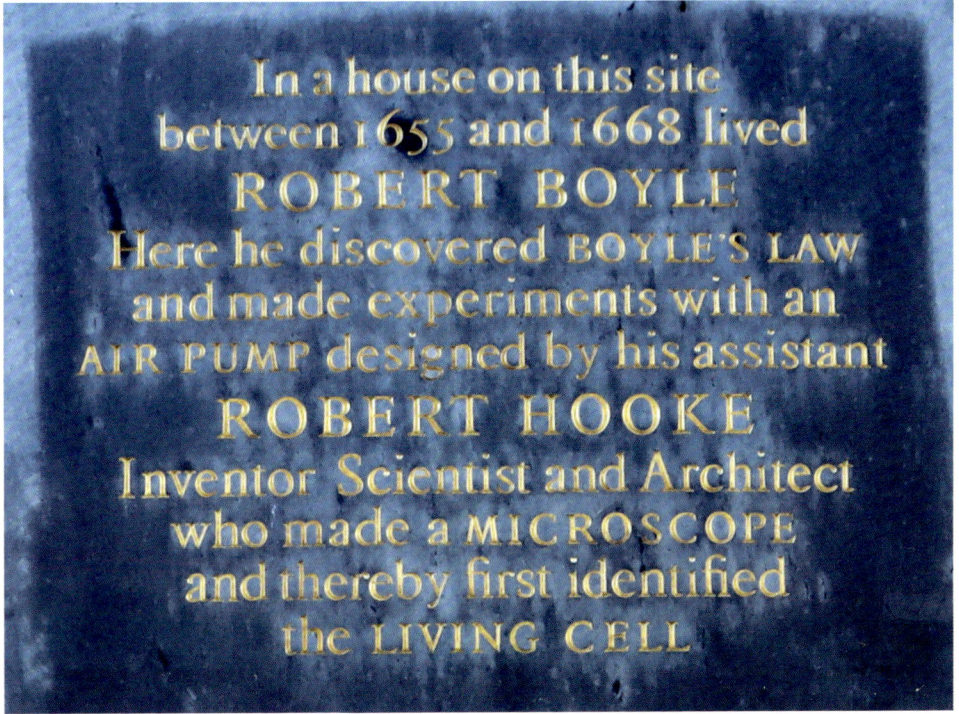

Figure 38. Plaque on the wall of University College, Oxford, commemorating the work at the site of Deep Hall of Robert Boyle and Robert Hooke.

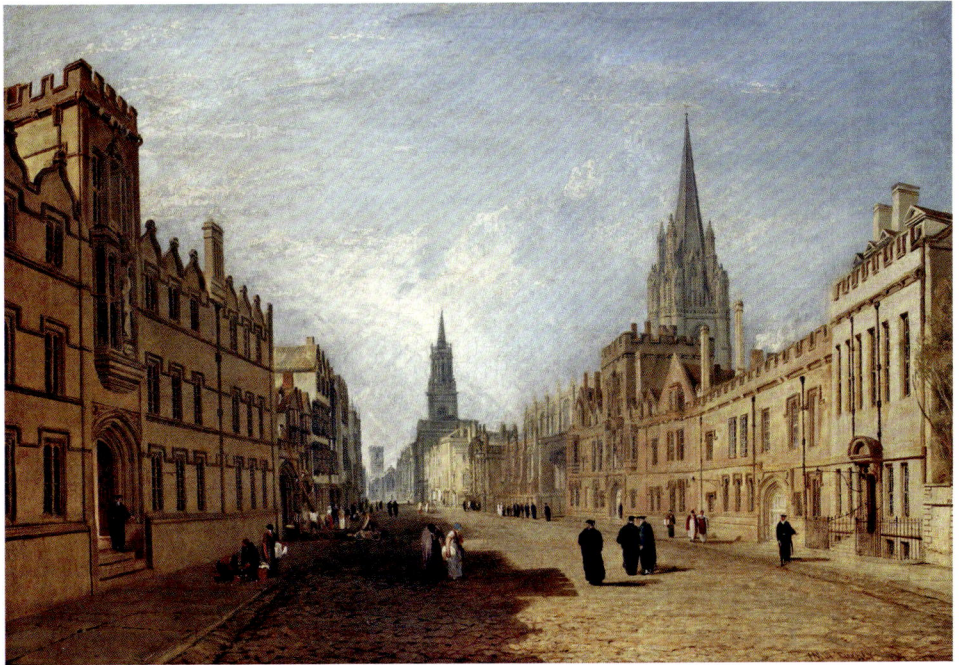

Figure 39. *High Street, Oxford* by J.M.W. Turner, 1809–10. Deep Hall on the left, adjacent to University College and opposite All Souls College, is seen receiving the attention of workmen, probably beginning its demolition. These were Boyle's lodgings.

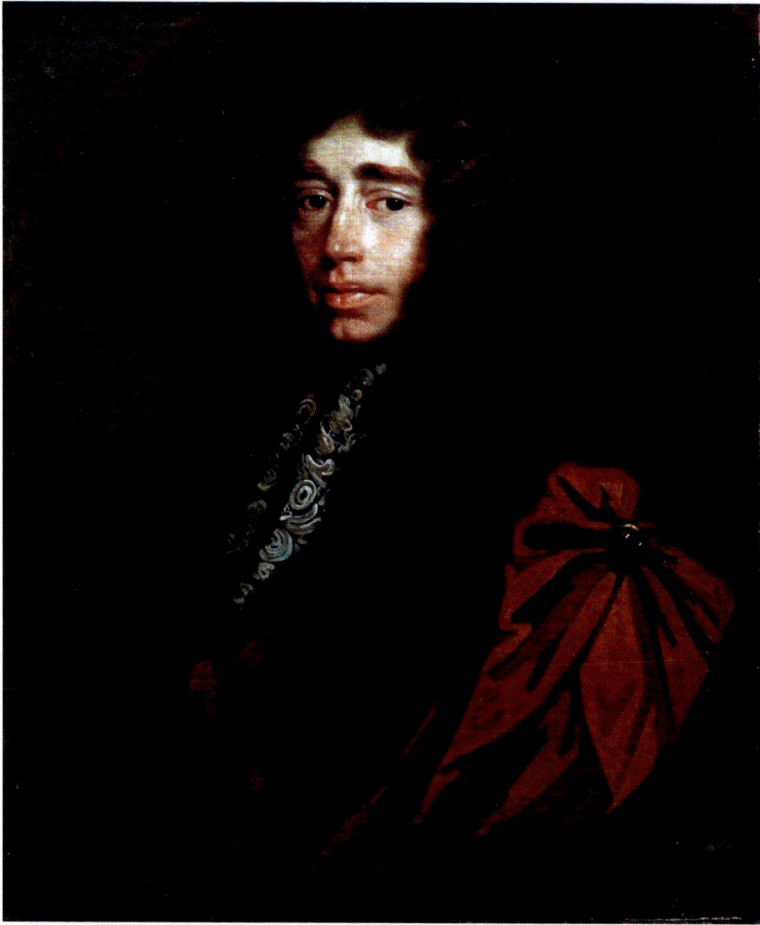

Figure 40. Could this be a portrait of Robert Hooke? *Portrait of a Man* in the style of Sir Peter Lely and Mrs Mary Beale with sitter aged 38 years is held in the store-room of the National Gallery of Denmark, which acquired the portrait in 1937.

Figure 41. Dr Gerry McCrum, Tutor in Engineering Science at Hertford College, Oxford. Always camera shy, Gerry was caught here on the day of his award of the degree of Doctor of Science.

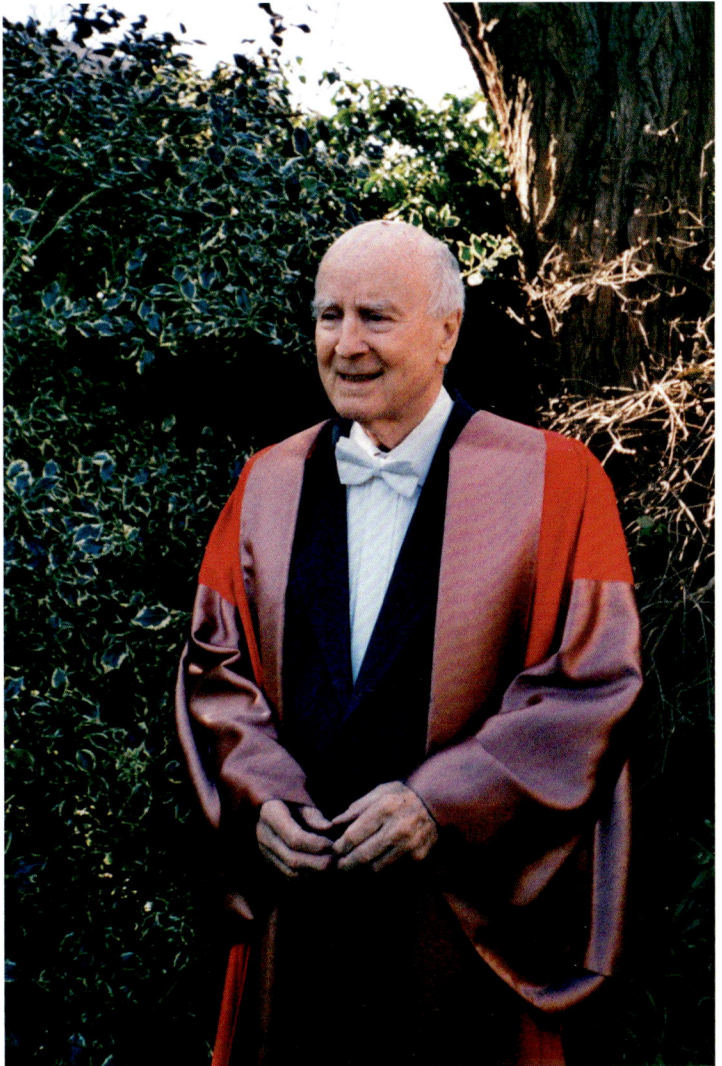

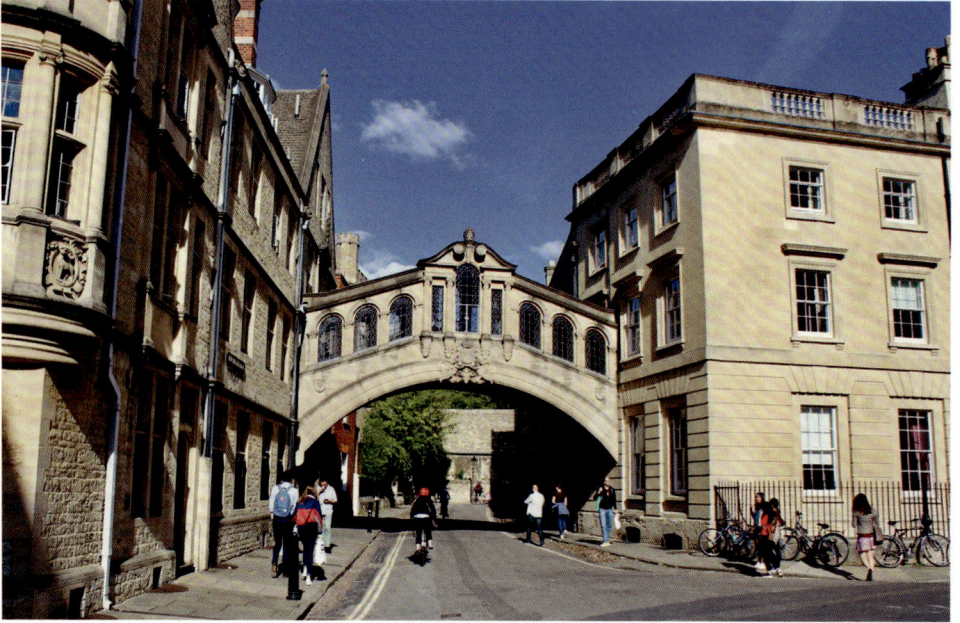

Figure 42. Hertford College buildings linked by its 'bridge of sighs', which sits across New College Lane. As a second-year undergraduate, the author occupied the first-floor corner bay window seen on the far left of the image. The bridge resembles Venice's Rialto Bridge, not the Bridge of Sighs of its Doge's Palace.

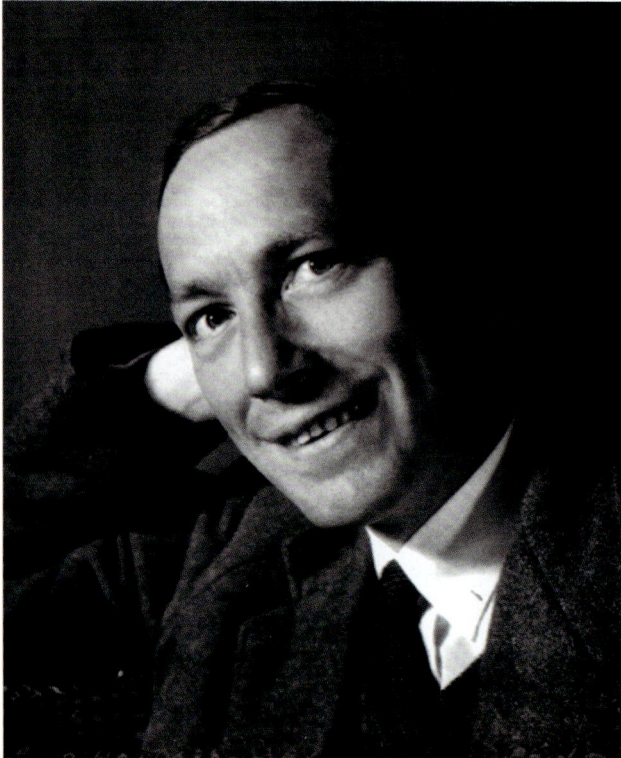

Figure 43. Dr Kenneth Hutton, founding headmaster of Hatfield Technical School, aged 38 in 1956. From a background in a public school and the University of Oxford, Hutton found himself from 1953 in charge of a new kind of co-educational state school which attempted to provide a mixture of technical and academic education.

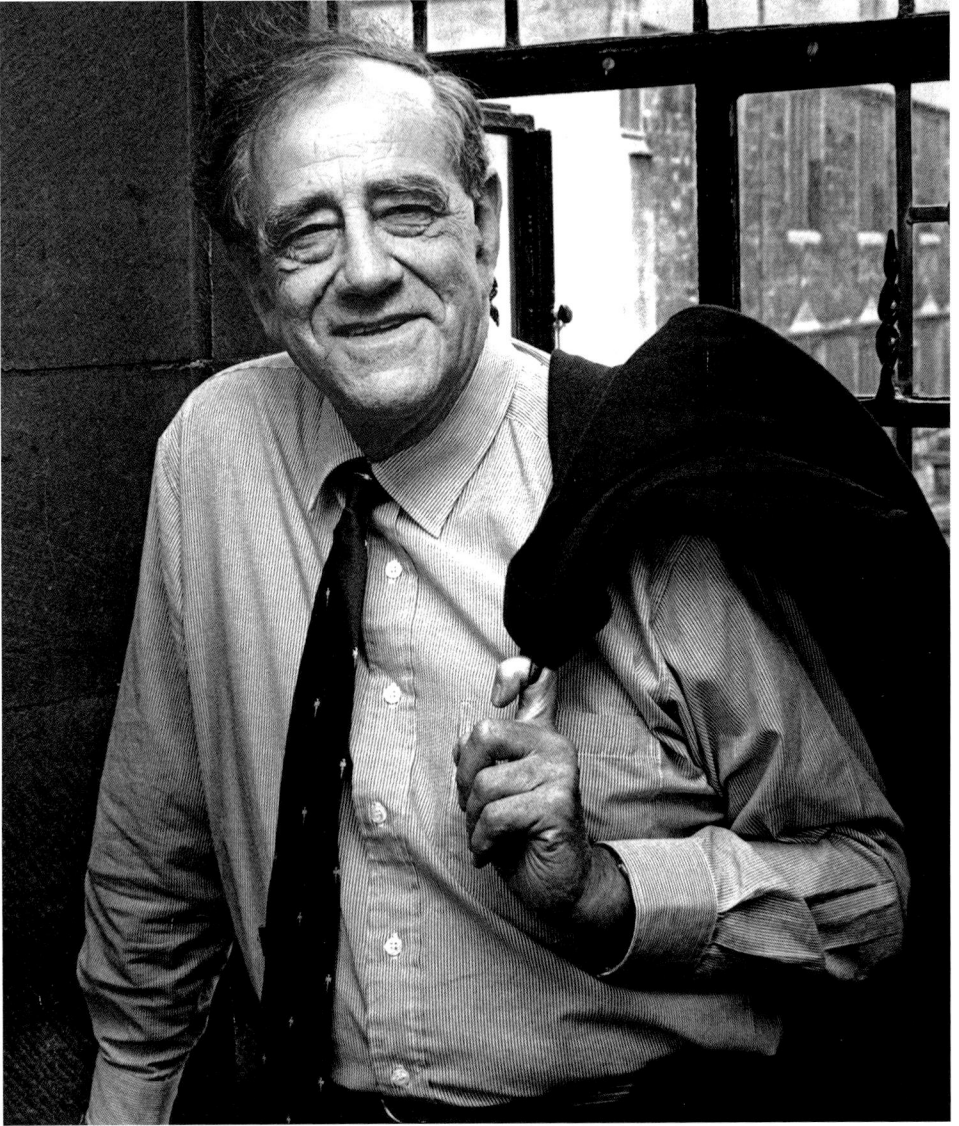

Figure 44. Dr Neil Tanner, physicist and Tutor for Admissions of Hertford College, Oxford, 1964–71 and 1980–9. Tanner was the driving force behind a novel scheme to attract state-educated schoolboys to come to study in Oxford.

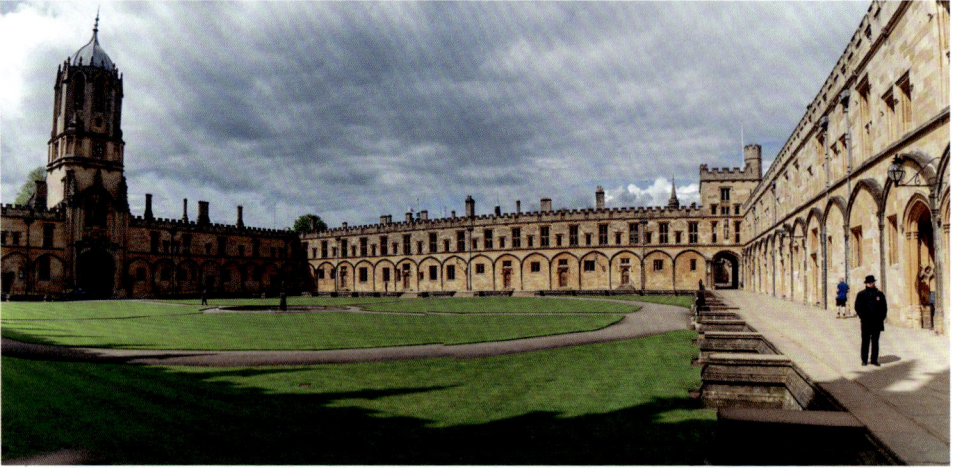

Figure 45. Christ Church, Oxford, a unique a mix of theological institution and secular place of learning. The houses around Tom Quad shown in this image are occupied by the Dean and canons of the chapter of the cathedral, the entrance to which is shown on the extreme right of the picture. Building of the quadrangle was commenced around 1525 when Cardinal Wolsey established Cardinal College and was further completed when Christ Church was founded by Henry VIII in 1546, though the planned cloisters never obtained their roof. The bell tower over the entrance gate was completed by Christopher Wren in 1682.

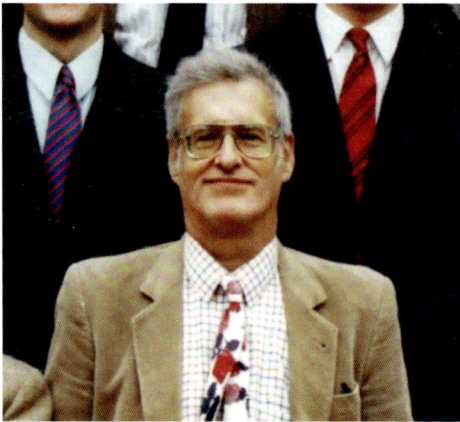

Figure 46. Dr Derek Bergel among senior colleagues at Merton College in 1991. Known for his expertise on the cardiovascular system, Bergel was the author's tutor in physiology at St Catherine's College. He later moved to become tutor at Merton.

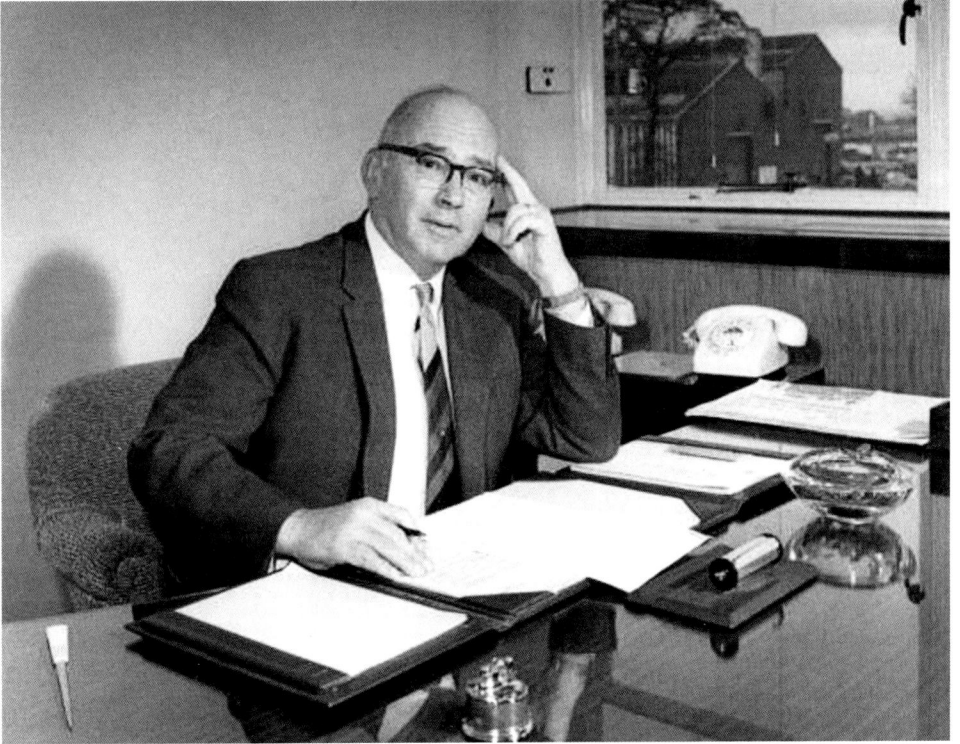

Figure 47. Medical philanthropist Ernest Foulkes at his desk in his company, Measuring and Scientific Equipment, which won a Queen's Award in 1966. Following the sale of the company in 1972 Foulkes endowed a foundation which has supported several hundred young scientists to study medicine.

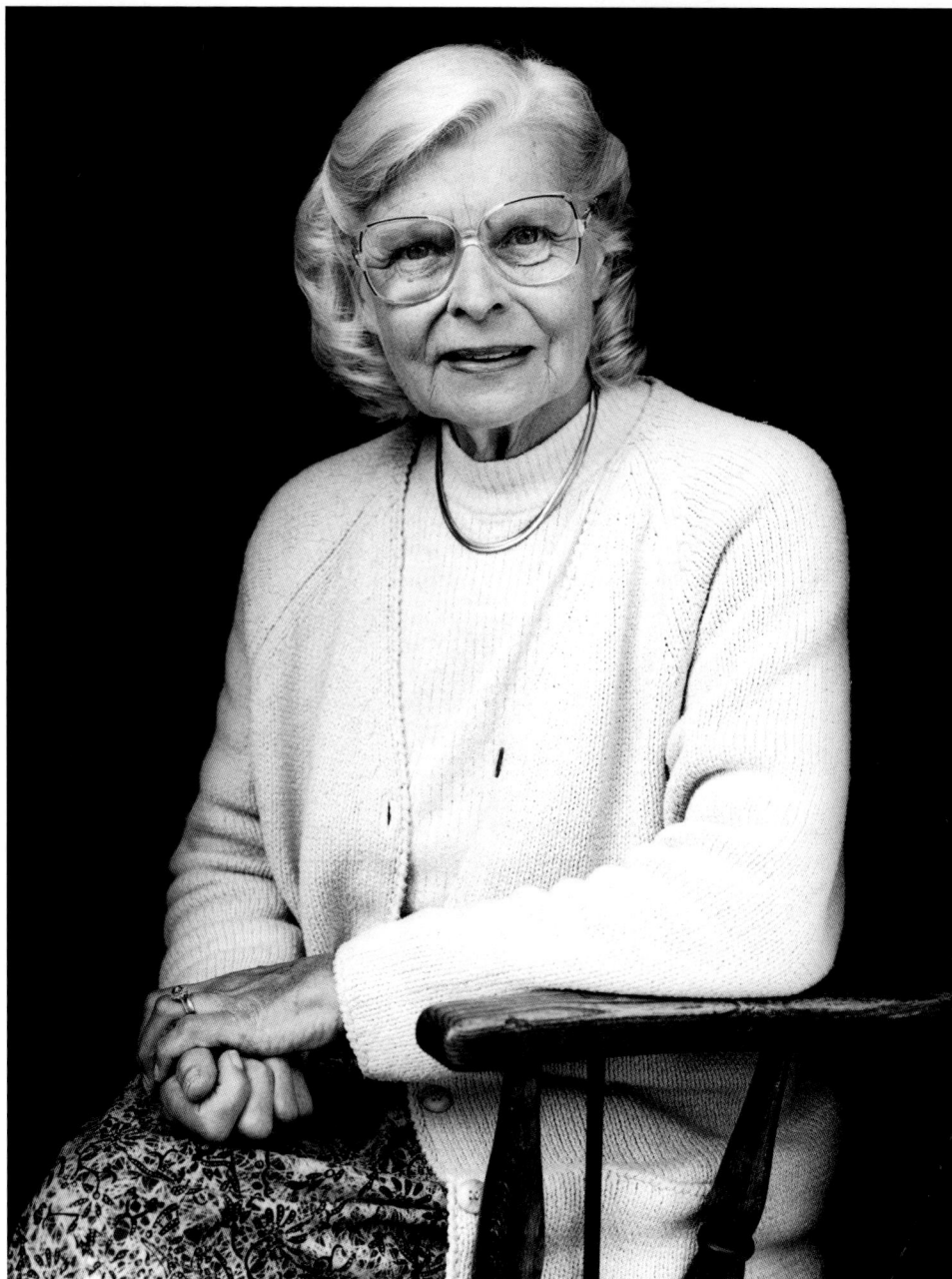

Figure 48. Dame Rosemary Rue photographed in 1996 by Nick Sinclair. Inspired by her own experiences of ill health and prejudice against women doctors, Dr Rue initiated a scheme in Oxford to help women doctors find part-time work and professional development in hospital medicine. The author found himself indebted to her as a lone male participant. She became President of the British Medical Association and a founding Fellow of Green College, Oxford.

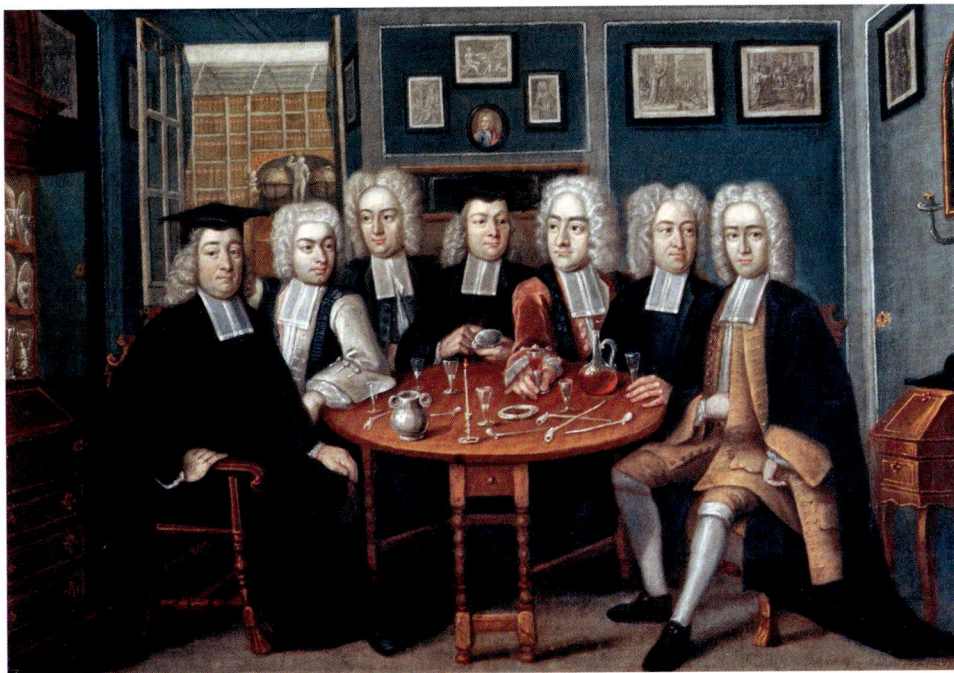

Figure 49. *Thomas Cockman (1675–1745), Master of University College, Oxford, and Fellows Sitting in the Old Master's Lodgings*, by Benjamin Ferrers (d. 1732). The successful party in the mastership dispute of the years 1722–9 is represented with Thomas Cockman in the centre, his brother John on the far left, and five supporting fellows. Cockman's dispute over the mastership with William Denison was finally resolved by the decision of a royal commission based upon the myth that the college had been founded by King Alfred the Great in the ninth century. The painting was acquired by the college in 2007 from descendants of John Cockman's son-in-law.

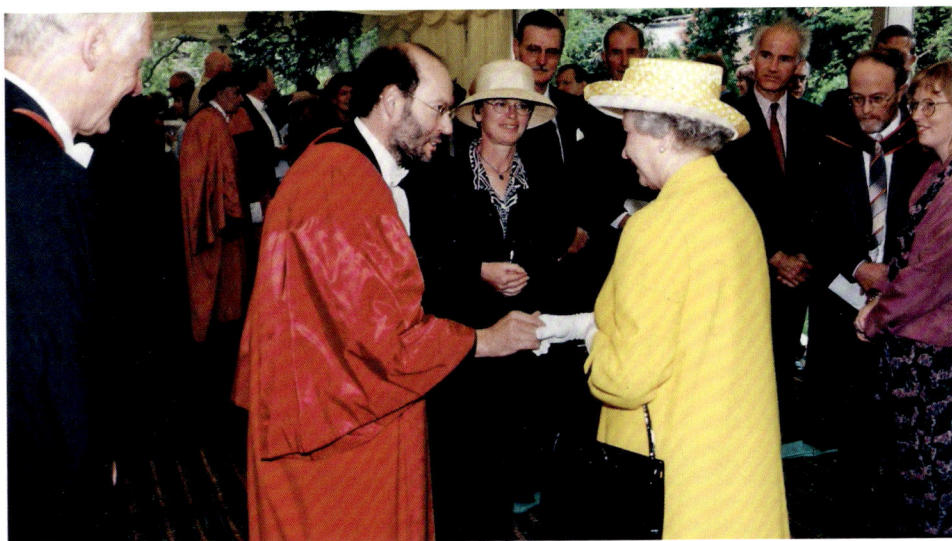

Figure 50. Visit of Her Majesty Queen Elizabeth II to University College on 21 May 1999 in the year of the college's 750th anniversary. Her Majesty is shown being greeted by the author and his wife, overseen from the left by the Master, Lord Butler.

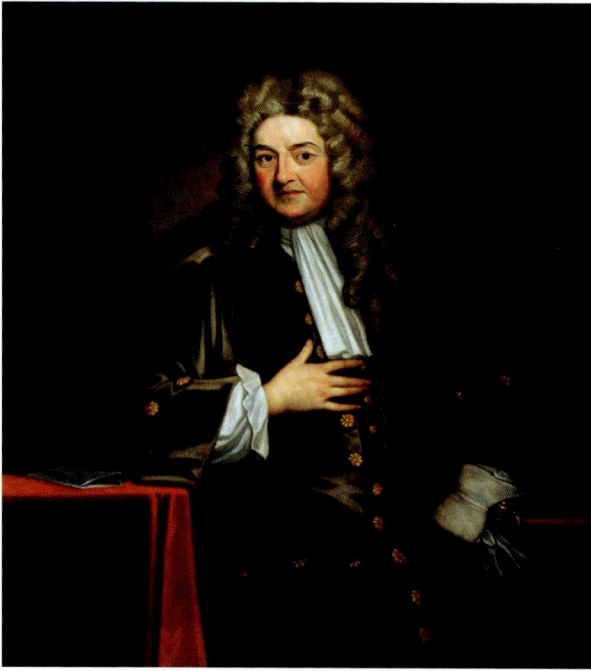

Figure 51. Portrait of John Radcliffe (1652–1714), (artist anonymous, after Kneller), undergraduate of Univ who became a successful and very wealthy doctor. He bequeathed money to build what is now Radcliffe Quadrangle in the college, to create two medical travelling fellowships and for several buildings in the University of Oxford.

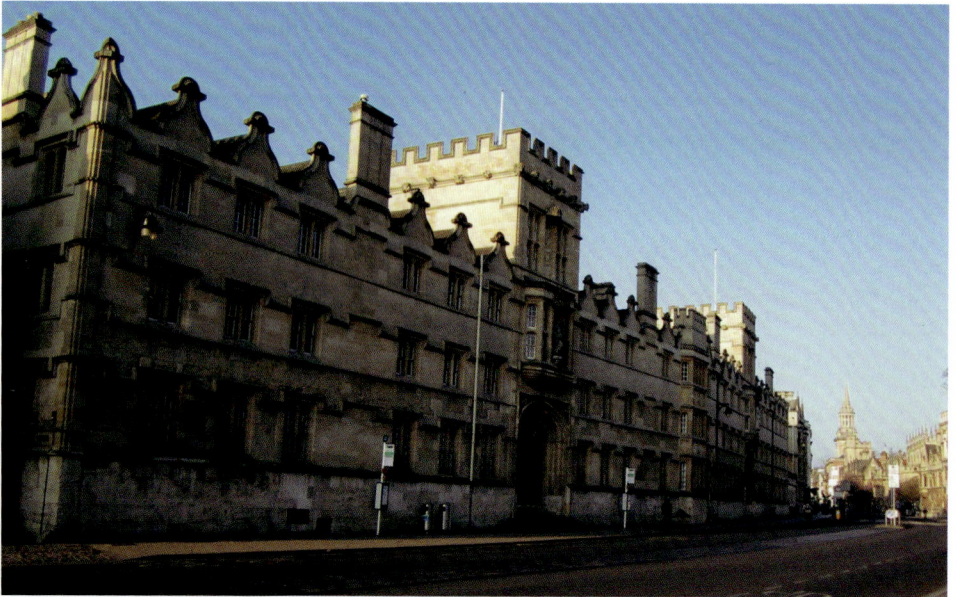

Figure 52. View from Oxford High Street of the Radcliffe Quadrangle of University College built from funds (£5,000) bequeathed to the college in Dr John Radcliffe's will of 1714. Radcliffe required that the new quadrangle should be "answerable to the front already built", which we see in the right-hand third of this image and which dates from nearly a century earlier. One amusing aspect of this 'quadrangle' is that barely a single room is truly rectangular because the structure follows a curve in the High Street.

almost any object whether alive or not) during some activity. To give an example from a living body, when I cycled from Hertford College to lectures in the engineering department, I performed *work* by turning the pedals and also gave off *heat* to the surrounding air, which was at a lower temperature. The loss of both together one could think of as a net reduction in the *internal energy* within my body. This comes from a store we associate with glycogen in muscles and fat (located we all know where). Interestingly, the rather poor efficiency with which the body conducts exercise results in the work done in cycling accounting for only about 20 per cent of the depletion of internal energy, heat loss being the other 80 per cent. We think of this as representing a mechanical efficiency in our muscles of 0.2, meaning that we are not very good at converting our store of internal energy into 'useful' work. When I got to my lectures, I found the tutor was often applying the first law of thermodynamics to car engines or gas turbines. Often these too had efficiencies of no more than 0.2. We were soon to learn a reason for this disappointing performance of both living and man-made machines: the second law.

The second law of thermodynamics touches not only on how inefficient our bodies are at (e.g.) cycling but also introduces us to the idea of *entropy*, which helps us to make progress understanding our body tissues. Physicists tell us that, when some heat H enters an object with temperature T then it can be useful to think of entropy increasing in the body by an amount H/T. Brace yourself for a statement that may seem at first so simplistic as to appear idiotic, but here we go. Let H be the heat moving from a hotter body with temperature T_{high} to a colder body with temperature T_{low}. If we follow the song's diktat that *heat cannot of itself pass from one body to a hotter body*, then it follows that the sum $[H/T_{low} - H/T_{high}]$ must always increase (because H/T_{low} is always a bigger number than H/T_{high}). There is no way that this can be juggled to give a negative number if both H and the Ts are positive numbers and the high temperature really is a larger number than the low temperature (you can try it if you like but you far better not-er!). This sum represents the change in entropy of the hot and cold bodies together, and we see that the entropy of the two together can *only ever increase*.

This statement might sound banal if it were not for the discovery by physicists that H/T is a precise quantitative measure of something inside an object that changes as heat flows in or out, namely the

degree of disorder or mixed-up-ness among the atoms and molecules
that constitute the body. These atoms and molecules busy themselves
in constant agitated motion and their disorder or mixed-up-ness is
greater at higher temperatures than at lower temperatures. In 1865,
well before the details of this disorder and motion of atoms and molecules were well appreciated, the scientist Rudolf Clausius invented
the name we use to describe it. He wanted to make it sound like
'energy' and decided to call it *entropy*, making use of Greek words ἡ
τροπή (*en-tropie*) to suggest an 'intrinsic transformation' that occurs
inside an object when heat flows in or out.[4] We can think of entropy
as a measure of something happening inside a body.

Now we know where the final line in the stanza of the song
comes from, even if Flanders and Swann did not give a very thorough
explanation: "Yeah, that's entropy, man!" And one thing our vocalists
failed to clarify is that the measure of temperature *T* that makes all
this fit together must be on a scale that goes from zero at the coldest
anything can be (minus 273 Celsius), and on upwards; this is called the
Kelvin scale. Normal human body temperature is 37 degrees on the
Celsius scale; on the Kelvin scale it is 310 degrees; just add 273.

So that is entropy. In the common imagination it is seen as something inscrutable and yet it is simple and pragmatic: its changes are
calculated by some heat divided by a temperature, two things that
are easily measured. Yet inscrutability cannot be denied because the
relationship between entropy as a measure of disorder among atoms
and molecules and the equations expressing that disorder is rather
impenetrable. We should not tackle it here; entropy is both simple
and complicated at the same time.

I am going to proceed to the Victorian era to tell how the laws
of thermodynamics helped to make sense of the odd behaviour of
animal tissues and then on to modern-day computational modelling
to find how entropy, in its role as a measure of disorder, has explained
how tissues can stretch at all.

Charles Roy and his five anomalies of body tissues

Back in 1880, thermodynamics was very much on the mind of Charles
Roy who was trying to get to the bottom of why animal tissues had
responses relating to heat that were the opposite of non-living materials. Roy was surprised by the fact that inanimate solids like metals

expand on heating and contract on cooling but animal tissues commonly did the opposite. A strip of human blood vessel moderately stretched and immersed in oil got *shorter* when *warmed* above room temperature and got *longer* when allowed to *cool* again. Vessels from a cow and sheep behaved in the same way.[5] These observations were to open up a whole new field of physiology.

Charles Smart Roy was a Scotsman who graduated in medicine from the University of Edinburgh in 1875. Young medics in those days could find themselves very quickly embroiled in the medical consequences of conflict: in 1876 he served as a surgeon in the Turkish Army in the Turko-Serbian war. Within a short period, he worked in Berlin, Strasbourg and Leipzig before moving to Cambridge in 1880, and then in 1881 to head a pathology laboratory in London. In 1884 he returned to Cambridge to become Professor of Pathology at the age of thirty. He had a short career, which was mainly in Cambridge, but he had an Oxford connection, illustrated by a photograph of him taken at the door of the Cambridge Pathological Laboratory with Oxford's Charles Sherrington in 1893 (Fig. 37).[6]

Sherrington was to go on to be Waynflete Professor of Physiology in Oxford in 1913, to receive the Nobel Prize for Physiology or Medicine in 1932, and to give his name to the Sherrington Building in Oxford in which I happen to be writing these lines. Roy was three years older than Sherrington and their careers shared some common tracks, including study in Cambridge, work in the laboratory of Professor Friedrich Goltz in Strasbourg, time as superintendents of the Brown Institute in London, and travel together to Spain in 1885 to investigate an epidemic of Asiatic cholera. Of time they spent in the building outside which they were photographed, Sherrington wrote of his companion: "I helped Roy in some experiments and recollect a physicist coming in and remarking on the clumsiness of our apparatus … Poor Roy was a very unpunctual person – he was failing then mentally and very forgetful … He was particularly dextrous with his fingers."[6] Indeed, it was the year before the photograph that Roy began to show signs of mental deterioration. He went on to die of a seizure aged only forty-three in 1897. Nevertheless, one might be envious of a scientifically very productive physiologist who, by the age of forty, could be said to be "a great traveller, an able linguist, an enthusiastic mountaineer, and a skilful sailor".[7]

Charles Roy's primary interest was in the function of the heart, circulation, kidney and spleen. Charles Sherrington was to make his name by elucidating the function of the nervous system. Their interests converged most productively in their 1890 paper together 'On the regulation of the blood-supply of the brain', in which they showed that "the blood-supply of any part of the cerebral tissue is varied in accordance with the activity of the chemical changes which underlie the functional action of that part".[8] That a relatively small region of brain can regulate its own blood flow is a central concept in modern neuroscience.

An enthusiastic climber and member of the Alpine Club, Roy was especially interested in whether the mountain sickness (as in Chapter Three) reported in 1892 by W. Martin Conway during an expedition to 23,000 feet (7,000 m) in the Karakoram could be attributed to heart failure or the "chemical change" of low oxygen on the brain and muscles.[9] His conclusion was that, at least as far as the heart was concerned, "there is no obvious reason why they should not have gone higher, if they could do it quietly enough and if they could choose their own times for going on and camping". This was a foresight into later research, which has confirmed that the heart continues to perform well, even at extreme altitude.

Roy became fascinated by the fact that animal tissues behaved in the opposite manner to non-living materials by contracting when warmed and expanding when cooled. It was during his time with Goltz in Strasbourg that he set about examining this behaviour in detail. In his paper of 1881 he presented this unexpected behaviour as a corollary that he *anticipated from the laws of thermodynamics* after observing another difference between living tissues and non-living materials; he had used one of Goltz's temperature-measuring devices (a "thermopile") to observe that animal tissues *give off heat when stretched* and *cool on recoil from stretch*. The 'ordinary rule' followed by inorganic materials Roy knew to be the opposite: they *become colder when stretched* and *become warmer when compressed*. So, in two ways, in a relationship first predicted by William Thomson in 1857 from the laws of thermodynamics, animal tissues showed the opposite behaviour to other materials.[10] Let's call these *Roy's anomalies numbers 1 and 2*. More were to come.

A further difference pops out of the pages of Roy's paper without much comment from him: animal tissues commonly *stretch a lot without breaking*. Roy's strip of human blood vessel (the aorta), which we met earlier, was originally extended by 32 per cent before starting the experiment, which showed how it shortened when heated and lengthened when cooled. Inanimate materials commonly stretch only a little before breaking and indeed, breaking them by stretching may be very difficult. Metals, stone, glass and modern-day plastics of our daily environment commonly deform very little in response to attempts to stretch them: not so some animal tissues, of which perhaps skin is the most accessible for observation. Skin stretches a lot without one having to pull too hard, a factor that aids much plastic surgery. The blood vessels, lungs and some ligaments do so too. I suggest for *Roy's anomaly number 3*: animal tissues tend to be *pliant*.

A fourth difference between animal tissues and inorganic substances to which Roy drew attention is that they do not obey Hooke's law, of which more in a moment. In fact, this difference exercised Roy to such an extent that it is the first feature of the "elasticity of animal tissues in general" that he mentions on the first page of his paper. Hooke's law, as summarised by Roy, is that "elongations produced by weights are proportionate to the weights employed". He asserted that "with animal tissues (excepting bone) this law does not hold good". This violation of Hooke's law Roy described as follows: "the increments in length, produced by the addition of successively increasing weights, diminish gradually in proportion to the weights employed". In other words, animal tissues get progressively more difficult to stretch.

This may sound like some trivial feature but much of significance is at stake. For body tissues the ability to resist stretch more vigorously as stretch gets greater can be thought of as a mechanism that prevents us becoming 'undone', to use the word with which the author of an account of an Antarctic expedition explains the condition known as scurvy.[11]

In scurvy, dietary deficiency of vitamin C leads to deterioration in the component of tissues that provides progressive resistance to stretch, *collagen*. We now know that many tissues contain fibres of collagen that are loose and crimped at low degrees of stretch and therefore have minimal influence on small extensions. However, the collagen fibres become taut at high stretch and then the taut collagen dominates the behaviour and limits further stretch. The expedition doctor onboard the *Belgica* and trapped in the ice of the Bellingshausen sea in the winter of 1898–9 noted that a diet of raw penguin meat alleviated the deterioration of body tissues in the crew. Fresh vegetables, a good source of vitamin C, were not available but raw meat substituted to some extent.

We see, therefore, that Roy's fourth anomaly of failure of tissues to obey Hooke's law was later to lead to a view of body tissues as composite materials containing different fibres, which have their own distinctive properties. Before I explore Roy's fifth anomaly, we need to take a detour into the seventeenth century to explore the background to Hooke's law and see how science was conducted at that time.

Robert Hooke: his location, his life and his law

Robert Hooke was intensely interested in tissues from living organisms but his law actually arose from preoccupation with something quite different, the building of a reliable timekeeper. The plaque on the High Street front of University College, Oxford, at which I have taught physiology for many years, introduces this most remarkable man (Fig. 38). It was set up in 1965 to celebrate the 300th anniversary of Hooke's most famous publication, his *Micrographia*, which included experiments conducted on the site.[12]

Born in 1635, son of the curate of Freshwater on the Isle of Wight where clocks, ships and rocks provided early childhood curiosities, Robert Hooke was apprenticed at the age of thirteen to the Dutch portraitist Peter Lely in London. He then took up schooling (using an inheritance from his recently deceased father) with Dr Richard Busby, headmaster of Westminster School.[13] Oxford's Christ Church now appears again in this account: Hooke was admitted there in 1653 as a chorister and 'servitor' to a wealthier student. Not long afterwards, in the winter of 1655–6, the aristocrat Robert Boyle set up lodgings in central Oxford and Hooke became his assistant. They were accommodated in a building that was a mixture of apothecary shop, guest house and laboratory. This building, known as Deep Hall, was owned by Christ Church but became the property of University College in the 1770s, hence the plaque we have on the college's wall.[14]

The site of Deep Hall is of considerable historical interest. The plaque suggests a confluence there of the physical and biological sciences, a division hidden in Hooke's day under the umbrella term 'natural philosophy'. We have found elsewhere that Deep Hall also witnessed a historic moment in anaesthesia (Chapter Six). It was demolished in 1809, an event captured in Turner's *High Street, Oxford* (1810), recently purchased by the Ashmolean Museum (Fig. 39); the site is now occupied by a statue of the poet Percy Bysshe Shelley.[15] This was set up in 1893 under a cupola representing the night sky and is accessible only via University College.[16] Current students may be most familiar with the location because it provides a blank wall along the High Street against which to queue for the popular mobile food vendor who parks there in the evenings.

Hooke was probably employed with Boyle at Deep Hall until the early 1660s when the centre of gravity of scientific discovery shifted to London: a "learned society", which gathered first after a lecture there by Wren in 1660 and received approval from King Charles II in 1663 as "The Royal Society of London for Improving Natural Knowledge". Boyle was a founder member who was happy for the inventive and dexterous Hooke to become the curator of experiments that were demonstrated at weekly meetings of the Society, and ultimately one of the Fellows. Hooke finally secured a modest income and accommodation as Gresham Professor of Geometry in London, one of the seven professors associated with what can be regarded as the first establishment of adult further education in the sixteenth century.[13] The extent to which Hooke made the transition from working-class servant to a status equivalent to the aristocratic virtuosi and gentleman scholars with whom he mixed is debatable.

Having settled in London, Hooke took an interest in something that had the potential to make him wealthy: the construction of a reliable timekeeper that would enable navigators at sea to identify their longitude with precision. It is here that we meet Hooke's law head-on. It was known that the time taken for a pendulum to complete one cycle of swinging (its period) could be used as a means of driving a clock 'escarpment' to enable fairly precise timekeeping. The period of swing of a pendulum depended upon its length. However, the period was increased by a small amount as the angle of the swing away from the vertical increased. For tiny angles the error is small; for swings of about 20 degrees it becomes an error of about 1 per cent. At sea, with the pitching and tossing in the boats of the time, the pendulum lost all its precision.

Hooke became an advocate of using a coiled spring instead of a pendulum, to overcome this source of error and to construct a device that could oscillate with a fixed period. He used a coiled metal spring attached to a stationary point in the timekeeper and the other end to a metal mass, which could oscillate around an axle. As the oscillation was dependent on the momentum and inertia of the mass, the period of the oscillations no longer depended on the position of a pendulum relative to the vertical. The reason for this is that the spring obeys Hooke's law: the force that the spring generates as the axle is twisted is in *exact* proportion to the angle through which the spiral spring is twisted. Add this advantage of a spring to the possibility of containing a spiral spring within a 'watch' that can be carried around, unlike devices containing a pendulum, and you have the potential to solve the longitude problem and make a fortune.

Historians have expended much time and effort on unravelling the relationships and correspondence linking Robert Hooke and the great Dutch scientist Christian Huygens to decide who might have priority over the discovery of the spring watch. In her entertaining account of the free flow of ideas between the Dutch Republic and England, Lisa Jardine reminds us that Huygens drew a sketch of a coiled spring in his notebook in January 1675 and wrote 'eureka' underneath it, and tells us that Huygens has long been credited with the invention of the spring watch.[17] In her book *Going Dutch* of 2008 she saw the question of priority as "still unresolved", noting that "Hooke's idea of using springs as isochronous regulators in place of pendulums was transmitted to Huygens" by members of the Society earlier, in 1665.

Excitement was raised among Hooke scholars by the unearthing of a "Hooke Folio". In 2006, Hooke's personal notes concerning the minutes of meetings of the Royal Society between 1661 and 1682 were found in a cupboard in Hampshire and were purchased by the Royal Society.[18] "It was one of those discoveries that historians of science dream of," wrote those who researched it, including Jardine. Among some 500 pages mostly in Hooke's hand (and never easy to read), one page stands out for our present theme. It is a draft of the minutes of the Society meeting of 23 June 1670 written by secretary Oldenburg and states: "The curator produced a pocket watch of a new contrivance devised by himself, which he affirmed should goe as equally as a pendulum ..." There are then notes pencilled in by Hooke (presumed to have been to help Oldenburg with an explanation), the beginnings of inking in the explanation by Oldenburg, and then a crossing-out of the whole section plus rubbing out of the pencil text. The official published Society minutes included nothing about the new device. These findings lend weight to the theory that Hooke's priority in the area of the spring watch was actually suppressed.

An intriguing aspect of the origin of Hooke's law tells us how protective scientists were of their priority claims (as we know they still are). On the first page of his publication in 1678 of *Lectures de potentia restitutiva, Or of Spring Explaining the Power of Springing Bodies* Hooke decodes an anagram that he had published two years earlier, not wishing at that time to let the cat out of the bag about what he had really discovered.[19] That was in the postscript of his 1676 book on "helioscopes and some other instruments", which was a bit of a rant about how his priority in a number of areas had not been recognised, and contains four anagrams of discoveries yet to be fully revealed. The anagram that interests us here is *ceiiinosssttuu*, said to be "The true Theory of Elasticity or Springiness".[20]

This is surely a very inventive way of both hiding a discovery and putting down a marker of having made it by a certain date! When decoded in *Of Spring* in 1678 the law ran as follows: *Ut tensio sic vis* or 'as the extension so the force' (*u* and *v* being interchangeable). Hooke's anagrams must have infuriated his scientific contemporaries even though their usage was well established in his day. One of the most famous anagrams is that of Galileo from 1610, which was 37 characters long and was used to both reveal and hide his discovery that Saturn appeared to be made of three bodies (we now recognise this as being the appearance of Saturn's rings). The anagram reached fame by being 'incorrectly' deciphered by Kepler as indicating that Mars has two moons, leading to the bizarre incident of Kepler deducing something that was eventually confirmed as true.[21]

Hooke's anagram put down a marker of discovery of Hooke's law in 1676. But he wanted everyone to know that he'd been thinking along these lines a lot earlier, probably while back in Oxford in 1660. In *Of Spring* he recounted that from the law:

appears the reason … why a Spring applied to the balance of a Watch doth make the Vibrations thereof equal, whether they be greater or smaller, one of which kind I shewed to the right Honourable the Lord Viscount *Brouncker*, the Honourable *Robert Boyle* Esq; and Sir *Robert Morey* in the year 1660. In order to have gotten Letters Patents for the use and benefit thereof.[19]

The patents did not happen, which may account for why the question of priority for the invention of the spring watch has persisted to the present day.

Recall that the failure of animal tissues to obey Hooke's law was what we can regard as *Roy's anomaly number 4* in our list of his differences between animal tissues and inorganic substances. This one Roy found "a very striking difference" but was unable to offer an explanation for it.[5] He did, however, make two suggestions: first, that a tissue such as the arterial wall "is marvellously well adapted to the circumstances under which it comes into play in the living animal". This suggestion came from his finding that large arteries were most compliant (i.e. most effective as a reservoir) at the arterial pressure normally found within them. He implied that this may be related to the deviation from Hooke's law, but did not demonstrate it. Second, he observed that his thermoelastic observations of animal tissues showed similarities with "caoutchouc" (natural rubber) and that the "molecular condition of animal tissues" might correspond to that of this naturally occurring substance. We shall see that Roy's *caoutchouc hypothesis* showed much foresight.

A diversion: what did Hooke look like?

Despite Hooke's role in science it has long been a source of irritation that we do not know what he looked like. He did possess a cantankerousness that may have persuaded the gentlemanly virtuosi among whom he worked to leave him off the wall even if a portrait had existed. He was, however, acquainted with the leading portraitists of his day. We have seen that he was briefly apprenticed to Sir Peter Lely. Hooke's incomplete but detailed diary recounts a visit to Lely on 27 December 1675. A closely associated portraitist and possible pupil of Lely, Mary Beale, worked in the style of Lely and was well known to Hooke. His diary of 20 April 1674 says: "At Boyles. He promised eye water and to sit at Mrs Beales. At Mrs Beales. Shavd and Cut hair at Youngs."[22] We note that Hooke was then thirty-eight years old. One reading of his words might be that he popped in to Beale to inform her that Boyle was planning to sit for a portrait with her. Another could be that a shave and cut might have been needed before sitting himself, especially if a wig was to be worn at the sitting. One does not have the impression that the busy day left time for a long sitting.

Boyle eventually made it for a sitting; the diary of 1 June 1675 states: "Mr Boyle promised to sit at Mrs Beales," and that of 8 June 1675 has the entry: "Dind with Mr. Boyle on pease. With Mr. Boyle to Mrs. Beal."[22] If a portrait of Boyle by Beale were ever completed, it is not now known, so we cannot tell if there were portraits of both Hooke and Boyle, now lost.

The archives have been scoured for a portrait of Hooke that may have hung in Gresham College, where the Royal Society was situated before moving to a new location after Hooke's death in 1703.[13, 23] Lisa Jardine thought she had identified a Hooke portrait and used it on the cover of her biography of Hooke but was soon caught out by the subject being identified as von Helmond.[24] Recently, Larry Griffing of Texas has made a case for Mary Beale's *Portrait of a Mathematician* being of Hooke.[25] Here the absence of a periwig, the presence of scientific instruments (arguably relating to Hooke's dispute with Newton), and details of the background scenery form part of Griffing's case. The problem with this attribution is the notion that Hooke would allow himself to be depicted in such an immature and wealthy dilettante manner. It would be interesting to know whether any information is to be found on the back of the portrait that might help with identification.

My own contribution to this search took me to the store-room of the National Gallery of Denmark in Copenhagen to look at both the front and the back of an unidentified *Portrait of a Man* in the style of Peter Lely and Mary Beale (Fig. 40).[26] This is an impressive portrait of a well-dressed and periwigged subject wearing a 1670s necktie. The subject looks out at us with the gravity and confidence of a person who knows his place in life but also displays an air of melancholy. However, its origins are unclear and it is not on display. The painting found its way to the museum from a Mrs Ellen Hansen of Copenhagen via the art dealer Ossip Kofman. How Mrs Hansen came upon it was unknown to the director of the gallery, Leo Swane, who described it in detail in 1939.[27] Swane had travelled to London in 1938 during an exhibition of seventeenth-century art and found nothing that came closer to the portrait than some later work by Sir Peter Lely, especially a close similarity to the portrait signed by Lely of the playwright William Wycherley (1640–1715), then in the National Gallery in London.

On the back of the Copenhagen portrait, in old writing, is to be

found: *Aetatis XXXVIII*. This Latin indicates that the age of the sitter
was thirty-eight. We know that Hooke visited Beale at that age. A
later inscription shows the coat of arms of the Rosenkranz family,
suggesting that it was once in their possession. Some would argue that
only titled or aristocratic gentlemen would be represented wearing a
periwig but the playwright Wycherley, with whose image the portrait
in question has been most closely identified, was a man of humble
origins and is bewigged in his Lely portrait. The artist Rita Greer has
made a career of painting imagined portraits of Robert Hooke in
many biographical settings, including Deep Hall; in all of these she
has seen fit to depict him with a wig or a very luxuriant youthful head
of hair.[28] Further investigation would need the expert opinion of an
art historian, or perhaps there may be a future revelation from some
as yet undiscovered source. Meanwhile, I like to imagine that Hooke
might have looked as dignified as the unidentified man in the store-
room in Copenhagen.

Rubber-like 'entropy elasticity' in body tissues and the paddywhack

The Boyle–Hooke plaque on the wall of University College tells us
that biological material interested Hooke: he observed the "cells"
in cork, a component of tree bark, illustrated in his *Micrographia* in
1665.[29] Indeed, this landmark book on a previously hidden microscopic
world concerns itself with biological materials from insects to blue
mould. We know from Hooke's *Of Spring* monograph that he had
been interested in organic "springy bodies" which included "Wood ...
Hair, Horns, Silk, Bones, Sinews ... and the like".[19] He was 200 years
too early to have come across another product of trees, the dried sap
in the form of *caoutchouc*, but we shall see that his speculations about
the vibrations of atoms were to have a direct bearing on its singular
properties. It was this amazing substance that was to provide a model
of arteries and other animal tissues.

   The tree product natural rubber displays a behaviour known as
entropy elasticity, which has provided an explanation for Roy's anoma-
lous behaviour of animal tissues. The reason for this is that the main
'stretchy' component of animal tissues is a substance known as *elastin*,
which displays an entropy elasticity that is the same as that of natural
rubber. It took 200 years for Hooke's law to be carefully applied to

animal tissues and a further hundred years for us to establish an explanation for Roy's observations on their strange thermoelastic behaviour.

My own involvement in this story came about because in 1974 my undergraduate tutor at Hertford College, Dr Gerry McCrum, was minded to recruit me to his laboratory for doctoral studies rather than let me take up a job offer from a company planning to build the Channel Tunnel. Norman Gerald McCrum (Fig. 41) was a 1951 graduate in physics of St Catherine's Society, Oxford (later St Catherine's *College*, and a college that I can also claim as one of my own since I later studied medicine there). McCrum's early career was in the United States and included research at DuPont, where he became expert in mechanical properties of new materials being developed by the company, such as nylon, polytetrafluoroethylene (PTFE) and Kevlar. In 1962 he moved to the Cavendish Laboratory in Cambridge where he developed new approaches to characterising the interrelationships between time- and temperature-dependence of the mechanical properties of the new materials. He came to Oxford in 1963 and developed an interest in the biological materials collagen and elastin. Gerry wanted the elastin 'entropy' problem investigated and Christ Church generously supported me with a senior scholarship for four years and also with a rooftop penthouse overlooking Tom Quad to encourage me.

It came as a surprise when Gerry (as I knew him) suggested early on in my doctoral project that I make a visit to a butcher's shop in Oxford's Covered Market. I was sent to find a large length of ligament from a cow known as the *ligamentum nuchae*, which Gerry knew to be a rich source of elastin. My asking with its Latin name did not succeed until the butcher realised that what I was asking for was the *paddywhack*, from which point he was very pleased to help. This ligament is a large midline structure at the back of the neck of animals and plays a major role in supporting the head when grazing. Had giraffes been available in Oxford's market an even more stunning specimen would have been available, but the paddywhack from a cow was quite long enough to provide samples several centimetres long. As the name suggests, it could be used to whack paddy, or give a spanking. The paddywhack is probably best known today as dog food, or at least dog entertainment. Dogs find dried yellow chunks of this ligament a tasty and lasting chew; both elastin, some 80 per cent of the ligament, and collagen, much of the remainder, take some demolition. The *ligamentum nuchae* in humans is much less impressive; we don't graze in quite the same manner although we do have a lot of elastin elsewhere in the body.

It looks as though we cannot escape Flanders and Swann, even with such an obscure piece of anatomy. They used a rewording of the well-known 'paddywhack' nursery rhyme song to tease General de Gaulle. The origins of 'This Old Man' appear to go back well into the nineteenth century. You may be intrigued to be introduced to the 'knick-knack' sound, which is the *playing the bones*, enthusiasm for which continues in the Rhythm Bones Society, which is very much alive in the United States.[30] A familiar version of the 'Old Man' song has ten stanzas; the first will do here as a reminder:

> This old man, he played one,
> He played knick-knack on my thumb;
> With a knick-knack paddywhack,
> Give a dog a bone,
> This old man came rolling home.

Flanders-and-Swann's corruption for the purpose of teasing the French and entertaining the British was entitled 'All Gall' and replaces 'paddywhack' with 'Armagnac' and other stirring suggestions.[31] Of General de Gaulle they sang:

> This old man, he played one,
> He played knick-knack at Verdun.
> Cognac, Armagnac,
> Burgundy and Beaune,
> This old man came rolling home.

My mission in Gerry's laboratory was to subject specimens of elastin to careful scrutiny. Would they get *shorter* when *warmed* above room temperature and get *longer* when allowed to *cool* again in the manner Roy had observed in his blood vessel? What did the laws of thermodynamics tell us about their molecular structure? This challenge was to occupy me for two of three years of doctoral studies. The mission may not sound complicated (or indeed gripping) but two hurdles stood in the way of detailed scrutiny and interestingly Roy had been ahead of the game in being aware of both of these. The first is that animal tissues contain water and *their properties depend upon how wet or swollen they are.* The second is that when a force is applied to stretch a tissue it takes time (sometimes a long time) for increase in length to occur. This can be thought of as a flow effect over time and is sometimes described as 'creep'. In short, Gerry was asking me to take these two phenomena into account – the effects of swelling and time – to find out what gives elastin those distinctive properties that Roy had discovered. To do this we had to take the argument to a molecular level in a manner that Roy was not equipped to do.

When a material, be it a metal or a ligament, is stretched, *work* is performed on the material. For most materials this work is *stored as internal energy* associated with the stretching of bonds between the atoms or molecules. For a few exceptional materials, including natural rubber and elastin, contrasting behaviour is seen. The work performed on stretching that material is not stored as internal energy, it is *given off as heat*. The change within the natural rubber or elastin is that the *entropy* of the material decreases (you will recall the change in entropy is $-H/T$). This signifies a decrease in the degree of disorder (mixed-up-ness) of the atoms or molecules of the material. In other words, most materials store lots of energy when stretched; natural rubber and elastin do not. They just become more organised internally, decrease their entropy, and give off heat.

This might not have interested people had it not been for what it tells us about the molecular structure of natural rubber and elastin. And let it not be thought that this topic is an intellectual backwater: the American chemist Paul Flory was awarded the Nobel Prize in Chemistry in 1974 for his work on the behaviour of large string-like molecules and it was his 1958 paper 'The elastic properties of elastin' that had provided preliminary evidence that elastin might be 'rubber-like' in displaying behaviour attributable to the disorder or entropy in *ligamentum nuchae.*[32]

The first task of new graduate students is to trawl over the work of the famous to look for subtleties and flaws that may have been missed, and this we did to dot the 'i's and cross the 't's of the earlier work. Indeed, the first year of my doctoral work on the *ligamentum*, 1974, was one of hot debate in which Flory reasserted his claim of rubber-like elasticity for elastin in the face of authors claiming something very different; these exchanges, especially with the most distinguished of his antagonists (Torkel Weis-Fogh), may have contributed to Weis-Fogh taking his own life in 1975.[33, 34]

At the heart of the matter was the notion that elastin might mimic natural rubber because of being made up of a network of long string-like molecules joined together at fairly infrequent points of 'cross-linking' (which stop the whole network falling apart). They would therefore be free to wriggle and writhe in a disordered manner, with the molecular motion we associate with thermal activity. We can think of this molecular mobility as conferring on the material a liquid-like deformability, which is constrained only by the cross-links between the strings.

One model of the individual molecules has been called 'random walk'. According to this, the shape taken up by a molecule looks, for a brief moment in time, like the path of a drunkard who takes many steps, each of which is random in its direction. For the drunkard this would clearly have to be in two dimensions on the ground; for the molecule it would be in three dimensions in space and represents the appearance of the molecule between the points where it is joined to other molecules at cross-links.

Consider a walk of 100 steps each of length 0.5 metres. A sober walker taking a straight line would cover a distance of 100 x 0.5 = 50 metres. How far would the drunkard travel in 100 steps from his starting point? A statistical calculation shows the answer to be on average $\sqrt{100}$ x 0.5 = 5 metres. (The reader can simulate random walks of this kind, using any number of random steps, with online software developed by Harukazu Yoshino of Osaka City University.[35]) If this mimics a string-like molecule in rubber then one can conclude that the material might stretch tenfold and, in doing so, the molecules go from the random-walk shape (with much disorder and entropy) to straight lines (which have only one shape and therefore minimum entropy). You may think that real rubbery materials rarely stretch to a tenfold extent, though reflecting on rubber bands, party balloons, rubber gloves or even condoms will remind one that this is not impossible. Using comparison with rubber we have a molecular explanation of how nature has been able to construct a pliant component of tissue (elastin) capable of stretching much more than other materials.

It came to be realised that if it is true that nature is capable of evolving rubber-like materials of this kind out of the *protein* molecules available for building a body, then something really remarkable has been achieved. This appeared all the more surprising because protein molecules, and their individual units of *amino acids* from which they are built, normally have a very high degree of architecture, allowing them to be building blocks with well-defined shapes, so one contrasting view was that it was unlikely that nature would build a molecule that was so ungainly as to be like the random walk of a drunkard.

Roy had noticed that body tissues dry out and change behaviour as they do so. His strategy for overcoming this problem was to immerse the specimen in olive oil so that "its condition as to moisture remained, therefore, unchanged during the experiment".[5] Flory also had a cunning way of studying *ligamentum nuchae*, which kept its volume fairly constant as its temperature changed: he immersed it in a mixture of glycol and water, in which it changed its volume very little over a wide range of temperature;[32] this simplified the equation he could use to analyse the behaviour. However, Flory's approach was rather unphysiological and possibly hid some internal energy changes that might accompany internal deviation from his 3:7 glycol:water mix occurring inside the elastin itself.

We set about studying elastin under the physiological condition of immersion in water. We took specimens of *ligamentum nuchae* from the butcher and pig's aorta from the abattoir. We used heat and chemical rinses to purify the elastin of these tissues, so removing the collagen and other material that others had left in place and which may have influenced their findings.

One striking thing about swelling needs a mention because it dominated all our measurements. When our elastin was cooled from 70°C to 0°C, its length (or any dimension) increased by 20 per cent. This represented a remarkable volume change of 73 per cent and was an astonishing verification of Roy's assertion that such tissues *expand on cooling*. The string-like molecules of elastin are capable of drawing in lots of water as they spread out, decreasing their entropy as they are cooled and give off heat. That is, the network of molecules behaves like a sponge. Around body temperature, elastin contains around 32 per cent of its weight as water.

Having taken this effect into account, we could identify a conclusion that agreed fairly well with the Nobel Prize-winning leader in the field. Flory had said that elastin was 100 per cent entropy elastic, storing no energy at all when stretched. We qualified this by finding

it to be 90 per cent entropy elastic while storing 10 per cent of the
work done in stretching it as internal energy.[36] In retrospect, publishing our findings in a paper with the title 'Elastin as a rubber' in a
journal with a large US audience may not have been the most apposite choice of words, the term 'rubber' having different connotations
across the Atlantic. Perhaps we should have gone for the word 'elastomer' instead.

However, elastin remains to some extent a mystery. Researchers continue to puzzle over whether elastin molecules contain some
more ordered regions, which could be associated with the 10 per cent
energy change that we observed.[37] Nature has produced other animal
tissues that are thought of as rubber-like, including the *resilin* associated with the ligaments in the wings of insects and *abductin* in the
hinges of shellfish. It would be easy to wander too far away from the
paddywhack if we were to explore the invertebrates, but an aside on
natural rubber helps to put our science into an intriguing historical
perspective.

The origins of rubber in South America

Natural rubber is a fascinating material. One might wonder how tree
sap became the mainstay of at least one aspect of civilisation: tyres for
motor transport (not to mention those party balloons, surgical gloves
and condoms). The French explorer and scientist Charles-Marie de
La Condamine was one of a team sent to South America by the Royal
Academy of Sciences of Paris in 1736. He observed Indians tapping
trees for a white resinous sap, which coagulated when exposed to air.
They worked it into torches that were resistant to being extinguished
by rain and that could burn for twelve hours. On hardening, the sap
would turn brown and pliant and the Indians moulded it into bottles to
carry water and other liquids.[38] In 1751 La Condamine gave a detailed
account to the Academy of how to recognise the trees and harvest the
sap, and suggested all sorts of uses for the novel (at least to the French)
material.[39] Boots and diving suits might be waterproofed; balloons
with a cannula attached might be an alternative to syringes; bouncing
balls could be made. The name of the material, *caoutchouc*, followed
the pronunciation by the indigenous population. By 1788, under that
name, *The New Royal Encyclopaedia* reported: "Of this gum, it is said,
the Chinese make elastic rings for lascivious purposes. Among us, it is

used by surgeons for injecting liquids, and by painters and others for rubbing out black lead pencil marks, and called India rubber."[40]

Caoutchouc is an unmodified natural product. It was not until 1839 that rubber as we know it today was created. In that year Goodyear discovered the process of vulcanisation, whereby the tree gum from *Hevea brasiliensis* could be converted into a highly pliant and deformable material but one with natural shape to which it would return spontaneously after being deformed. Vulcanisation introduces cross-links between the long string-like molecules; this leaves the molecules free to wriggle around and change shape between those cross-links but provides a network of interconnections, which prevents the molecules from flowing indefinitely as they would in a liquid. The long string-like molecules are made from individual links consisting of carbon and hydrogen atoms (polyisoprene). Before vulcanisation the gum can be thought of as *plastic* in the technical sense that its original shape is lost under prolonged loading. In fact, the untreated gum behaves as *elastic* for short loadings but not under very prolonged loads. A ball of gum will bounce when dropped on hard ground, but if left sitting on the ground for a very long time will tend to flow into a flat puddle.

So distinctive are the properties of this vulcanised substance that the term 'rubber-like' has come to refer to a state of matter, analogous to solid, liquid or gas. Experiments on natural rubber have shown the degree to which it is entropy elastic. It is very similar to elastin in this respect; when stretched, about 15 per cent of the work done on stretching it is stored as internal energy and 85 per cent is given off as heat. One view taken by materials scientists is that we should regard an 'ideal' rubber-like state as being 100 per cent entropy elastic; the word *elastomer* is sometimes used to describe this state. In that sense, natural rubber is only 85 per cent elastomer! Interestingly butyl rubber, one of the synthetic rubber-like materials, is probably the closest to being 'ideal' in the sense used here: it is 97 per cent entropy elastic.[41]

Molecules in motion

Robert Hooke was enthusiastic about material substances being as much about motion as about particles. In his monograph of 1678 *Of Spring* he wrote:

> I suppose then the sensible Universe to consist of body and motion. By Body I mean somewhat receptive and communicative of motion or progression ... for neither Extension nor Quantity, hardness nor softness, fluidity nor fixedness, Rarefaction nor Densation are the properties of Body, but of Motion or somewhat removed ... These two do always counterbalance each other in all the effects, appearances, and operations of Nature, and therefore it is not impossible but that they may be one and the same; for a little body with great motion is equivalent to a great body with little motion as to all its sensible effects in Nature.[19]

This is a very modern view of the nature of matter.

He goes on in that publication to illustrate his argument by asking the reader to:

> imagine a very thin plate of Iron, or the like, a foot square, to be moved with a Vibrative motion forwards and backwards the flat ways the length of a foot with so swift a motion as not to permit any other body to enter into that space within which it Vibrates, this will compose such an essence as I call in my sense a Cubick foot of sensible body.

He even proposes a possible frequency with which such movements might take place: one million per second. One might speculate that those early experiments in Oxford with the air pump celebrated on the plaque on the High Street (Fig. 38) contributed to the notion that not only gases consist of particles under motion. Hooke seems to have viewed all structures as consisting of much open space.

That early work with Boyle in Oxford led to the notion that the pressure of a gas varies inversely with its volume, assuming that its temperature does not change: 'Boyle's law'. The concept of particles having motion that increases with the reduction in volume seems to have been a basis for this law. The case has been made by Bernard Cohen that precedence should possibly have gone to Hooke himself, on the grounds that Hooke was the first experimentally to verify a pre-existing proposal of this relationship, even though Boyle published it.[42] Were that to have been the case, we should have two 'Hooke's laws', not the present one.

Physicists now think of the atoms that constitute molecules as vibrating with barely imaginable frequencies of more than 100 million million times per second (10^{14} Hertz) – rather faster than Hooke envisaged. The wonders of modern computation and imaging have been used by Sarah Rauscher and Régis Pomès from the University of Toronto to show us what the wriggling of elastin molecules might look like if slowed down to a speed we can follow. In their paper on the liquid structure of elastin, they have computed the motion of a bundle of twenty-seven elastin-like stringy molecules wrapped together with 39,000 water molecules to give us a video of the action.[37] Each molecule is depicted in its own colour. Over one minute (our time) we can watch the jerks, twitches and wriggles filling the one-tenth of a millionth of a second (molecular time) taking us in twenty-seven colours down close to those individual motions of the atoms that make up the molecular strings. It is not to be missed.

The string-like molecules of elastin and natural rubber make up a network that has properties of both a solid and a liquid. They are solids in the sense that they deform only to a limited degree; they are like liquids in that, when they are stretched, the molecules freely slide or flow over each other until constrained from further excursions by their cross-links. Before stretching the molecules look like the 'random walks' we visited earlier; when fully stretched the molecules are more nearly lying in straight lines. The extent to which the molecules are cross-linked affects the degree to which they are free to behave like long random walks. In fact, elastin usually does not like to be stretched to more than twice its length; the variable extensibility of rubber products in daily life, according to their degree of cross-linking, is well known to us: compare rubber bands with rubber erasers.

The liquid-like sliding of molecules in natural rubber and elastin can occur only if the *temperature is high enough* to keep the molecules in motion. The jerks, twitches and wriggles of the elastin molecules modelled by the Toronto researchers required the thermal motion of the molecules to be great enough for them not to 'freeze'. The same is true of natural rubber even though its polyisoprene molecules have a very different detailed structure from the protein molecules of elastin.

For elastin, unlike natural rubber, there is a second absolute requirement for the liquid-like sliding of molecules: the presence within the elastin of *enough water molecules* to lubricate the motion. The need for water inside elastin arises from a property of protein molecules being attracted to water. In contrast the polyisoprene molecules of natural rubber abhor water and distance themselves from it; they can remain in motion without it.

We are about to discover what happens to elastin and rubber when the temperature falls below what is required to keep the molecules in motion. For elastin, the same change occurs if the water content becomes inadequate. Both materials undergo a transition from being pliant and deformable to being like glass. For a body tissue a transition to being like glass is clearly not such a good idea.

Viscoelasticity: when molecular motion slows

The hybrid liquid–solid behaviour of elastin and natural rubber is a property we may think of as precarious because it can make the material more likely to fail if it is cooled. The slowing of the sliding motion of molecules by lowering the temperature causes the materials to display increasingly *viscous* behaviour, requiring time to complete any motion. We could list this as number five of Charles Roy's anomalies of animal tissues that set them apart from other materials.

> When, for example, a strip of arterial wall, hung up by one extremity is stretched, by means of weights attached to its lower end, it does not at once attain the full degree of expansion which will finally be produced by the weight employed, but, after having stretched rapidly to a certain length, it continues and with increasing slowness to elongate, until a point is reached at which the elasticity of the tissue exactly balances the weight used, and the two opposing forces are in equilibrium.[5]

Roy was not aware of any mention of this phenomenon in the physiological literature in English. He chose to describe it as the *elasticity after-action*, following the name used by Wilhelm Weber in 1835 to describe experiments on another biological material, silk: *elastische Nachwirkung*.[43] The favoured term for this property is now *viscoelasticity*. For Roy, the time-dependent behaviour was both a nuisance and intriguing. He was concerned that a long wait would be required for a specimen to reach "equilibrium" and that his specimens might dry out or even putrefy in the time required. He compromised by leaving five to ten minutes between measurements. *Roy's anomaly number 5* has become a whole field of materials science in its own right.

For Gerry McCrum and me too, this viscoelasticity was a prominent feature of the behaviour of elastin, which needed to be considered in the search for an accurate measure of entropy elasticity. Two to three hours of waiting were barely sufficient to convince us that Roy's 'equilibrium' had been reached when elastin was stretched, and so a process of stretching and then waiting, or 'annealing', at a high temperature (where the viscous behaviour was less marked), before exploring behaviour at lower temperatures, was adopted.[44]

Natural rubber had long been known to show viscoelasticity, and this becomes more pronounced as its temperature is lowered into a band known as the *glass-transition zone*, at the lower end of which rubber becomes brittle like glass. The zone for natural rubber is 20–30 degrees wide and a precise *glass-transition temperature* can be defined in the middle of the zone; for rubber it is about −70°C. Across the transition zone, as the temperature falls, the resistance to stretch put up by rubber (we call this the *Young's modulus*) increases a thousand-fold from that of pliant rubber to that of rigid glass. One of the consequences of this is that rubber can split or shatter if deformed fast; rapid stretching leads to the development of high stresses and a greater tendency for failure.

Since the glass-transition temperature for rubber is a temperature around those sometimes recorded near the poles, there has been concern in the Nunavut medical community about the storage of rubber condoms in extreme cold temperatures. On a more serious note, it was concluded that the disaster striking the *Challenger* Space Shuttle in 1986 was due to the extremely low launch temperature causing some rubber-like seals in the fuel tanks to be close to, or within, their glass-transition zone, and to fracture, permitting the escape of fuel.

Our Oxford studies showed that body temperature is within the glass-transition zone of elastin. This means that we have to think of body tissues as viscoelastic and in that sense flowing over time in response to the activities of the body, not just responding abruptly.[44] The duration of a heartbeat is far shorter than the time required for elastin in the arterial wall to reach an equilibrium degree of stretch. Movements of the lung elastic fibres with breathing are similarly fast, as can be the stretching of ligaments attached to joints. In all these settings the resistance the tissue offers to being stretched depends upon the speed with which it is being stretched, which in turn may affect its vulnerability to damage or failure.

Equally important for the pliant behaviour of elastin is its need to remain well hydrated with water. It needs to be both warm and wet. The paddywhack supplied for veterinary use is dried and dogs find it a challenging toy to chew; indeed, suppliers tend to warn that it is unsuitable for puppies. Dried *ligamentum nuchae* from the pet shop is a reminder to us that the extent to which elastin in its glass-transition zone is very dependent not only on its temperature but on how much water it contains. The requirement for water in elastin to remain rubber-like was especially well studied in Italy.

A fine early study of this phenomenon was published in 1968 by Lorenzo Gotte of the University of Padua, described in a biographical commemoration as "a pioneer of elastin".[45] He and his colleagues found that totally dry elastin had its glass transition at a temperature of about 185°C while elastin with 38 per cent water had the transition at about 0°C.[46] For the normal ~30 per cent water content the transition was around room temperature. In one experiment at room temperature (23°C) they demonstrated that the stiffness of elastin (its Young's modulus) increased 100-fold as the water content fell from 39 per cent to 28 per cent.[46] It follows that there are two ways in which to encourage the elastic tissues of your body to change from being rubber-like to being glass-like, or at least very viscous in their response to movement or stretch. One is to cool them down; the other is to dry them out.

Skin turgor: at last an explanation

It was to the properties of skin that my thoughts turned to try to understand the well-known but mysterious clinical sign of 'skin turgor'. In 1981 I wrote a paper for *The Lancet* to try to persuade the clinical world that the viscoelastic properties of elastin provided an explanation for a well-known bedside sign of dehydration: loss of skin turgor.[47] From time immemorial the appearance and texture of skin has helped physicians in their assessment of a patient's condition. A sign variously described as 'tenting', 'the sign of the ridge', 'loss of turgor' and 'inelastic skin' is helpful in assessing dehydration in patients. This sign consists of delay in the return of skin to its normal flat position after being raised for a few seconds by pinching between the examiner's fingers. Recoil of the skin after a modest degree of stretch is known to be achieved by fibres of elastin in the skin. Collagen is also present but it only becomes taut at higher degrees of extension, beyond which skin strongly resists further extension.

Healthy skin typically recoils within a couple of seconds after being pinched. In dehydration it may take much longer. An estimate from the published data on elastin suggested to me that a decrease of only 3.4 per cent in the wet weight would be expected to lead to a forty-fold slowing of the viscoelastic recoil, an estimate now cited in clinical guidance.[48, 49] An example of poor skin turgor in a seventy-four-year-old man lacking about 10 litres of body fluid and showing an approximately forty-second delay in the recoil of the skin of the abdomen can be seen in online images in the *New England Journal of Medicine*.[50] Caution is needed in the interpretation of this sign in the elderly because age alone can enhance the viscoelastic delay in the recoil of the skin due to the reduction in water content of elastin that occurs with increasing age.[47, 51]

Elastic fibres elsewhere in the body are less accessible than those in skin. Charles Roy concluded his study of 1881 by writing that "the elasticity of the arteries is much more readily modified by diseases affecting the general nutrition than is usually imagined". Regarding ageing he wrote: "With old age the elasticity of the arteries is found greatly modified in its characters, becoming less and less fitted to enable the arteries to fulfil their function in the economy."[5] The skin-turgor sign seems likely to be indicative of changes elsewhere in the elastin fibres of the body if they experience the exaggerated viscoelastic behaviour associated with ageing and disease.

Charles Roy: a role model

I have described *Roy's five anomalies* as we have followed his exploration of differences between animal and inanimate materials: contraction on heating; warming on stretching; pliancy; failure to obey Hooke's law; viscoelasticity with rubber–glass transition.

For medical students the stretchiness of body tissues has typically been close to the bottom of the list of topics which engender excitement. Near the top of the list has been 'Starling's law of the heart', the concept that the vigour with which the heart contracts depends upon the pressure to which it is filled by blood coming from the veins. This is associated with Ernest Starling (whom we met in Chapter Three) and his experiments on the dog's heart published in 1914.[52] What sadly goes unrecognised by most students and teachers of physiology is that Charles Roy described this phenomenon thirty-five years earlier in a detailed study on the frog heart in Berlin before he moved on to his body-tissue experiments in Strasburg.[53] Starling did not acknowledge Roy's contribution. Roy extensively cited those who had conducted similar experiments in the years before his own, and arguably gave the clearest account.[54, 55]

In this chapter I have celebrated Roy's observations on animal tissues. Like him, we have used the laws of thermodynamics to probe their strange behaviour. The laws have enabled us to progress to a molecular view of highly mobile molecules for which we traced one origin in Robert Hooke's seventeenth-century writings about "body and motion".

The elastin component of many body tissues has been found to have rubber-like behaviour that is precarious because of the proximity of tissue conditions of temperature and water content to a transition zone in which the pliant, stretchy elastin becomes more time-dependent in its behaviour, and consequently more resistant to deformation, more brittle and at greater risk of failure. There is more work to be done to relate these properties further to 'hardening of the arteries', loss of lung elastic tissue in chronic lung diseases, and those frequent musculo-skeletal injuries and deficiencies that are part of everyday life for many.

Had Roy's early death at the age of forty-three not taken him from the Cambridge Pathology Laboratory (Fig. 37) he might well have studied other animal tissues using the "clumsy" apparatus he shared with Sherrington, and offered more tantalising observations to interest us.

CHAPTER EIGHT

INHABITED RUINS[1]

Seven Colleges and an NHS Locker

Cause to be grateful

In 1971, in what seemed like time travel, I found myself deposited in mediaeval Oxford following a childhood daily home-school routine in buildings no older than the 1950s. I was unfamiliar with fan vaulting, gargoyles and crenellations. Imagine the surprise of finding yourself living within yards of a 'bridge of sighs' (Fig. 42), across which was the morning route to breakfast, which led on to the dining hall via a broad spiral staircase modelled on France's Château de Blois. True, the bridge and staircase were replicas constructed in the years 1887–1914, but the college had its origins in 1283, a dizzyingly long time back for a newly arrived eighteen-year-old.[2] Hertford College was the first of seven Oxford colleges of which I was to become a member. I have yet to meet anyone who claims a higher number so perhaps I am unique in this respect.

In this chapter I explore how it came about that Oxford provided me with an environment in which to immerse myself not only in architecture that enlivened my interest in history but also in the inspiring collection of scientific and medical endeavours and achievements I have explored in the preceding chapters. In this story several figures stand out: innovators and philanthropists who established new ways for academic life to flourish. These people profoundly influenced my life, like that of many others. In recounting a little about their lives and motivations I aim to express my gratitude.

A novel kind of school

First, I would like to visit a mentor from my school. Dr Kenneth Hutton was the founding headmaster of a distinctive institution known as Hatfield Technical School, where I spent seven formative years. Hutton had been educated at Winchester and Oxford and came to the headship as an experienced chemistry teacher, a speaker of Russian and German, and a passionate organist (Fig. 43). Though having little experience of the state school system, he brought an energy and enthusiasm to presiding over a brand-new, well-resourced, rare breed of school.[3]

While in 1940 the 'phoney war' moved to the 'blitz' and increasing depletion of Britain's manpower and infrastructure, in 1941 the British government, possibly somewhat optimistically, chose the President of St John's College Oxford, Cyril Norwood, to chair a report on "post-war education". The very wordy Norwood Report begins with five lines from Plato in the original Greek lauding education as ranking "foremost among blessings" and goes on to recommend restructuring state secondary school education to include "Technical Schools" alongside "Grammar Schools" and "Modern Schools". We read that "the function of the secondary Technical School should be primarily to give a training for entry into industry and commerce at the age of 16+ to meet the demands of local industrial conditions and, wherever possible and expedient, to offer facilities for advanced work from 16 to 18".[4] For all three types of school three elements of education were defined as: "(i) training of the body, (ii) training of character, (iii) training in habits of clear thought and clear expression of thought in the English language" (Welsh was not neglected), but one is hard-pressed to find in the report what the defining elements of a 'technical' education might be.

The Education Act of 1944 introduced this tripartite structure as envisaged in the Norwood Report but even by the 1960s few technical schools had been established; in 1965 only 3 per cent of all pupils in maintained secondary schools in England and Wales were to be found in technical schools, and that percentage was halved five years later.[5] In Hatfield, Hutton had his own ideas about what a technical school might promote, though it has been suggested that he had wanted it to be a grammar school.[6] This might explain the unique hybrid it actually became.

It was a co-educational school, opened in 1953 as the right-hand wing of a striking expanse of new buildings, the technical side of education being spurred on by generous provision of workshops and laboratories. The left-hand wing was Hatfield Technical *College*; its close proximity to the school provided an added stimulus to advanced activities: I recall using the Elliot computer in the college for a school project; this involved yards of punched-tape, as the input–output to a computer was at the time. In the school both sexes had access to metal-work (lathes and even a forge), woodwork and technical drawing. German was available for study from year one, with Russian, French, Italian, Spanish and Latin in later years. All pupils were to learn to swim in their first year and boys received a term of cooking lessons in their second year "so that they could fend for themselves".[6] Hutton himself participated in the then-novel practice of teaching eleven-year-olds about sexual intercourse.[3] Whether leaving school able to build a radio but knowing almost no chemistry could be regarded as a good 'technical' outcome for me, I remain unsure. My lack of chemistry at that stage is ironic given that Hutton himself not only published school chemistry texts but also a much-reprinted Pelican Original called *Chemistry: The Conquest of Materials,* of which I became aware only much later.[7]

In Chapter Three we met, in a previous time in Oxford, an admissions liaison between the future Everest climber George Mallory, then (in 1911) a history master at Charterhouse, and the Balliol College history don Francis Urquhart. This was a means by which school-masters could recommend pupils suitable for study at university. My departure from Hatfield and arrival in Oxford followed a similar arrangement: Dr Hutton's school was on the radar of an Oxford don, Dr Neil Tanner.

Hertford College: a new road to Oxford

Neil Tanner was an innovator in widening access to an Oxford education (Fig. 44). His name has been given to a break with tradition that shook up Oxford's dons: the 'Tanner scheme'.[8]

My view of this scheme as a participant was as follows: Mr Slaney, the then headmaster at Hatfield School, asked me into his office one day in 1970 and enquired whether I might like to pursue my interest in mathematics and physics by going to Oxford to study engineering. Not wishing to cause any embarrassment by declining, I soon found myself being driven by my university-naïve parents to a meeting (could it have constituted an interview?) with Dr McCrum, the engineering tutor at Hertford College. I was swallowed by a large armchair in his room, 'Old Buildings Staircase 1', as I was asked about how atoms might pack together to form a crystal.

A few days later, a letter arrived offering me a place to read Engineering Science, as Oxford (I felt strangely) called the subject. This was conditional upon obtaining two passes (grade E or above) at A level. The college perspective perhaps tells us more about what was going on. Neil Tanner was a feisty Australian physicist who had become Tutor for Admissions in 1964. With a few experimental exceptions, involving tiny numbers of students from maintained schools in targeted regions, admission to Oxford and Cambridge colleges at that time required sitting an entrance examination, for which independent (private) schools usually provided special tuition as part of a third year of sixth-form studies. Speaking in 1970 of grammar-school headmasters, Tanner noted how "unhappy" they were "about the Oxbridge prospects of their favourite pupils. They argued that they could neither staff an Oxbridge coaching organisation nor persuade their pupils to stay for a seventh term in the sixth-form, and for these reasons were at a disadvantage."[9]

Furthermore: "At the time Hertford was not the most affluent of colleges academically speaking and with more than its fair share of angry young Fellows, was in the rare state, for an Oxford college, of being ready for change."[9] In 1968 the college went public with a plan to admit up to a quarter of its newcomers on the basis only of school recommendation and an interview, "whereupon there descended upon the College's collective heads all things mentionable and unmentionable. ... angry words were spoken, and Hertford was condemned by a massive majority."[9] Those applying to be admitted this way were free to attempt the entrance examination for the benefit of obtaining a small financial award, as I chose to do in 1970.

This scheme ran until 1985 and admitted about 450 undergraduates. The college, along with four others, went 'mixed' and admitted women from 1975, agreeing to defer including women in the Tanner scheme by two years so as not to upset the women-only colleges. Analyses showed the academic results of Hertford College to be rocketing upwards: "one of the most talked-about transformations in the standing of a college in the modern history of the university".[8]

Since then the entrance examination has first been abandoned and then reintroduced in many formats, and questions about the propriety of different routes of admission have never been absent from an annual round of collegiate heart-searching. I was in the thick of this later as Tutor for Admissions for my then college University College ('Univ') for several years. Individual colleges continue to explore their own initiatives for harvesting those of potential or proven academic ability in combination with fairness (often thought of in terms of compensation for 'disadvantage'). In 2020 one scheme, Opportunity Oxford, spread to the whole university from a trial in my college.[10] This is likely to be a never-ending story of adaptation, reflecting changing social mores, cultural battles within society and political manipulation.

Neil Tanner was more than a revolutionary tutor for admissions. In 2015, six years after his death, Arthur McDonald of the Sudbury Neutrino Observatory Ontario was awarded the Nobel Prize for Physics in the name of the team as a whole, which included the Oxford group that Neil Tanner had led.

The tutorial: an old way of teaching

Neil Tanner helped to transport me into a world of bridge structures, fluid flows, control loops and electrical circuits; this was to be solid grounding for my later exposure to the medical science of physiology.

I noted earlier my arrival in the mediaeval world of old buildings; was the method of teaching as ancient as the buildings around me? From my first week the 'tutorial' loomed large and for years set the pace of academic work and consequently of everything else. The tutorial is a distinctive form of teaching in which a tutor meets frequently with a student over most of the course of their study either on their own or in a small group. In his history of the University of Oxford, Laurence Brockliss traces the origin of this practice to the way students were accommodated 500 years ago.

> Oxford and Cambridge were Europe's only universities where town and gown were segregated: as in the fifteenth century, all members of the two universities had to reside in a college or hall. This had a profound effect on the way arts tuition developed across the period. ... The colleges appointed their own lecturers in the main branches of the course, especially in the subjects covered by the BA [Bachelor of Arts] curriculum, and insisted that each undergraduate was looked after by a personal

tutor. The Oxbridge tutorial system that had come into being by
the end of the sixteenth century was unique. … only at Oxford
and Cambridge was every student following the first part of the
arts course put under the care of an older member of the university, who was supposed to police behaviour, look after his
finances, and closely supervise his academic progress.[11]

Given how rare such teaching is in other universities, it is interesting to explore further how the tutorial developed. My own student
experience, eventually embracing the study of both engineering and
then medicine, was that written work was invariably set for a weekly
hour-long tutorial, and that in the tutorial I was either alone with
the tutor or was taught with one other student. Sometimes I faced
two such tutorials in a week in different topics with different tutors.
Brockliss identifies several steps in the evolution of such teaching.
One is associated with radical reforms that took place in the university leading up to the Oxford University Act of Parliament in 1854:

Tutors, before mid-nineteenth century, seldom set written work.
It was the custom in the 1830s for the undergraduates as a body
to be given an essay or theme to do each week, but the respon-
sibility for setting and marking their efforts lay with the dean.
It was only by the 1840s … that the task began to be usurped by
some of the younger tutors, who developed it into a much more
individually tailored exercise.[11]

One of the most famous pioneering tutors was Benjamin Jowett
of Balliol College. He became a tutor in 1842 and held the office until
he became Master of Balliol from 1870 until his death in 1893. The
reformers' efforts contributed to the broadening of the intake of
students to the middle classes and of the syllabus beyond reading
classical literature to include mathematics and the physical sciences.
A change in emphasis was also taking place from the tutorial seen
as a nurturing of students' souls by ordained Anglican fellows to a
more liberal homosocial relationship in which Hellenism, especially
an appreciation of Plato, played a role.[12] The weekly regularity of
tutorial hours was probably established in the 1870s, when contracts
were established between colleges and tutors. Over 150 years since
then the standard contractual arrangement has changed little, with

a humanities tutor teaching for some twelve hours per week and a science tutor six hours per week. Tutors often shared duties between college and university, and so the hours varied according to other responsibilities.

The nature of the work may surprise some. A few tutors in the humanities continue the nineteenth-century tradition of having the student read an essay aloud in the tutorial, commenting on the content as it is read, or upon completion. It is from such an arrangement that stories arise of students not knowing how to respond when a tutor falls asleep as they read. The more widespread practice now is for work to be handed in in advance of the tutorial and returned with comments at the meeting.

A tutorial in physical sciences such as engineering is commonly based upon a sheet of problems in which the language of discourse is mathematics. The typical week's work consists of a sheet of ten problems. Each requires the formulation of the problem and its solution in mathematical terms. We might be dealing, for example, with the speed with which a wave travels down a channel of water, or whether a concrete bridge can sustain a given load. Infrequently the week's assignment may involve some prose, a description perhaps of the principles underlying a nuclear reactor.

I recall that as engineering students we developed a strategy designed to suit both ourselves and our tutor. Of ten increasingly challenging problems we might decide to complete about seven and claim to need the tutor's help to complete the remaining three. This meant not having to work too hard in advance of the tutorial and thereby giving the tutor something to do to fill the time! After all, completing the ten problems might embarrass a tutorial partner or leave little to discuss in the tutorial. Later, as a tutor in engineering, I had to cope both with students who completed virtually none of the work and with those who had sailed through the complete problem sheet. This involved having some interesting extension material up one's sleeve for the able and interested.

My observation has been that some older tutors found this problem-based teaching more challenging than younger tutors, themselves fresh from the very same exams in which such problems were set. As you might imagine, there was always a scramble for the 'solutions' to problem sheets, the contents of which tended to change only slowly as years went by, sometimes incorporating novel problems from examination papers. The 'solution sheets' circulated clandestinely and tutees thought it best to keep quiet about their use.

On the whole, I think it is fair to say that the undergraduate course material in the physical sciences has remained focused on textbooks in which are found solutions to classical problems which have long been available. It was and remains rare to consult original scientific literature in the early years of these courses. One might provocatively liken them to the reading of the classical texts before the mid-nineteenth century but regard the material as more useful for solving engineering problems.

What needs further explanation is that our problem-solving was not only extracted from textbooks and clandestine solution sheets. Most mornings at 9 a.m. a long trail of undergraduates could and can be seen heading in the direction of the science area for the first lecture of the day, one of maybe a dozen or so in the week. Unlike attendance at tutorials, presence at lectures is not compulsory but for perhaps the majority of students is an established part of soaking up a syllabus presented in a systematic manner. Students rarely seen at lectures are often the ones who find themselves unable to satisfy the examiners and so make an early departure from their studies.

Wycliffe Hall: among the bishops-to-be

Colleges naturally compete to attract student applications. One of the ways they do this is to offer inexpensive accommodation. Recent years have seen colleges build the equivalent of whole villages in their bid to house an increasing intake. In the early 1970s Hertford College was able to offer me only two years of accommodation for my three-year course, both close to the 'bridge of sighs'.

In the third year, my peers studying engineering set up home together in shared rented housing. I was more of a loner and took the offer of a garret accessible only by ladder in the roof of a theological college. Wycliffe Hall is one of Oxford's permanent private halls, founded in 1877 and named after the fourteenth-century Bible translator John Wycliffe, who spent much of his life in Oxford. The hall's accommodation was assembled from red-brick Victorian private houses and a convent, which accounts for its collection of nooks and crannies, some of which may once have been servants' quarters. My tiny hideaway was too modest to be suitable for the ordinands and was rented out for a small fee. Here I was secluded with my engineering textbooks between breakfasting with future bishops and sometimes observing their rituals in chapel before supper. One day my social horizons were broadened when I observed from my garret window one of the theology tutors holding a tutorial on a rooftop balcony with all participants naked in the summer sun. One is reminded of the Hellenism of the late-Victorian tutorial.

The distractions of the internet and the profusion of social meeting places with which we are familiar today did not then exist and being isolated some distance from the popular King's Arms pub encouraged me to perform well in my Finals and set me on a course to become a tutor myself, though my own tutorials have never been held without clothing.

Christ Church: under the eyes of King Henry VIII

The manner in which science is recorded and recognised may surprise some. The big names who receive credit for discoveries are often not those who conduct the experiments for which they are lauded. Graduate students, often studying for a doctorate, spend long hours with sophisticated machinery pursuing the suggestions of their desk-bound or conference-bound seniors, so senior scientists are always on the lookout to recruit research students.

Thus it was that my undergraduate engineering tutor at Hertford College, Dr Gerry McCrum, persuaded me not to follow my two early objectives – becoming a schoolteacher or helping to build the Channel Tunnel – and instead become one of his small team of research students. The question I faced in 1974 was how to fund three years of doctoral research. The answer came in the form of a generous scholarship; several of the wealthier Oxford colleges offer support to those wishing to start an academic career in the form of Senior Scholarships (the term 'Senior' distinguishing them from scholarships awarded to undergraduates). I was fortunate to secure one for four years, which also provided accommodation in Christ Church.

It was a culture shock as I moved from the attic of a relatively modest Victorian theological college to a flat in arguably the grandest theological college in the country, originally founded by Cardinal Wolsey in 1525 (Fig. 45). This unique institution combines the Dean and canons of Oxford's cathedral chapter with a college that is similar to the thirty or so other colleges in Oxford in admitting students to study a wide range of subjects in both the sciences and humanities. The Dean is the head of the college and the cathedral acts as the college chapel.

I was now attending the same college as Robert Hooke and enjoying the view from my balcony of the bell tower built by Christopher Wren. The living company was as engaging as the long-deceased: a strong educational feature of Oxford colleges is the mix one experiences of students and staff from the full breadth of academic subjects. I could breakfast with my astrophysicist doctoral-student colleague and then have dinner with canons and dons (at Christ Church, confusingly called 'Students') under the gaze of founder Henry VIII in Oxford's largest dining hall.

My life was not all socialising. My years at Christ Church were spent in research as described in Chapter Seven and I combined this with being a tutor in engineering at Hertford College. Gerry McCrum was both my 'line manager' at the head of a small team of tutors and also my doctoral supervisor. He was a superb mentor who created sound working conditions in which to conduct experiments and provided rigorous academic supervision. This opportunity to study and research under a world authority is a major factor in making Oxford so rewarding.

In the pre-word-processor age Gerry taught me an eccentric way of writing a scientific paper, which lasted me for a decade and helped me assemble a book: the paper-scroll washing-line technique. Gerry would write a paper by hand in the form of a long scroll of sheets of paper stapled together top to bottom, and suspended about his office on lengths of string. Insertions and deletions were conducted by cutting out and stapling in sections until the final draft took the form of a scroll several or many feet long like washing on the lines filling his office. This would then be passed to his secretary (academics had secretaries in those days) for preparation in courier script on a typewriter. Our first paper together was published in *Nature*; I think I can see it to this day in draft hanging across Gerry's office.

After three years of research and a couple of publications it was time to submit a thesis and navigate the ordeal of having it examined. The supervisor of a doctoral student gets labour free of charge for several years, in return for which they have an important favour to make in return; they have to nominate examiners who are likely to award the candidate a pass. The exam is usually conducted as follows: the candidate writes a thesis, typically two to three hundred pages of text and figures. This begins with acknowledgements in which the student usually says what a wonderful supervisor they have had, then reviews the field of past work, and finally gets into the method and results meat of the original contribution claimed by the candidate. If the candidate wants to show off, a couple of published papers which resulted from the work may be bound into the volume.

The examiners then hold an oral *viva voce* examination, commonly lasting a couple of hours or more and in some universities conducted in gowns, hoods, bow ties and mortarboards. The oral examination has three aims. The first is to explore whether the candidate has a sound knowledge of the field of work. Second, examiners check whether the thesis is the candidate's own work. The third aim is to confirm that the student has made an original contribution. The examiners write a report for the university, in which they make a recommendation: pass, fail, lower degree, or come again later.

I have known some embarrassments in this process. Supervisor and friends may gather around with champagne after the viva to congratulate the candidate only later to find that the candidate has not passed. As examiner, I once found a thesis so poorly written that I reported to the university in question that I regarded it 'un-*viva*-able'. I was encouraged to demit as examiner soon to find that the candidate passed with other examiners with no concerns. Once we found that a thesis was not from the hand of the candidate presenting it. Generally, though, my experience has been that scientific doctoral theses represent dedication to a topic amounting to many years of work and make a commendable original contribution to their field.

In 1977 my doctoral supervisor recommended Dr Derek Bergel to be an examiner (Fig. 46). One can think of him as a latter-day Charles Roy, to whose genius some of Chapter Seven of this book is devoted. Like Roy, Bergel was fascinated by the properties of arteries. In 1960, after qualifying in medicine at St Bartholomew's Medical Centre, Bergel wrote his PhD thesis entitled 'The visco-elastic properties of the arterial wall', needless to say citing Roy.[13] Bergel came to Oxford in 1968 and took up a fellowship at St Catherine's College where he tutored in medicine. Of his classic text of 1972, *Cardiovascular Fluid Mechanics*, it has been suggested that "William Harvey would have taken delight in reading."[14] I concur.

Bergel and his co-examiner recommended that my doctoral thesis, 'Rubber-like elasticity in the body',[15] be given the thumbs-up and later in the autumn of 1978 I found myself a pre-clinical medical student at St Catherine's College, writing essays for none other than Derek Bergel. He had generously agreed to admit me to the medical course on the understanding that I got myself qualified for entry; I had no biology or chemistry. Off I went to the Oxford College of Further Education (I do not count this as my eighth Oxford college) to take classes for O-level biology. For chemistry, the University of Oxford deemed appropriate a 'Qualifying Examination in Zoology for Medical Students', for which I was a lone candidate. I scraped through on a viva characterised by a large dose of sympathy from the examiners for schooling that had left me ignorant of the properties of glycerol.

Ernest Foulkes, medical philanthropist

Medicine studied as a graduate required fees that were beyond my means. I had to look for financial support. It was an elderly industrialist called Ernest Foulkes who came to my rescue; receipt of a fellowship from Ernest Foulkes, with its associated financial help, led to my opportunity to study medicine.

Born in Frankfurt in 1902, Foulkes followed school by studying at the Technische Hochschule in Berlin where he specialised in factory planning. In 1929 he obtained a doctorate in engineering. Observing the rise of Nazism, he left Germany for Spain in 1933, where he was joined by his fiancée, Senta. They married, soon found that the Spanish political climate was becoming as threatening as that in Germany, and so in 1936 they came to Britain. Starting out with minimal resources but much determination, Foulkes established a manufacturing company, Machine Shop Equipment (MSE), to make machine tools, which were then increasingly in demand. In spite of this, when war with Germany broke out in 1939, bureaucracy decreed that he be interned on the Isle of Man[16] as a 'friendly enemy alien' while Senta retained her freedom and worked to get him an early release after one year.[17]

After the war MSE billed itself as Measuring and Scientific Equipment and established itself as a leader in producing centrifuges for laboratory use. In 1966 MSE won one of the first Queen's Awards to Industry for export achievement. In Figure 47 we see Foulkes in the

1960s sitting at his desk in the company office in Crawley. In 1972 MSE was sold to Fisons; the sale enabled Foulkes to establish a foundation for the "training of scientists and others to study medicine and of medical and other men and women to study science and/or technology".[18] The first seven fellowships of the Foulkes Foundation were awarded in 1975 and a further eight in 1976; mine was one of nine awarded in 1977, the year in which Foulkes became CBE. All awards in those years, and many subsequently, have been to scientists with a doctorate or master's degree who wished to study medicine. When an assessment of the impact of Foulkes' philanthropy is undertaken (as surely, after fifty years, it soon must be), it will be fascinating to find out what careers have ensued for the 500 or so beneficiaries.

St Catherine's College: smoke-filled tutorials

St Catherine's College was my next culture shock. Still living in Christ Church, I made my way across the town to have tutorials with Bergel in a modernist college resembling a glasshouse. St Catherine's was founded in 1962 and its renowned buildings were designed by the Danish architect Arne Jacobsen. Added to the architectural novelty for me was that Bergel was rarely detached from his pipe and his pipe was often alight. Tutorials were characterised by a cycle of lighting and extinguishing, and consequently periods of smoke filling Bergel's tiny Jacobsen-style room. These were wonderful occasions in which I was beginning to learn some physiology, soon to be supplemented by teaching in neuroscience by Dr John Morris; he sometimes saw me in the anatomy department where a background odour of the formaldehyde used to preserve dead bodies made a not-too-pleasing alternative to tobacco smoke.

Earlier in this chapter we met the admissions initiative of Neil Tanner, which brought me and some hundreds of state-educated boys and girls to Oxford. It is interesting to note that St Catherine's has its origins in a similar admissions initiative 100 years earlier, in 1868, when a 'Delegacy for Unattached Students' was formed. This arrangement, created in response to the recommendation of a royal commission of 1852, enabled students to be members of the university without being a member of a college, thus avoiding the prohibitive costs of Oxford college living.[19] Several thousand students benefited from the 'delegacy' route into Oxford, including John Vane (later,

Sir John), winner of the 1982 Nobel Prize in Physiology or Medicine, who came to Oxford in 1946 to study pharmacology.

The medicine tutorial: nowhere to hide

I earlier depicted the tutorial in the physical sciences as heavily focused on the weekly 'problem sheet', for which the language of discourse was mathematics. On starting medicine, I came to see that the tutorial in that faculty was a different beast. The language of discourse was prose rather than mathematics, often assisted by anatomical diagrams or graphs displaying data. Even in the few areas of physiology or pharmacology to which mathematical rigour can be applied, asking medical students to write equations rather than words is usually greeted with the sentiment that maths was left behind at school and is now long forgotten.

A weekly essay remains the tradition, with the tutor hoping that the student will formulate something in their own words and express their engagement with the topic, rather than cutting-and-pasting from a textbook or online material, or using the fruits of artificial intelligence. The student might be asked to explain the mechanism by which a nerve cell transmits a pulse of electrical information from toe to spinal cord, or to describe the rationale behind the drug treatment of asthma. It would be common for a first-year undergraduate to be directed to textbooks to research an essay topic of this kind but soon the emphasis shifts towards papers in the scientific journals, which we might call primary sources.

This essay is then fair game for interrogation. The tutor can explore whether it is the student's own work and what level of understanding they bring to the topic. It is this 'nowhere-to-hide' property of the Oxford essay-based tutorial that can make it such a robust vehicle for learning in depth. For some with the skill it can be a practice ground for bluffing as camouflage for woeful preparation, as has been reported to be the case for some of our recent political leaders by their then tutors.[20]

In the medical sciences the transition to primary sources in scientific journals occurs mainly in the second year of a three-year pre-clinical course and by year three the reading is almost exclusively from primary sources. One of the consequences of this high degree of specialisation is the more limited extent to which an individual tutor might attempt to teach the syllabus. In the physical sciences it is common for a tutor to cover a large proportion of a student's tutorial topics well into a third year of a course. In the medical sciences third-year students tend to be tossed from one tutor to another, visiting several colleges and departments in the process of receiving a succession of individual tutors' one and only tutorial on the topic of that tutor's research. Sadly, the mediaeval continuity of a tutor seeing their tutee frequently for most of the course has now disappeared as far as third-year medicine is concerned.

I should explain to future patients of these 'tossed' third-year students that the material necessary to qualify as a doctor is largely taught and examined around a detailed syllabus in the first and second years of a medical course. There is no future in a student thinking that they can focus on the heart while neglecting the gut. The third year, in contrast, is a kind of 'intercalated bachelor's degree' in which the unwritten syllabus is as wide as human biology itself and the student free to pursue a subject they find of interest. It is here that we see many undergraduates in their third year of medicine reaching a remarkable level of knowledge of topics of research after only a week or two of study.

I should further explain that the three pre-clinical years are followed by three years of clinical study, based in the hospital setting, to make a total of six. Here the emphasis is on a series of rotations through attachments to specialities such as surgery, ophthalmology, obstetrics and general practice.

Because I already had a degree, albeit in engineering, I was spared the 'intercalated' third year of medical studies and in 1979 made my way to learning clinical medicine in the Oxford hospitals for three years. Still a member of St Catherine's College, my visits there were more social than didactic because the teaching of clinical medicine is centred in hospital wards. We wore white coats and had stethoscopes, ophthalmoscopes, and paper notebooks bulging from our pockets. A new kind of 'nowhere-to-hide' bedside tutorial took place in which teaching, sometimes regrettably by humiliation, by feared senior doctors supplemented teaching by instruction. Small groups of student doctors were attached to 'firms' led by two or three consultants, whose juniors ('registrars') were expected to take us aside for seminars on everything from how to manage the acute abdomen to investigating the pyrexia of unknown origin.

In the final year a wonderful opportunity presented itself of travelling to a developing country for two months to see medicine in a completely different setting from the wards of Oxford's brand-new John Radcliffe Hospital. I travelled to Hiranpur, a mission hospital in Bihar state in India, to see a world of advanced diseases and traumas that were almost unthinkable in the UK. I saw the external signs of cancers and infections that had progressed to cause bodily destruction. Injuries included the results from falling into cooking fires, or from high up in trees, or from the outside of railway carriages. I was struck by how little of what I had learned was of value to the local people.

I returned to the challenge of a year of what we then called a 'house doctor' (1982–3), consisting of six months working on a surgical firm and six months on a medical firm. This was a period of rapid learning 'on the job', working ridiculously long hours and trying hard not to do more harm than good.

Mission impossible: becoming a part-time doctor

My house-doctor year permitted a little time in which to continue tutoring in engineering at Hertford College but I wanted to get back to doing research. The question was how to become a part-time doctor to make time for science. The answer came in the form of innovation fought for by Dr (later, Dame) Rosemary Rue. If Neil Tanner was the academic who shook up Oxford's admissions for students from state schools, it was Rosemary Rue who revolutionised opportunities for women to work as doctors and, paradoxically, in doing so, provided me, a man, with the opportunity to be both physiologist and doctor.[21] Figure 48 shows a portrait of her commissioned by the *British Medical Journal*.

We can think of Rue as battle-trained for the remarkable outcome she was to bring about. As a child she lived in London but was evacuated to Totnes during the Second World War, where she was bed-bound with tuberculosis in isolation for nearly a year; this experience inspired her to study medicine. You might think that the London School of Medicine for Women (the Royal Free Hospital) would have been precisely geared to the needs of women when she entered there in 1945 but sadly it was not; she had to resign from the course in 1949 on account of wishing to marry but was able to continue her medical studies in Oxford, which, perhaps surprisingly, appeared at first to have been more enlightened in this respect. However, the authorities later dismissed her from a post in an Oxford community hospital when they discovered that she was married and a mother to boot. Accordingly, she moved to general practice in 1951.

In 1954 Rue had the misfortune of becoming the last case of paralytic poliomyelitis in Oxfordshire.[22] She was in hospital for five months and it took ten years of rehabilitation and five major operations before she could walk without help. One is struck by her account of the challenges of trying to carry a medical bag, of the impossibility of navigating long hospital corridors and stairs, and of being the subject of "pitying but also disapproving" onlookers who were not accustomed to seeing badly disabled people.[22] She slowly rebuilt her career, leading to health authority management in Hertfordshire and then in the Oxford 'region' as it was then termed, and she eventually became the overall regional manager.

It was in Oxford that she identified many "women who had qualified, who had gone off to have families and who simply weren't welcomed back to the profession".[22] In 1965, with approval and finance from the regional board, Rue identified four women to work as supplementary part-time hospital doctors, and the number soon increased to thirty-three.[23] Known locally as the 'Oxford married women's part-time scheme', this grew until 1981 when a paper reported that 249 doctors had passed through the scheme and a further 120 were then in training.[24] It is a fascinating feature of this report that, although the theme addressed is "part-time training to enable women doctors to develop their potential more fully" and "part-time posts for doctors with domestic commitments", no mention is made of whether men were included in the statistics.[24] Nevertheless, in 1983 I joined the scheme, first to work part-time in the accident service and then to train mostly part-time in anaesthetics for six years while continuing my physiology research. Whether I was the first male of the 500 or so participants at that stage, I cannot establish; I have never identified another male participant from that time. I may have had a unique opportunity, in that sense at least.

Rosemary Rue's innovation eventually expanded into a national scheme using the terms "flexible" or "less-than-full-time" (LTFT) training. It is notable that even nationally the opportunity for men to adopt a career as a part-time doctor still appears to be very limited; one study found only 3 per cent of men in hospital specialities who were classified as LTFT ten years after graduation.[25] The percentage in training grades during the few years after graduation is likely therefore to be miniscule. I note with interest that current eligibility criteria for entry to such training include ill health, disability, carer responsibilities, and factors pertaining to sport and religion. These would not have justified my participation; I was allowed in the long term to be a half-time hospital doctor in training and a half-time physiologist. Rosemary Rue's innovation enabled the anaesthetic department to 'take a chance on me' making good. But there was a big catch; in those years, the full-time contract for junior doctors in Oxford was a ninety-two-hour week. This meant that the contract for a half-time job was for a forty-six-hour week. My physiology had to be squeezed in but went ahead somehow.

Rosemary Rue went on to play a major role in regional hospital development, including the establishment of a dedicated women's hospital in which I was to work as an anaesthetist for many years after completing my training.

Linacre College and the daughters of penicillin

The next port of call in my tour of colleges takes us a little closer to things medical. Named after Thomas Linacre, founder of the Royal College of Physicians in the early sixteenth century, Linacre College is a graduate-only mixed institution with a strong medical and international tradition. It was founded in 1962, taking over the building vacated as St Catherine's Society moved to its 'Jacobsen' site to become St Catherine's College. Linacre itself moved on in 1977 to sit close to St Catherine's by the Cherwell river, where it now commands a wonderful position in an expanse of green sports fields.

In 1983 after my house jobs my eye was caught by Linacre's advertisement of its EPA Cephalosporin Junior Research Fellowships. Junior research fellowships are offered by many colleges in order to support young academics soon after completing their doctorates. In Linacre's case the name tells us that their origins lie in one of Oxford's most wonderful medical stories: the discovery of the daughters of penicillin.

'EPA' stands for Edward Penley Abraham who came to Queen's College, Oxford, to study chemistry in 1932. He took a first-class degree and then a doctorate before pursuing both science and his future wife in Scandinavia in the years 1938–9, escaping back to Oxford at the beginning of the war. He joined the team of Howard Florey, later Nobel laureate for his work on penicillin, playing a role in the production and purification of this anti-microbial agent for its use in humans in 1941.[26] In the post-war years Abraham continued to work on anti-microbial agents, one of which was identified in the culture of an organism from a sewage outfall in the Bay of Naples called *Cephalosporium acremonium*. In 1955 the new drug was announced under the name cephalosporin C and found to have the particular benefit of treating some infections that were resistant to penicillin. This was the first of many generations of cephalosporin drugs, which have proven to be of immense value; we may think of them as daughters of penicillin and one of the quieter glories of Oxford science. Finding that, as an employee of the University of Oxford, he stood to benefit personally from patents associated with cephalosporins, Abraham generously set up several charitable funds to receive benefits from the discoveries, one of which was the EPA Cephalosporin Fund established in 1970 "for education, and research in medicine chemistry and biology, in the University and colleges of Oxford, KES, and the Royal Society". With 'KES' he was remembering his King Edward School VI, Southampton.[26]

Several colleges were to benefit. The closest to the Sir William Dunn School of Pathology, where the work was based, was its immediate neighbour on the Cherwell, Linacre College. I was delighted to be appointed to a fellowship in a college with such historic medical links but also a refreshingly modern and friendly atmosphere. This is a college in which the common room is shared between students and staff, and in which pushchairs with young children are to be seen at mealtimes, in striking contrast to the formality of those dinners at Christ Church presided over by the portrait of Henry VIII. Linacre has acquired a particularly strong reputation for the construction of elegant eco-friendly buildings on its Cherwell base while recently receiving some opprobrium for its plan to change its name from that honouring the great physician to that of a donor offering the college £155 million.[27] It will be interesting to see whether the name of Thomas Linacre does indeed disappear from among the Oxford colleges.

Lincoln College: penicillin's further reaches

Howard Florey of penicillin fame came to Oxford to take up the post of Professor of Pathology in 1935. Established university chairs such as this are associated with a college fellowship and the Pathology chair had become associated with Lincoln College. After the success of penicillin in the war years and of a shared award of the Nobel Prize in Physiology or Medicine in 1945, Florey obtained a benefaction of £50,000 from Lord Nuffield to establish three fellowships at Lincoln College.[28] I have noted in Chapter Six the enthusiasm with which Nuffield supported anaesthesia in the 1930s following his dental traumas. This post-war benefaction of 1948 was to commemorate penicillin. One of the fellowships was made available for Edward Abraham who later, in 1960, was elected to a professorial fellowship.

In 1984 I was privileged to be elected to a Nuffield Medical Fellowship at Lincoln College and thereby found myself in a line of descent from Abraham, whom I met in the college on several occasions before he died in 1999. Abraham had a strong affection for Lincoln; he set up the first and largest of his trust funds in 1967 so that Lincoln would be especially favoured and the Rector of Lincoln was a trustee ex officio. Brockliss notes that Abraham was able to donate £30 million to Lincoln and the Dunn School by 2000,[11] while Jones estimated in 2014 that Abraham's three trust funds together had a capital base of well over £150 million.[26]

Lincoln College was founded in 1427 and has its main site on the junction of Oxford's High Street and Turl Street, with limited room for expansion. In contrast to Oxford's largest college, St Catherine's with about 960 students, it is one of the smaller colleges with about 640 students.[29] Of these the proportion of graduate students is unusually high at around 50 per cent, which may be related to the building in around 2005, in Museum Road away from the main site, of Lincoln's EPA Centre with forty-eight rooms for graduate students, another extension of Edward Abraham's remarkable philanthropy.

As I look back to my arrival at Lincoln College in 1984 I am surprised that the penicillin trail should have led to the college wishing to support my rudimentary work on artificial lungs (Chapter One). The deed of the fund specified that preference should be given to candidates "who offer to conduct research in experimental pathology and bacteriology (the subjects whose study provided the fundamental knowledge of penicillin)".[30] I like to think that they saw seeds of promise in my motive of finding a new treatment for lung failure; they also gave me the opportunity to teach their undergraduates in medicine and physiology while working as a doctor, a grounding for later becoming a full tutor in medicine elsewhere. I think that it was during my Lincoln years that I gathered my thoughts most productively on how to hold those 'no-place-to-hide' essay-based tutorials in my room on Turl Street and how to conduct experiments with more dextrous fingers in the university's biomedical engineering centre where my experiments were based in my post-doctoral years. It was also during those years that I fell in love with anaesthesia and all its paraphernalia.

Clinical anaesthesia: an NHS locker with tea bags

The life of Oxford colleges is replete with meeting a broad range of people in shared meals, tutorials and lectures, or while pottering around the 'inhabited ruins'. From their arrival, undergraduates meet peers reading a large range of subjects and having a broad span of sporting and cultural interests. The relationships so begun often last a lifetime. My own batch of continuing friendships from student years includes contemporaries who studied history, modern languages, theology, physics and art, as well as, inevitably, many who studied engineering and medicine. The different constituencies are grouped socially into 'common rooms', leading to JCR, MCR and SCR for the junior, middle and senior members of a college, yet these are not rigidly segregated groups. The tutorial is only one of the ways in which there is engagement and exchange of ideas across the different ages and seniorities.

By way of contrast I find remarkable the minimal attention the health service gives to the communal needs of its participants. If we try to draw a parallel with the common room of colleges we might look to the 'doctors' mess' as a candidate. Here is, or at least was, a location where medical staff congregated and which provided professional support as well as a social scene.[31] Colleagues who were junior doctors in the late 1970s give accounts of the mess typically having domestic staff who cooked them breakfast, lunch and dinner, of the mess being where other doctors provided tips on how to manage patients, and how it was a centre of discussion of rotas, higher exams and battling burnout. One colleague recalls an event that contributed to his decision to leave the NHS for an academic career: it was the replacement in 1984 by Gloucester Royal Infirmary of freshly prepared hot food on the evening shift by a slot machine delivering cold pizza.

My first year as a hospital doctor was 1982 and I never benefited from any doctors' mess. My own experience has been much more that of the 'NHS locker', a small metal cabinet in which one is able to store some items of clothing and one or two how-to-be-a-doctor manuals.

In 2019 the General Medical Council reviewed doctors' working conditions in its report 'Caring for doctors Caring for patients'. The authors observed:

> Doctors repeatedly mourned the loss of the doctors' mess. Such facilities offered a space for doctors to share their difficult experiences in the course of their work, to learn from each other, to provide social support and to laugh and relax. They ensured that doctors could eat well during the course of their work, rather than having to make do with fast food or no food at all – particularly on night shifts.[32]

The report acknowledged that the doctors' mess was lost to history but recognised the need for a substitute in which a range of staff could meet. "With multidisciplinary working, we are not proposing a return to doctors' messes but a staff canteen, separate from facilities for patients, where doctors can eat with each other and other staff. This creates a sense of being valued, respected and supported by their organisations."[32]

Unfortunately, even where such a canteen exists, the nature of an anaesthetist's schedule means that visiting it is likely to be a rare or never event. The day, and sometimes also the night, is full of a succession of cases in which the anaesthetist attends the patient while the surgeon operates but also works without a break while the surgeon does not operate; he or she recovers the preceding patient following one operation and then prepares the next patient for surgery. Further, for most of my career the canteen has been in a separate building far away and it was unthinkable to the schedule (and the surgeons) that I would take myself off to find food. But theatre suites did and do contain a 'rest room' of sorts where a few minutes of repose can sometimes be sought between cases. Here the provision is usually limited to tea bags, instant coffee and milk, though recent years saw a plan to withdraw the tea bags on grounds of economy and ask staff to make their own arrangements. Such are the economies of NHS life.

Big meetings of doctors there were. As the bureaucracy and monitoring enveloping doctors increased, especially around 2000–5, the years of the enquiry into Harold Shipman's murder of patients, departmental meetings of doctors every few months became mandatory. The traditional format was 'morbidity and mortality', in which patients were discussed and commonly a guest lecturer updated us on an area of research. For anaesthetists, who spend much of their working lives isolated from their anaesthetic colleagues, these were valuable opportunities to discuss and learn. An almost invariably bleak feature was that refreshments at these meetings, if they occurred, were only available from sponsorship by a pharmaceutical company or equipment manufacturer manning a display stand, building into the gatherings the potential for conflict of interest, which we have been increasingly trying to avoid.

What gatherings there were became especially important as learning opportunities as from 1989 I continued my anaesthetic practice beyond being a 'junior doctor' in training to working part-time as 'clinical fellow' and then later 'consultant' in the Nuffield Department of Anaesthetics. After completing training, the lot of an anaesthetist is often that of a lone mariner at sea among other kinds of medical staff. Keeping up to date with developments in the field requires special effort. Towards the end of my clinical duties I was mandated to participate in seventeen separate online or in-house training courses, some annually, not one of which I found directly relevant to the conduct of anaesthesia. This meant passing seventeen different assessments even before thinking about whether to use gas-and-air to put a patient to sleep. In these years the NHS locker became a store for all sorts of items to help one sail through a demanding shift; biscuits were to be found there and also a back-up supply of tea bags to cover any deficit in the rest room.

For much of my career, my aim has been to build my working week from three components: patients, students and experiments. I was fortunate that, as I finished my years of training as an anaesthetist, something new came along that helped to put these layers together.

University College: medical tutor

In the spring of 1989 I went on holiday to Wales and was therefore out of contact with the rest of the world, as one was in the days before mobile phones and the internet. This was the morning after my interview for a lectureship in Oxford. These posts took the form of a 'joint appointment' between a department of the university and a college; both had to agree on the outcome despite having their own individual requirements of the appointee. The interview process started with a short talk to the staff of the University Laboratory of Physiology, where the questions suggested that my pictures of artificial lungs hardly cut the mustard among the department's explorers of the inner workings of the living cell; the head of department, the renowned Professor Colin Blakemore, had frowned. Later there had been an interview across a dark baize table in a wood-panelled seventeenth-century room in University College ('Univ'), where some concern was expressed that I had no actual degree in physiology. One of those present, later a colleague and friend, recalls a friendly and positive conversation but one with searching questioning.

There were also two trials by eating. One involved the logistics of assimilating a crumbly bread roll and being interrogated in face-to-face encounters while standing up and also holding a drink. The other was being presented with the full regalia of a college evening dinner in which swordfish was served, while I and the other candidates eyed each other suspiciously. In my case there was a strong sense of being out of one's depth. The job was clearly going to go to one of the card-carrying physiologists around the table. So the next day my wife and I set off early for Wales with the children in the back of the car. It was time to think about the beach and move on from regretting not having answered those difficult questions any better.

A phone call reached me on my return home. They were clearly put out that I had assumed no need to be contacted while on holiday but, despite this, they kindly offered me the job. In fact, two physiology jobs were going that day, so there were two lucky applicants. One was indeed a real physiologist, and also a woman who was appointed to a women's college. She went on to be honoured by Queen Elizabeth. I just remained grateful for the good company and the exceptional innovators and philanthropists who had helped me to get the interview in the first place.

From this point on, my encounters with fascinating aspects of physiology took on a new pace. Now I had to understand enough of a wide range of the syllabus to be able to explain it to students, the acid test for scientists. The new job would contain 'students' and 'experiments'; Professor Blakemore, no longer frowning, also kindly made provision for me to continue to practise anaesthesia, so the third element, 'patients', was satisfied too. It was a dream ticket for an interesting job.

There can be no better fortune in life than to fall in with good company. My good fortune was to find myself among scientists in Oxford who not only conducted their research with the enthusiasm and the disinterest you need to make solid progress, but also (on the whole) enjoyed passing their insights on to a younger generation. Being given a job in physiology was my biggest boost to having a go at science. The lectureship came with an appointment as tutor at Univ, the college claiming to be Oxford's oldest. My mediaeval experience of Oxford took a further step back to even earlier dates. This was the college that was first 'founded' by Alfred the Great and then 'unfounded' by him, as it were, one thousand years later. This requires explanation.

The college that was not founded by King Alfred

In 1722 the long-standing Master of Univ, Arthur Charlett, succumbed to a stroke, leaving the institution bitterly divided as to who should succeed him. It fell to ten fellows of the college to conduct an election but no agreement could be reached as to which of several historic statutes applied to voting. The result was a bitter stalemate lasting seven years in which two rivals both claimed the mastership.[33]

Colleges have 'Visitors' who are deemed to be the final arbiter in disputes that cannot be settled internally. Unfortunately, this dispute extended to disagreement about who was the college's Visitor. For one group, supporting William Denison (a fellow), it was the 'Chancellor of Oxford as represented by the Hebdomadal Council' of the university. For the other group, supporting Thomas Cockman (a former student) the Visitor was argued to be the king, George I.

The claim by one party that the king was Visitor stemmed from the college being seen as a royal institution founded by King Alfred, a notion then itself with a long history. Alfred was king of England from 886 until his death in 899.[34] A dispute over ownership of land in

1381 had led the fellows of University College to send a petition to the
king (Richard II) which referred to the college as the 'foundation of
the University of Oxford founded by King Alfred'. This linked Alfred,
famous for his support of learning, with establishing the University
of Oxford, which Univ's archivist Robin Darwall-Smith says was a
logical assumption at that time.[33] It was in a later petition to Richard
II, in 1384, that Alfred is first claimed as the college's founder, and this
was because the clerk drafting the document had misread the 1381
petition and erroneously written that the *college*, and not the *university*, was a royal foundation.[35]

So this mythical founding by King Alfred became the weapon of
Thomas Cockman and his supporters in his bid for the mastership in
the 1720s. In 1729, after seven years of wrangling, a final 'Visitation'
of the college was held by 'Commissioners' in London and Cockman
was declared the true Master of University College. Interestingly this
immediately followed publication in 1728 by a former fellow, William
Smith, of the first scholarly, if indigestible, history of the college with
a full title that clearly lays out its position: *The Annals of University-
College. Proving William of Durham the True Founder: and Answering All
Their Arguments Who Ascribe It to King Alfred.*[36] The case is a compel-
ling example of human folly, showing how a decision with important
consequences can be made on the basis of a fiction accepted by intelli-
gent people. In this case the outcome was favourable; Darwall-Smith
describes Cockman as "one of the most sympathetic characters in
this whole history", who restored the stability of the college.[33]

A favourite college portrait from this period is that of Thomas
Cockman and his supporters by the artist Benjamin Ferrers (Fig. 49).
To us today it is almost cartoon-like in its depiction of the winning
party and yet so replete with detail of the Master's lodgings that we
feel transported to the room and are tempted to take the celebratory glass of the (might it have been?) madeira being pushed towards
the viewer by the Master's immediate neighbour while Cockman
takes snuff. We note the spread of clay pipes and are reminded of
the Oxford tradition of 'dessert', in which dons gather after dinner to
drink port or madeira and take snuff from the 'anatomical snuff box'
between the tendons at the base of the thumb.

Though sadly not founded by Alfred, the college I joined as tutor
does lay claim to being Oxford's oldest, based upon the bequest in
1249 by William of Durham to the University of Oxford to invest

in land to support four Masters of Arts studying theology, probably following the model of a *collège* in Paris. Other colleges have claimed precedence on the grounds of being first to house scholars on their current site (Balliol, ~1263) or being the first functioning Oxford college (Merton, 1274).[11] There is something inspiring about working in an institution with a history as long as ours. The 750th anniversary in 1999 was a memorable event for which the Master, Lord Butler, commissioned Darwall-Smith's *History*, we received a visit from Queen Elizabeth (Fig. 50), and a series of distinguished visiting lecturers made us feel both long established and engaged with the issues of the modern world.

Dr John Radcliffe: Oxford's greatest medical alumnus

My appointment in 1989 to teach at Univ gave me my seventh Oxford college. I was now at the college that, some three centuries earlier, had admitted a student who became the most munificent of all Oxford's medical benefactors, Dr John Radcliffe (Fig. 51). Debate surrounds the precise date of his birth but it is likely that he was admitted to University College in 1665 at the age of thirteen following schooling in Wakefield.[37] The study of Latin, Greek, grammar and logic will have occupied four years leading to his Bachelor of Arts degree, at which juncture he decided to study further, showing an inclination towards 'physick' as medicine was then known (though we notice the 'k' being used less as the seventeenth century leads to the eighteenth). The tradition was that the BA degree could be followed by further study towards a Master of Arts degree to be taken seven years after 'matriculation', i.e. commencement of studies. An MA was a prerequisite for later taking a medical degree. In Radcliffe's day it was possible to take a fellowship en route to the MA. Accordingly, in 1670 at the age of eighteen, he was elected to a Yorkshire Fellowship at Lincoln College, the post providing opportunity for teaching as well as study, as was the case with my fellowship at Lincoln three centuries later. During his time at Lincoln, in 1675, Radcliffe took the degree of Bachelor of Medicine.

In describing the education Oxford provided for future physicians, Radcliffe's biographer Joseph Nias listed the minimal teaching available (including discussion of Hippocrates and Galen, and walking around the Botanic Garden) and noted "the whole forming slender provision for instruction in the rudiments of an important profession".[38] It seems to have been this lack of appropriate instruction that led him as the first item in his will to make provision for students of medicine to learn abroad: "yearly six hundred to two persons out of the university of Oxon when they are Masters of arts and enter'd on the physic line ... for the space of ten years and no longer, the halfe of which time at least, they are to travel in parts beyond sea, for their better improvement".[38]

Some 160 Radcliffe Travelling Fellows have been appointed since Radcliffe's death in 1714 and many have made substantial contributions to developments in medicine. Until 1858 these appointments remained two at a time for a maximum of ten years. Since then they have been appointments for three and later two years, most recently with an emphasis on medical research, often undertaken in developing countries.[39] If this alone were Radcliffe's medical legacy it would rank as one of Oxford's most significant. The estate he left has exceeded this by far. It included £5,000 for a doubling of the size of University College by the building of a second quadrangle "answerable to the front already built and for the building of the Masters lodgings and chambers for my two travailing [sic] fellows", the inside of the new lodgings being revealed in the Cockman painting in Figure 49.[38] This architectural specification led to the remarkable construction soon after Radcliffe's death of an almost identical quadrangle to one built nearly a century before, a sentiment for conservatism with which one senses our present king would be in favour (Fig. 52). Further to this magnificent building the will made provision for the Radcliffe Camera library and the trustees of his estate were eventually able to fund the Radcliffe Infirmary and Observatory.

It is notable that Radcliffe left no funds for Lincoln College.[40] He fell out with this, his second alma mater, because of the mode of his departure from it in 1677. By that date a fellow, he had failed to become ordained in holy orders in the manner specified by the college's statutes and was obliged to take his medical practice into the town, eventually leaving in 1684 to begin his flourishing practice in London, which led to him becoming physician to King William III and Queen Anne and to financial success.

Radcliffe's first biographer, William Pittis, writing the year after his death, was clear that his reputation preceded him to London. One factor was his management of smallpox cases in Oxford: "by giving his Patients Air ... and not stoving them up, as was done by the *Galen-ists* of those Days, resc'd more than a hundred from the Attacks of Death, which gave Wings to his Reputation".[41] One particular aristocratic patient seems to have had a disproportionately large effect on his reputation:

> But what fixed it in a higher Orb, and bore it up above the Reach of any one of his Competitors, was, a remarkable Case in the Cure of the Lady *Spencer*, at *Yarnton*, some few miles from Oxford ... and he was not two Years Batchelor of Physick, when there was scarce any Family of Credit that was not beholden to him for the Preservation of one, or more Lives.

Oxford may have provided little in the way of practical teaching of medicine but clearly had the potential for a pragmatic ambitious young physician to begin to make a fortune. How apposite it is that so much of that wealth found its way back to the city for educational purposes.

Pittis lets us into a secret, which reveals why Radcliffe's fortune made its way to Oxford rather than to any heirs: a lucky escape from parenting another man's child, which appears to have put him off marrying for life:

> In 1693, the Doctor, who 'till then had shewn Tokens of the greatest Aversion to Matrimony, by the Solicitation of his Friends, was induc'd to think of altering his Condition; and the Daughter of a certain wealthy Citizen, that shall remain nameless, was pitch'd upon for that end ... But *Hymen* had otherwise intended; for the Father's Book-keeper ... by a Sort of illegal Familiarity, which in Process of Time made the design'd Bride very sick, and discover'd an Amour that could not be any longer conceal'd from such penetrating Eye's as the Doctor's.[41]

In spite of further temptations as "several Ladies frequently feign'd themselves ill, to be visited by him", in 1694 Radcliffe

> laid a Plan for his succeeding Benefactions to the Place of his Education ... as may be seen from his answer to a Man of Fashion, who, after asking him, *Why he did not marry some young*

Gentlewoman, to get Heirs by? Had, by Way of Reply, *That truly he had an old one to take Care of, which he intended should be his Executrix.*

And so came the monies to Univ and the University of Oxford.[41]

Replete with funds, in 1907 University College established a "Prize for the Furtherance of Medical Science in the University, to be known as the Radcliffe Prize".[38] I was fortunate to be awarded this upon completion of my medical degree at St Catherine's College in 1982. I like to think that in 1989 Univ may have taken this as a good omen when deciding to appoint me to be a fellow and tutor. The prize has allowed me to feel a direct beneficiary of Radcliffe's generosity; in return I keep his portrait on the wall of my teaching room at Univ.

Meeting ingenious physiologists past and present

In the Preface to this book I set myself the task of attempting to explain why the academic environment of Oxford provides rich opportunities for encountering 'ingenious modern physiologists', noting that David Macbride had turned to one in 1772 to help him understand why a patient's blood might settle to reveal a 'buffy coat' on its surface. My own roll call of historic inspirational physiologists associated with Oxford includes William Harvey, Robert Hooke, John Scott Haldane, Florence Buchanan, Mabel FitzGerald, Robert Macintosh and Dan Cunningham. They are ever present in their portraits, artefacts, plaques, street names and even their devices.

In this and the preceding chapters I have tried to show the reader how medical science builds on the work of our predecessors in order to advance. This requires that those predecessors are men and women of significant achievement but also that among them are those who are capable of perceiving the potential in young men and women and who make the effort to encourage them or to create the conditions under which that potential can bear fruit.

Innovators such as Neil Tanner, Ernest Foulkes and Rosemary Rue have devised novel strategies to identify individuals who can benefit from educational, scientific and medical opportunities. Benefactors, including John Radcliffe, Lord Nuffield and Edward Abraham, have enabled a community and an environment in which disinterested exploration of science can be conducted by students and young academics taught and supervised by their tutors, lecturers and professors.

More than this, the individual career also sometimes needs an element of luck. I count myself indeed lucky to have benefited from the wisdom, support and encouragement of those I have described, who laid for me the foundations of a fascinating and rewarding career in medical science. The concentration in Oxford of this conglomeration of support and inspiration is frankly astonishing. The department from which I write (Physiology, Anatomy & Genetics) has been ranked by the QS World University Rankings world number one for Anatomy & Physiology for each of the last four years.[42] This makes me acutely aware that we make scientific progress not only because of our own abilities and efforts but also by the support of our seniors and contemporaries.

This is a continuing process: there will be future Huttons, McCrums and Bergels and, we hope, Abrahams and Nuffields to help them flourish and, no doubt, future Dorringtons able to pay tribute to how they were helped. By this means medical science advances and in doing so improves our ability to help those sick people who pass through our hands, which above all constitute medicine's raison d'être.

NOTES

Preface

1. Macbride, D., *A Methodical Introduction to the Theory and Practice of Physic* (London: W. Strahan, T. Cadell, 1772), 677 pp.
2. Dorrington, K., 'More on the history of the ESR', *The Lancet*, 1(8538) (1987), p. 930.
3. Rivière, L., *The Universal Body of Physick, in Five Books; Comprehending the Several Treatises of Nature, of Diseases and Their Causes, of Symptoms, of the Preservation of Health, and of Cures* (London: Philip Briggs, 1657), 422 pp.
4. Lemoine, M. and T. Pradeu, 'Dissecting the meanings of "physiology" to assess the vitality of the discipline', *Physiology*, 33(4) (2018), pp. 236–45.
5. Smith, T.G., et al., 'Commercial air travel and in-flight pulmonary hypertension', *Aviation, Space and Environmental Medicine*, 84(1) (2013), pp. 65–7.

1. Murder in Main Quad

1. Kurusz, M., 'May 6, 1953: the untold story', *ASAIO Journal*, 58(1) (2012), pp. 2–5.
2. Romaine-Davis, A., *John Gibbon and His Heart–Lung Machine* (Philadelphia: University of Pennsylvania Press, 1991), 251 pp.
3. University College Archives, *Anecdotes* (2007).
4. Dewsbery, S., *University College Record* (2013), pp. 130–2.
5. Levine, J., *The Secret History of the Blitz: Chancers, Outcasts and Unsung Heroes – Life in the Shadows During Britain's Darkest Days* (London: Simon & Schuster, 2016), 357 pp.
6. University College, *Governing Body Minutes*, UC:GB4/A1.11, 16 November 1940.
7. Hessel, E.A., 2nd, 'History of cardiopulmonary bypass (CPB)', *Best Practice & Research: Clinical Anaesthesiology*, 29(2) (2015), pp. 99–111.
8. Melrose, D.G., ' A Mechanical heart–lung for use in man', *British Medical Journal*, 2(4827) (1953), pp. 57–62.
9. Aird, I., et al., 'Assisted circulation by pump-oxygenator during operative dilatation of the aortic valve in man', *British Medical Journal*, 1(4874) (1954), pp. 1284–7.
10. Melrose, D.G., et al., 'Elective cardiac arrest', *The Lancet*, 269(6879) (1955), pp. 21–2.

11. Bellhouse, B.J. and F.H. Bellhouse, 'Mechanism of closure of the aortic valve', *Nature*, 217(5123) (1968), pp. 86–7.

12. Melrose, D.G., et al., 'The membrane oxygenator; some aspects of oxygen and carbon dioxide transport across polyethylene film', *The Lancet*, 1(7029) (1958), pp. 1050–1.

13. Bellhouse, B.J., et al., 'A high efficiency membrane oxygenator and pulsatile pumping system, and its application to animal trials', *Transactions of the American Society for Artificial Internal Organs*, 19 (1973), pp. 72–9.

14. Melrose, D.G., et al., 'Oscillating silicone membrane tubes: a new principle of extracorporeal respiration', *Biomedical Engineering*, 7(2) (1972), pp. 60–6.

15. Spratt, E.H., et al., 'Evaluation of a membrane oxygenator for clinical cardiopulmonary bypass', *Transactions of the American Society for Artificial Internal Organs*, 27 (1981), pp. 285–8.

16. Karlson, K.E., et al., 'Laboratory and clinical-evaluation of a membrane-oxygenator with secondary flows in the blood channels', *World Journal of Surgery*, 6(3) (1982), pp. 358–61.

17. Dorrington, K.L., et al., 'Oxygen and CO_2 transfer of a polypropylene dimpled membrane lung with variable secondary flows', *Journal of Biomedical Engineering*, 7(2) (1985), pp. 89–99.

18. Sykes, M.K., et al., 'Pulmonary changes after extracorporeal circulation in dogs', *British Journal of Anaesthesia*, 38(6) (1966), pp. 432–45.

19. Helmsworth, J.A., et al., 'Clinical use of extracorporeal oxygenation with oxygenator-pump', *Journal of the American Medical Association*, 150(5) (1952), pp. 451–3.

20. Bartlett, R.H., 'Esperanza: the first neonatal ECMO patient', *ASAIO Journal*, 63(6) (2017), pp. 832–43.

21. Toomasian, J.M., et al., 'National experience with extracorporeal membrane oxygenation for newborn respiratory failure. Data from 715 cases', *ASAIO Transactions*, 34(2) (1988), pp. 140–7.

22. Bartlett, R.H., et al., 'Extracorporeal circulation in neonatal respiratory failure: a prospective randomized study', *Pediatrics*, 76(4) (1985), pp. 479–87.

23. 'UK collaborative randomised trial of neonatal extracorporeal membrane oxygenation. UK Collaborative ECMO Trial Group', *The Lancet*, 348(9020) (1996), pp. 75–82.

24. Arensman, R.M. (author) and J.D. Cornish (ed), *Extracorporeal Life Support* (Boston; Oxford: Blackwell Scientific, 1993), xvii, 375 pp.

25. Kolobow, T., et al., 'An alternative to breathing', *Journal of Thoracic and Cardiovascular Surgery*, 75(2) (1978), pp. 261–6.

26. Trahanas, J.M., et al., '"Treating lungs": the scientific contributions of Dr Theodor Kolobow', *ASAIO Journal*, 62(2) (2016), pp. 203–10.

27. Dorrington, K.L., et al., 'Extracorporeal oxygen and CO_2 transfer of a

polypropylene dimpled membrane lung with variable secondary flows: partial bypass in the dog', *Journal of Biomedical Engineering*, 8(1) (1986), pp. 36–42.

28. Gattinoni, L., et al., 'Low-frequency positive-pressure ventilation with extracorporeal CO_2 removal in severe acute respiratory failure', *Journal of the American Medical Association*, 256(7) (1986), pp. 881–6.

29. Dorrington, K.L., 'Extracorporeal gas exchange in acute respiratory failure', *British Medical Journal (Clinical Research Edition)*, 296(6616) (1988), pp. 151–2.

30. Gardaz, J.P., et al., 'Physiological profile during venovenous perfusion in dogs using a polypropylene membrane lung with secondary flows', *Journal of Biomedical Engineering*, 10(1) (1988), pp. 74–81.

31. Sinclair, M.E., et al., 'Anticoagulation by ancrod for carbon dioxide removal by extracorporeal membrane lung in the dog', *Journal of Thoracic and Cardiovascular Surgery*, 97(2) (1989), pp. 275–81.

32. McRae, K.M. and K.L. Dorrington, 'Haemolysis during *in vitro* CO_2 removal from human blood using a membrane lung', *Journal of Biomedical Engineering*, 11(5) (1989), pp. 369–74.

33. Dorrington, K.L., et al., 'A randomized comparison of total extracorporeal CO_2 removal with conventional mechanical ventilation in experimental hyaline membrane disease', *Intensive Care Medicine*, 15(3) (1989), pp. 184–91.

34. Dorrington, K.L. and F. M. Ratcliffe, 'Effect of a single inflation of the lungs on oxygenation during total extracorporeal carbon dioxide removal in experimental respiratory distress syndrome', *Intensive Care Medicine*, 17(8) (1991), pp. 469–74.

35. Ratcliffe, F.M., K.L. Dorrington and M.K. Sykes, 'Optimum airway pressure during apnoeic oxygenation with extracorporeal carbon dioxide removal in experimental respiratory distress syndrome', *British Journal of Anaesthesia*, 61 (1988), 499P–500P.

36. Morris, A.H., et al., 'Randomized clinical trial of pressure-controlled inverse ratio ventilation and extracorporeal CO_2 removal for adult respiratory distress syndrome', *American Journal of Respiratory and Critical Care Medicine*, 149(2 Pt 1) (1994), pp. 295–305.

37. Peek, G.J., et al., 'Efficacy and economic assessment of conventional ventilatory support versus extracorporeal membrane oxygenation for severe adult respiratory failure (CESAR): a multicentre randomised controlled trial', *The Lancet*, 374(9698) (2009), pp. 1351–63.

38. Morris, A.H., et al., 'Counterpoint: Efficacy of extracorporeal membrane oxygenation in 2009 influenza A(H1N1): sufficient evidence?', *Chest*, 138(4) (2010), pp. 778–81; discussion pp. 782–4.

39. Park, P.K., H.J. Dalton and R.H. Bartlett, 'Point: Efficacy of extracorporeal membrane oxygenation in 2009 influenza A(H1N1): sufficient evidence?' *Chest*, 138(4) (2010), pp. 776–8.

40. Combes, A., et al., 'Extracorporeal membrane oxygenation for severe acute

respiratory distress syndrome', *New England Journal of Medicine*, 378(21) (2018), pp. 1965–75.

41. Extracorporeal Life Support Organization (ELSO). World's Largest Registry of ECMO Runs and ECLS Centers. www.elso.org/default.aspx

42. Barbaro, R.P., et al., 'Extracorporeal membrane oxygenation support in COVID-19: an international cohort study of the Extracorporeal Life Support Organization registry', *The Lancet*, 396(10257) (2020), pp. 1071–8.

43. Dorrington, K.L., *Anaesthetic and Extracorporeal Gas Transfer*. Oxford Medical Engineering Series (Oxford: Clarendon Press, 1989), 274 pp.

44. Young, J.D., et al., 'Femoral arteriovenous extracorporeal carbon dioxide elimination using low blood flow', *Critical Care Medicine*, 20(6) (1992), pp. 805–9.

45. Mi, M.Y., M.A. Matthay and A.H. Morris, 'Extracorporeal membrane oxygenation for severe acute respiratory distress syndrome', *New England Journal of Medicine*, 379(9) (2018), pp. 884–7.

46. Kolobow, T., 'The artificial lung: the past. A personal retrospective', *ASAIO Journal*, 50(6) (2004), pp. xliii–xlviii.

47. Ali, J. and A. Vuylsteke, 'Extracorporeal membrane oxygenation: indications, technique and contemporary outcomes', *Heart*, 105(18) (2019), pp. 1437–43.

48. Ciardha, N.O. and K. Royds, 'A clinical perfusion scientist: the job and the role in ECMO during the Covid-19 pandemic', *Physiology News*, 121 (2021), pp. 38–9.

49. Group, R.C., et al., 'Dexamethasone in hospitalized patients with Covid-19', *New England Journal of Medicine*, 384(8) (2021), pp. 693–704.

50. Hattenstone, S., 'The G2 interview. Michael Rosen on his Covid-19 coma: 'It felt like a pre-death, a nothingness', *Guardian*, 30 September 2020.

2. Mabel's Barometer

1. FitzGerald, M.P., 'The changes in the breathing and in the blood at various high altitudes', *Philosophical Transactions of the Royal Society B*, 203 (1913), pp. 351–71.

2. Torrance, R.W., 'Mabel's normalcy: Mabel Purefoy FitzGerald and the study of man at altitude', *Journal of Medical Biography*, 7(3) (1999), pp. 151–65.

3. Tissot van Patot, M., 'The science and sagacity of Mabel Purefoy FitzGerald', *Physiology News*, 100 (2015), pp. 26–31.

4. Haldane, J.S. and J.G. Priestley, 'The regulation of the lung-ventilation', *Journal of Physiology*, 32(3–4) (1905), pp. 225–66.

5. FitzGerald, M.P. and J.S. Haldane, 'The normal alveolar carbonic acid pressure in man', *Journal of Physiology*, 32(5–6) (1905), pp. 486–94.

6. Miscellaneous, 'The catastrophe of the Zenith', *American Journal of Science and Arts*, 9 (1875), pp. 481–2.

7. Tissandier, G., '*Le voyage à grande hauteur du ballon "Le Zenith"*', *La Nature*, 100 (1875), pp. 337–44.

8. Bert, P. (trans. M.A. Hitchcock and F.A. Hitchcock) *Barometric Pressure: Researches in Experimental Physiology* (Columbus, OH: College Book Co., 1943), 89 pp.

9. Tissot van Patot, M., 'A higher calling. How a noblewoman from England changed the face of high-altitude medicine', *Telluride Magazine,* Winter/Spring (2019–20), pp. 76–8.

10. Haldane, J., 'A rapid method of determining carbonic acid in air', *Journal of Hygiene,* 1 (1901), pp. 109–14.

11. FitzGerald, M.P., 'Further observations on the changes in the breathing and the blood at various high altitudes', *Proceedings of the Royal Society B,* 88(602) (1914), pp. 248–58.

12. Douglas, C.G., J.S. Haldane, Y. Henderson & E.C. Schneider, 'Physiological observations made on Pike's Peak, Colorado, with special reference to adaptation to low barometric pressures', *Philosophical Transactions B,* 203 (1913), pp. 185–318.

13. Lloyd, B.B., 'Daniel J.C. Cunningham: Oration at His Funeral Service' in P. Zapata, C. Eyzaguirre and R.W. Torrance (eds), *Frontiers in Arterial Chemoreception* (New York & London: Plenum Press, 1996), pp. 39–43.

14. RAMC, *224th Parachute Field Ambulance in Operation Overlord.* www.pegasusarchive.org/normandy/war_224pfa.htm

15. Lloyd, B.B., M.G. Jukes and D.J. Cunningham, 'The relation between alveolar oxygen pressure and the respiratory response to carbon dioxide in man', *Quarterly Journal of Experimental Physiology and Cognate Medical Sciences,* 43(2) (1958), pp. 214–27.

16. Cunningham, D.J.C. and B.B. Lloyd (eds), *The Regulation of Human Respiration: The Proceedings of the J. S. Haldane Centenary Symposium held in the University Laboratory of Physiology, Oxford* (Oxford: Blackwell Scientific Publications, 1963), 591 pp.

17. Taube, H.W.L., *Dissertationem inauguralem de vera nervi inter costalis origine* (Göttingen, 1743), 20 pp.

18. De Castro, F., 'The discovery of sensory nature of the carotid bodies' in C. Gonzalez, C.A. Nurse and C. Peers (eds), *Arterial Chemoreceptors* (Berlin: Springer, 2009), pp. 1–18.

19. Vial, D.D., 'A tribute to Fernando De Castro on the centennial of his birth' in P. Zapata, C. Eyzaguirre and R.W. Torrance (eds), *Frontiers in Arterial Chemoreception* (New York: Plenum Press, 1996), pp. 1–11.

20. Bascom, D.A., et al., 'Changes in peripheral chemoreflex sensitivity during sustained, isocapnic hypoxia', *Respiration Physiology,* 82(2) (1990), pp. 161–76.

21. Bascom, D.A., et al., 'Effects of dopamine and domperidone on ventilation during isocapnic hypoxia in humans', *Respiration Physiology,* 85(3) (1991), pp. 319–28.

22. Pedersen, M.E., K.L. Dorrington and P.A. Robbins, 'Effects of haloperidol on

ventilation during isocapnic hypoxia in humans', *Journal of Applied Physiology*, 83(4) (1997), pp. 1110–15.

23. Pedersen, M.E., K.L. Dorrington and P.A. Robbins, 'Effects of somatostatin on the control of breathing in humans', *Journal of Physiology*, 521 (Pt 1) (1999), pp. 289–97.

24. Nagyova, B., K.L. Dorrington and P.A. Robbins, 'Effects of midazolam and flumazenil on ventilation during sustained hypoxia in humans', *Respiration Physiology*, 94(1) (1993), pp. 51–9.

25. Pandit, J.J., et al., 'Effects of subanaesthetic sevoflurane on ventilation. 1: Response to acute and sustained hypercapnia in humans', *British Journal of Anaesthesia*, 83(2) (1999), pp. 204–9.

26. Nagyova, B., K.L. Dorrington and P.A. Robbins, 'Effect of low-dose enflurane on the ventilatory response to hypoxia in humans', *British Journal of Anaesthesia*, 72(5) (1994), pp. 509–14.

27. Nagyova, B., et al., 'Influence of 0.2 minimum alveolar concentration of enflurane on the ventilatory response to sustained hypoxia in humans', *British Journal of Anaesthesia*, 78(6) (1997), pp. 707–13.

28. Nagyova, B., et al., 'Comparison of the effects of sub-hypnotic concentrations of propofol and halothane on the acute ventilatory response to hypoxia', *British Journal of Anaesthesia*, 75(6) (1995), pp. 713–18.

29. Pandit, J.J., et al., 'Competitive interactions between halothane and isoflurane at the carotid body and TASK channels', *Anesthesiology*, 133(5) (2020), pp. 1046–59.

30. Bisgard, G.E., M.A. Busch and H.V. Forster, 'Ventilatory acclimatization to hypoxia is not dependent on cerebral hypocapnic alkalosis', *Journal of Applied Physiology*, 60(3) (1986), pp. 1011–15.

31. Engwall, M.J. and G.E. Bisgard, 'Ventilatory responses to chemoreceptor stimulation after hypoxic acclimatization in awake goats', *Journal of Applied Physiology*, 69(4) (1990), pp. 1236–43.

32. Howard, L.S. and P.A. Robbins, 'Ventilatory response to 8 h of isocapnic and poikilocapnic hypoxia in humans', *Journal of Applied Physiology*, 78(3) (1995), pp. 1092–7.

33. Tansley, J.G., et al., 'Changes in respiratory control during and after 48 h of isocapnic and poikilocapnic hypoxia in humans', *Journal of Applied Physiology*, 85(6) (1998), pp. 2125–34.

34. Donoghue, S., et al., 'Ventilatory acclimatization in response to very small changes in PO_2 in humans', *Journal of Applied Physiology*, 98(5) (2005), pp. 1587–91.

35. Dawkins, R. and Y. Wong, *The Ancestor's Tale: A Pilgrimage to the Dawn of Evolution* (London: Orion, 2004), 528 pp.

36. Shmakova, L., et al., 'A living bdelloid rotifer from 24,000-year-old Arctic permafrost', *Current Biology*, 31(11) (2021), pp. R712–3.

37. Martinón-Torres, M., et al., 'Earliest known human burial in Africa', *Nature*, 593(7857) (2021), pp. 95–100.

38. Loenarz, C., et al., 'The hypoxia-inducible transcription factor pathway regulates oxygen sensing in the simplest animal, *Trichoplax adhaerens*', *EMBO Reports*, 12(1) (2011), pp. 63–70.

39. Rytkonen, K.T., 'Evolution: Oxygen and early animals', *Elife*, 7 (2018).

40. Donnelly, S., 'Why is erythropoietin made in the kidney? The kidney functions as a critmeter', *American Journal of Kidney Diseases*, 38(2) (2001), pp. 415–25.

41. Jaakkola, P., et al., 'Targeting of HIF-α to the von Hippel-Lindau ubiquitylation complex by O_2-regulated prolyl hydroxylation', *Science*, 292(5516) (2001), pp. 468–72.

42. Bishop, T. and P.J. Ratcliffe, 'Genetic basis of oxygen sensing in the carotid body: HIF2α and an isoform switch in cytochrome c oxidase subunit 4', *Science Signaling*, 13(615) (2020), pp. 1–2.

43. Eckardt, K.U., et al., 'Rate of erythropoietin formation in humans in response to acute hypobaric hypoxia', *Journal of Applied Physiology*, 66(4) (1989), pp. 1785–8.

44. Smith, T.G., et al., 'Pulmonary artery pressure increases during commercial air travel in healthy passengers', *Aviation, Space and Environmental Medicine*, 83(7) (2012), pp. 673–6.

45. Smith, T.G., et al., 'Commercial air travel and in-flight pulmonary hypertension', *Aviation, Space and Environmental Medicine*, 84(1) (2013), pp. 65–7.

46. https://www.nobelprize.org/prizes/medicine/2019/ratcliffe/photo-gallery/

3. Ills of the Hills

1. Dorrington, K.L., 'No medical equipment at Goûter Refuge', *High Mountain Sports*, 223 (June) (2001), p. 76.

2. Golding, S., *Oxford University on Mont Blanc: The Life of the Chalet des Anglais* (London: Profile Books, 2022), 320 pp.

3. Bishop, M.C., *Memoir of Mrs Urquhart* (London: Kegan Paul, Trench, Trübner & Co., 1897), 391 pp.

4. Bailey, C., 'The treasures of the humble', *Alpine Journal*, 50(257) (1938), pp. 189–98.

5. Mathews, C.E., *The Annals of Mont Blanc* (London: T. Fisher Unwin, 1898), 368 pp.

6. Vincent, C., et al., 'Detection of a subglacial lake in Glacier de Tête Rousse (Mont Blanc area, France)', *Journal of Glaciology*, 58(211) (2012), pp. 866–78.

7. Benson, G.R., 'Notes – chiefly from the narrative of his guides – relating to the death of R. L. Nettleship'. balliolarchivist.wordpress.com/2014/08/13/exhibition-archive-rl-nettleship/

8. O'Connor, W.J., *Founders of British Physiology: A Biographical Dictionary*,

1820–1885 (Manchester and New York: Manchester University Press, 1988), 278 pp.

9. Fye, W.B., 'Ernest Henry Starling, his law and its growing significance in the practice of medicine', *Circulation*, 68(5) (1983), pp. 1145–8.

10. Starling, E.H., 'On the absorption of fluids from the connective tissue spaces', *Journal of Physiology*, 19(4) (1896), pp. 312–26.

11. Starling, E.H., *The Fluids of the Body* (Chicago: W.T. Keener & Co., 1909), 186 pp.

12. Glover, G.H. and I.E. Newson, 'Brisket disease (dropsy of high altitudes)', *Bulletin 204*, Agricultural Experiment Station of the Agricultural College of Colorado (1915), p. 24.

13. Maggiorini, M., 'High altitude-induced pulmonary oedema', *Cardiovascular Research*, 72(1) (2006), pp. 41–50.

14. Hochstrasser, J., A. Nanzer and O. Oelz, '*Das Höhenödem in den Schweizer Alpen. Beobachtungen über Inzidenz, Klinik und Verlauf bei 50 Patienten der Jahre 1980–1984*', *Schweizerische Medizinische Wochenschrift*, 116 (1986), pp. 866–73.

15. Weibel, E.R. and D.M. Gomez, 'Architecture of the human lung', *Science*, 137(3530) (1962), pp. 577–85.

16. Weibel, E.R., 'The ultrastructure of the alveolar-capillary membrane or barrier' in A.P. Fishman and H.H. Hecht (eds), *The Pulmonary Circulation and Interstitial Space* (Chicago and London: University of Chicago Press, 1969), pp. 9–25.

17. Hall, W.D., 'Stephen Hales: theologian, botanist, physiologist, discoverer of hemodynamics', *Clinical Cardiology*, 10(8) (1987), pp. 487–9.

18. White, C.R. and R.S. Seymour, 'The role of gravity in the evolution of mammalian blood pressure', *Evolution*, 68(3) (2014), pp. 901–8.

19. West, J.B., 'Role of the fragility of the pulmonary blood–gas barrier in the evolution of the pulmonary circulation', *American Journal of Physiology (Regulatory, Integrative and Comparative Physiology)*, 304(3) (2013), pp. R171–6.

20. Johansen, K., 'Heart and circulation in gill, skin and lung breathing', *Respiration Physiology*, 14(1–2) (1972), pp. 193–210.

21. Maggiorini, M., et al., 'High-altitude pulmonary edema is initially caused by an increase in capillary pressure', *Circulation*, 103(16) (2001), pp. 2078–83.

22. Vejlstrup, N.G. and K.L. Dorrington, 'Intense slow hypoxic pulmonary vasoconstriction in gas-filled and liquid-filled lungs: an *in vivo* study in the rabbit', *Acta Physiologica Scandinavica*, 148(3) (1993), pp. 305–12.

23. Holdsworth, D.A., et al., 'Iron bioavailability and cardiopulmonary function during ascent to very high altitude', *European Respiratory Journal*, 56(3) (2020), p. 1902285.

24. Sylvester, J.T., et al., 'Hypoxic pulmonary vasoconstriction', *Physiological Reviews*, 92(1) (2012), pp. 367–520.

25. Lang, M., et al., 'Hypoxaemia related to COVID-19: vascular and perfusion

abnormalities on dual-energy CT', *Lancet Infectious Diseases*, 20(12) (2020), pp. 1365–6.

26. Reeves, J.T., et al., 'Physiological effects of high altitude on the pulmonary circulation', *International Reviews of Physiology*, 20 (1979), pp. 289–310.

27. Dirken, M.J.N. and H. Heemstra, 'Alveolar oxygen tension and lung circulation', *Quarterly Journal of Experimental Physiology*, 34(3–4) (1948), pp. 193–211.

28. Dirken, M.J.N. and H. Heemstra, 'The adaptation of the lung circulation to the ventilation', *Quarterly Journal of Experimental Physiology*, 34(3–4) (1948), pp. 213–26.

29. Dorrington, K.L., et al., 'Time course of the human pulmonary vascular response to 8 hours of isocapnic hypoxia', *American Journal of Physiology (Heart and Circulatory Physiology)*, 273(3 Pt 2) (1997), pp. H1126–34.

30. Talbot, N.P., et al., 'Contrasting effects of ascorbate and iron on the pulmonary vascular response to hypoxia in humans', *Physiological Reports*, 2(12) (2014), e12220, pp. 1–9.

31. Merz, T.M. and J.P. Hefti, 'Humans at extreme altitudes', *BJA Education*, 21(12) (2021), pp. 455–61.

32. Fullick, A., J. Locke and P. Bircher, *A Level Biology for OCR* (Oxford: Oxford University Press, 2015), 707 pp.

33. Kent, M., *Advanced Biology*, 2nd edn (Oxford: Oxford University Press, 2013), 632 pp.

34. Dorrington, K.L. and J.D. Young, 'Development of the concept of a liquid pulmonary alveolar lining layer', *British Journal of Anaesthesia*, 86(5) (2001), pp. 614–17.

35. von Neergaard, K., '*Neue Auffassungen über einen Grundbegriff der Atemmechanik*', *Zeitschrift für die gesamte experimentelle Medizin*, 66 (1929), pp. 373–94.

36. Gil, J. and E.R. Weibel, 'Improvements in demonstration of lining layer of lung alveoli by electron microscopy', *Respiration Physiology*, 8(1) (1969), pp. 13–36.

37. Bachofen, H., et al., 'Experimental hydrostatic pulmonary edema in rabbit lungs: morphology', *American Review of Respiratory Disease*, 147(4) (1993), pp. 989–96.

38. Basset, G., C. Crone and G. Saumon, 'Significance of active ion transport in transalveolar water absorption: a study on isolated rat lung', *Journal of Physiology*, 384 (1987), pp. 311–24.

39. Basset, G., C. Crone and G. Saumon, 'Fluid absorption by rat lung in situ: pathways for sodium entry in the luminal membrane of alveolar epithelium', *Journal of Physiology*, 384 (1987), pp. 325–45.

40. Gjedde, A., P.M. Gross and A.J. Hansen, 'In memoriam: Christian Crone,

M.D., Ph.D. (1926–1990)', *Journal of Cerebral Blood Flow and Metabolism*, 13(1) (1993), pp. 3–4.

41. Vejlstrup, N.G., C.A.R. Boyd and K.L. Dorrington, 'Effect of lung inflation on active and passive liquid clearance from in vivo rabbit lung', *American Journal of Physiology (Lung Cellular and Molecular Physiology)*, 267(4 Pt 1) (1994), pp. L482–7.

42. Dorrington, K.L. and C.A.R. Boyd, 'Active transport in the alveolar epithelium of the adult lung: vestigial or vital?' *Respiration Physiology*, 100(3) (1995), pp. 177–83.

43. Sartori, C., et al., 'Salmeterol for the prevention of high-altitude pulmonary edema', *New England Journal of Medicine*, 346 (2002), pp. 1631–6.

44. Cogo, A., et al., 'Italian high altitude laboratories: past and present', *High Altitude Medicine and Biology*, 1(2) (2000), pp. 137–47.

45. Mosso, A., *Life of Man on the High Alps* (London: T. Fisher Unwin, 1898), 342 pp.

46. Ainslie, P.N. and A.W. Subudhi, 'Cerebral blood flow at high altitude', *High Altitude Medicine and Biology*, 15(2) (2014), pp. 133–40.

47. Croft, Q.P.P., et al., 'Variations in alveolar partial pressure for carbon dioxide and oxygen have additive not synergistic acute effects on human pulmonary vasoconstriction', PLoS ONE, 8(7) (2013), p. e67886.

48. West , J.B., et al., 'Pulmonary gas exchange on the summit of Mount Everest', *Journal of Applied Physiology: Respiratory Environmental & Exercise Physiology*, 55(3) (1983), p. 678–87.

49. Hackett, P.H. and R.C. Roach, 'High-altitude illness', *New England Journal of Medicine*, 345(2) (2001), p. 107–14.

50. Ferrazzinin, G., et al., 'Successful treatment of acute mountain sickness with dexamethasone', *British Medical Journal (Clinical Research Edition)*, 294(6584) (1987), pp. 1380–2.

51. Liu, C., et al., 'Dexamethasone mimics aspects of physiological acclimatization to 8 hours of hypoxia but suppresses plasma erythropoietin', *Journal of Applied Physiology*, 114(7) (2013), pp. 948–56.

52. Smith, T.G., et al., 'Effects of iron supplementation and depletion on hypoxic pulmonary hypertension: two randomized controlled trials', *Journal of the American Medical Association*, 302(13) (2009), pp. 1444–50.

53. Talbot, N.P., et al., 'Intravenous iron supplementation may protect against acute mountain sickness; a randomized, double-blinded, placebo-controlled trial', *High Altitude Medicine and Biology*, 12(3) (2011), pp. 265–9.

54. Blücher, Evelyn, Princess, *An English Wife in Berlin* (London: Constable, 1920), 336 pp.

55. Bell, G., Letter from Gertrude Bell to her father, dated 21 August 1900, Newcastle University, Gertrude Bell Archive. gertrudebell.ncl.ac.uk/letters. php

56. Richalet, J.-P., 'The scientific observatories on Mont Blanc', *High Altitude Medicine and Biology*, 2(1) (2001), pp. 57–68.

57. Golding, S. and P. Gillman, 'George Mallory and Francis Urquhart: an academic friendship', *Alpine Journal*, (2017), pp. 231–8.

58. Hsia, C.C.W., D.M. Hyde and E.R. Weibel, 'Lung structure and the intrinsic challenges of gas exchange', *Comprehensive Physiology*, 6(2) (2016), pp. 827–95.

4. Deceits of the Heart

1. Hughes, J.T., 'Miraculous deliverance of Anne Green: an Oxford case of resuscitation in the seventeenth century', *British Medical Journal (Clinical Research Edition)*, 285(6357) (1982), pp. 1792–3.

2. A Scholler in Oxford, *Newes from the Dead. Or, A True and Exact Narration of the Miraculous Deliverance of Anne Greene* (Oxford: Leonard Lichfield, 1651), 10 pp.

3. Molnár, Z., 'Thomas Willis (1621–1675), the founder of clinical neuroscience', *Nature Reviews Neuroscience*, 5(4) (2004), pp. 329–35.

4. Herring, N. and D.J. Paterson, *Levick's Introduction to Cardiovascular Physiology*, 6th edn (Boca Raton, London, New York: CRC Press, 2018), 426 pp.

5. Hemmeter, J.C., 'The history of the circulation of the blood; contributions of the Italian anatomists and physiologists; their bearing upon the discovery by Harvey', *Johns Hopkins Hospital Bulletin*, 170(May) (1905), pp. 165–78.

6. Arcieri, J.P., *The Circulation of the Blood and Andrea Cesalpino of Arezzo* (New York: S.F. Vanni, 1945), 193 pp.

7. Bishop, G., 'Geronimo Fabrizio, Latinised as Hieronymus Fabricius ab Aquapendente, S J (1537–1619). Circulation of the blood, before William Harvey', in G. Bishop, *Jesuit Pioneers of Modern Science and Mathematics* (Gujarat Sahitya Prakash, 2005), pp. 153–67.

8. Harvey, W., *Exercitatio anatomica de motu cordis et sanguinis in animalibus* (An Anatomical Exercise on the Motion of the Heart and Blood in Living Beings). An English translation with annotations by C.D. Leake (Menassa, WI: Collegiate Press, 1928), 155 pp.

9. Iimura, A., Y. Nakamura and M. Itoh, 'Anatomical study of distribution of valves of the cutaneous veins of adult's limbs', *Annals of Anatomy*, 185(1) (2003), pp. 91–5.

10. Gladstone, E., 'Johann Sigismund Elsholtz: Clysmatica Nova (1665): Elsholtz' neglected work on intravenous injection: Part III', *California and Western Medicine*, 39(2) (1933), pp. 119–23.

11. Gladstone, E., 'Johann Sigismund Elsholtz: Clysmatica Nova (1665): Elsholtz' neglected work on intravenous injection: Part IV', *California and Western Medicine*, 39(3) (1933), pp. 190–3.

12. Lewisohn, R., 'The citrate method of blood transfusion after ten years. A retrospect', *Boston Medical and Surgical Journal*, 190(18) (1924), pp. 733–42.

13. Dorrington, K.L. and M.C. Frise, 'Lessons of the month 1: Learning from

Harvey; improving blood-taking by pointing the needle in the right direction',
Clinical Medicine, 19(6) (2019), pp. 514–18.

14. Dorrington, K.L. and J.K. Aronson, 'Failed phlebotomy? Think William
Harvey', *British Medical Journal*, 349 (2014), p. g5232.

15. Franklin, K.J., *A Facsimile Edition of Richard Lower's Tractatus de Corde London
1669*, prefaced by an Introduction and Translation, in R.T. Gunther (ed.) *Early
Science in Oxford,* vol. IX (Oxford, printed for the subscribers, 1932), 426 pp.

16. 'WHO guidelines on drawing blood: best practices in phlebotomy', World
Health Organisation (2010), 109 pp.

17. Lahiru, 'How to take blood with an intravenous cannula – a novel technique
for the smallest veins!' www.youtube.com/watch?v=mZKddr1jbm4

18. Åstrand, P.-O., et al., 'Cardiac output during submaximal and maximal work',
Journal of Applied Physiology, 19(2) (1964), pp. 268–74.

19. Marx, H.J., et al., 'Maintenance of aortic pressure and total peripheral
resistance during exercise in heat', *Journal of Applied Physiology*, 22(3) (1967),
pp. 519–25.

20. Lind, A.B. and G.W. McNichol, 'Muscular factors which determine the
cardiovascular responses to sustained and rhythmic exercise', *Canadian Medical
Association Journal*, 96(12) (1967), pp. 706–13.

21. Pescatello, L.S., et al., 'Short-term effect of dynamic exercise on arterial blood
pressure', *Circulation*, 83(5) (1991), pp. 1557–61.

22. Buchanan, F., 'The physiological significance of the pulse-rate', *Transactions of
the Junior Oxford University Scientific Club*, 34 (1910), pp. 351–65.

23. Krogh, A. and J. Lindhard, 'The regulation of respiration and circulation
during the initial stages of muscular work', *Journal of Physiology*, 47(1–2) (1913),
pp. 112–36.

24. Parkes, M.J., 'Evaluating the importance of the carotid chemoreceptors in
controlling breathing during exercise in man', *BioMed Research International*,
(2013), 893506.

25. Herigstad, M., G.M. Balanos and P.A. Robbins, 'Can human cardiovascular
regulation during exercise be learnt from feedback from arterial
baroreceptors?' *Experimental Physiology*, 92(4) (2007), pp. 695–704.

26. Wood, H.E., M. Fatemian and P.A. Robbins, 'A learned component of the
ventilatory response to exercise in man', *Journal of Physiology*, 553(Pt 3) (2003),
pp. 967–74.

27. Scharhag, J., et al., 'Athlete's heart. Right and left ventricular mass and
function in male endurance athletes and untrained individuals determined
by magnetic resonance imaging', *Journal of the American College of Cardiology*,
40(10) (2002), pp. 1856–63.

28. Hammond, H.K., et al., 'Heart size and maximal cardiac output are limited
by the pericardium', *American Journal of Physiology (Heart and Circulatory
Physiology)*, 263 (1992), pp. H1675–81.

29. Dorrington, K.L. and M.C. Frise, 'Sir George Johnson FRCP (1818–96), high blood pressure and the continuing altercation about its origins', *Experimental Physiology*, 106(9) (2021), pp. 1886–96.

30. Hall, J.E., et al., 'In Memoriam. Arthur C. Guyton (1919–2003)', *Physiologist*, 46(3) (2003), pp. 126–8.

31. Guyton, A.C. and T.G. Coleman, 'Long-term regulation of the circulation: interrelationships with body fluid volumes', in E.B. Reeve and A.C. Guyton (eds), *Physical Bases of Circulatory Transport: Regulation and Exchange* (Philadelphia: W.B. Saunders, 1967), pp. 179–201.

32. Guyton, A.C., 'The surprising kidney-fluid mechanism for pressure control – its infinite gain!', *Hypertension*, 16 (1990), p. 725–30.

33. Guyton, A.C. and T.G. Coleman, 'Quantitative analysis of the pathophysiology of hypertension', *Circulation Research*, 24(5 Suppl) (1969), pp. 1–19.

34. Dorrington, K.L. and J.J. Pandit, 'The obligatory role of the kidney in long-term arterial blood pressure control: extending Guyton's model of the circulation', *Anaesthesia*, 64(11) (2009), pp. 1218–28.

35. Foëx, P. and J.W. Sear, 'Hypertension: pathophysiology and treatment', *Continuing Education in Anaesthesia Critical Care & Pain*, 4(3) (2004), pp. 71–75.

36. Ritter, J.M., et al., *Rang and Dale's Pharmacology*, 9th edn (Elsevier, 2020), 808 pp.

37. Cain, A.E. and R.A. Khalil, 'Pathophysiology of essential hypertension: role of the pump, the vessel, and the kidney', *Seminars in Nephrology*, 22(1) (2002), pp. 3–16.

38. Digne-Malcolm, H., M.C. Frise and K.L. Dorrington, 'How do antihypertensive drugs work? Insights from studies of the renal regulation of arterial blood pressure', *Frontiers in Physiology*, 7(320) (2016), pp. 1–19.

39. Mahajan, S., et al., 'Hemodynamic phenotypes of hypertension based on cardiac output and systemic vascular resistance', *American Journal of Medicine*, 133(4) (2020), pp. e127–39.

40. Hall, J.E. and M.E. Hall, *Guyton and Hall Textbook of Medical Physiology*, 14th edn (Philadelphia: Elsevier, 2020), 1152 pp.

5. A Spoonful of Sugar

1. Bates, C., 'Eyes wide open: patient has open-heart surgery while he is awake', *Daily Mail*, 12 February 2010. www.dailymail.co.uk/health/article-1250507/Eyes-Wide-Open-Patient-open-heart-surgery-awake.html

2. Fzaïcou, M.A., *'Auto-observation d'une auto-opération de hernie sous la rachi-strychno-stovaïnisation'*, *La Presse Médicale*, 12 (1911), pp. 105–9.

3. Lee, J.A., R.S. Atkinson and M.J. Watt, *Sir Robert Macintosh's Lumbar Puncture and Spinal Analgesia: Intradural and Extradural* (New York: Churchill-Livingstone, 1985), 352 pp.

4. Anonymous, 'The Leeds poisoning case', *Lyttelton Times*, 16 August 1856, p.8.
5. Jonnesco, T., 'Remarks on general spinal analgesia', *The British Medical Journal*, 2(2550) (1909), pp. 1396–401.
6. Wohlgemuth, H., *'Bessere Ausbildung in der Narkose and Anästhesie'*, *Deutsche Medizinische Wochenschrift*, 34 (1908), pp. 1595–6.
7. Wohlgemuth, H., *'Internationaler Chirurgenkongress Abgehalten in Bruessel vom 21–27 September 1908'*, *Wiener Medizinische Wochenschrift*, 51 (1908), pp. 2812–15.
8. Brickner, W.M., 'Jonnesco's contribution to spinal anesthesia', *American Journal of Surgery and Gynecology*, 24 (1910), pp. 24–5.
9. Jonnesco, T., 'Concerning general rachianesthesia', *American Journal of Surgery and Gynecology*, 24 (1910), pp. 33–4.
10. McGavin, L., 'Remarks on eighteen cases of spinal analgesia by the stovaine-strychnine method of Jonnesco', *The British Medical Journal*, 2 (1910), pp. 733–6.
11. Cook, G.C., *Disease in the Merchant Navy: A History of the Seamen's Hospital Society* (Boca Raton, FL: CRC Press, 2019), 632 pp.
12. Anonymous, 'Spinal analgesia', *The British Medical Journal*, 2 (1909), p. 1542.
13. Anonymous, 'Obituary: Arthur Edward James Barker, F.R.C.S. (England and Ireland), Professor of Surgery, University College Hospital Medical School, Consulting Surgeon to Queen Alexandra's Military Hospital, Millbank, Surgeon to University College Hospital, Colonel, Army Medical Service', *British Journal of Surgery*, 4(13) (1916), pp. 11–13.
14. Barker, A.E., 'A report on clinical experiences with spinal analgesia in 100 cases, and some reflections on the procedure', *The British Medical Journal*, 1(2412) (1907), pp. 665–74.
15. Lee, J.A., 'Arthur Edward James Barker 1850–1916. British pioneer of regional analgesia', *Anaesthesia*, 34(9) (1979), pp. 885–91.
16. Barker, A.E., 'A second report on clinical experiences with spinal analgesia: with a second series of one hundred cases', *The British Medical Journal*, 1(2457) (1908), pp. 244–9.
17. Doenitz, A., *'Die Hoehenausdehnung der Spinalanalgesie'*, *Münchener Medizinische Wochenschrift*, 53 (1906), pp. 2341–3.
18. Kroenig, B. and C.J. Gauss, *'Anatomische und physiologische Beobachtungen bei dem ersten Tausend Rückenmarkanäthesien'*, *Münchener Medizinische Wochenschrift*, 54 (1907), pp. 1969–74.
19. Barker, A.E., 'A third report on clinical experiences with spinal analgesia: with a third series of one hundred cases', *The British Medical Journal*, 2(2486) (1908), pp. 453–5.
20. Carrie, L.E.S., 'The spread of local anaesthetic solutions in the glass spine', YouTube (2014). www.youtube.com/watch?v=XQ7zh5rdu6o
21. Stoneham, M.D., et al., 'Oxford positioning technique improves haemodynamic stability and predictability of block height of spinal

anaesthesia for elective caesarean section', *International Journal of Obstetric Anesthesia*, 8(4) (1999), pp. 242–8.

22. Carrie, L.E.S., 'Spinal and / or epidural blockade for Caesarean section' in F. Reynolds (ed.), *Epidural and Spinal Blockade in Obstetrics* (London: BaillièreTindall, 1990), pp. 139–50.

23. Carrie, L.E.S., 'An inflatable obstetric anaesthetic "wedge"', *Anaesthesia*, 37(7) (1982), p. 745–7.

24. Bier, A., '*Versuche über Cocainisirung des Rückenmarkes*', *Deutsche Zeitschrift für Chirurgie*, 51 (1899), p. 361–9.

25. Goerig, M. and H. Bohrer, '*Die totale Spinalanästhesie nach Jonnesco*', *Anästhesiologie Intensivmedizin Notfallmedizin Schmerztherapie*, 31(1) (1996), pp. 46–8.

26. Tarcoveanu, E. and N. Angelescu, 'A European surgeon: Thoma Ionescu (Thomas Jonnesco) – founder of the Romanian school of surgery (1860–1926)', *Acta Chirurgica Belgica*, 109(6) (2009), pp. 824–8.

27. Cox, J.J., et al., 'An SCN9A channelopathy causes congenital inability to experience pain', *Nature*, 444(7121) (2006), pp. 894–8.

28. Sula, A., et al., 'The complete structure of an activated open sodium channel', *Nature Communications*, 8 (2017), p. 14205.

29. Goldberg, Y.P., et al., 'Loss-of-function mutations in the Nav1.7 gene underlie congenital indifference to pain in multiple human populations', *Clinical Genetics*, 71(4) (2007), pp. 311–9.

30. Niu, H.L., et al., 'Inhibition of Na$_v$1.7 channel by a novel blocker QLS-81 for alleviation of neuropathic pain', *Acta Pharmacologica Sinica*, 42(8) (2021), pp. 1235–47.

31. Jenkins, J.G. and M.M. Khan, 'Anaesthesia for Caesarean section: a survey in a UK region from 1992 to 2002', *Anaesthesia*, 58(11) (2003), pp. 1114–18.

32. Stamer, U.M., et al., 'Change in anaesthetic practice for Caesarean section in Germany', *Acta Anaesthesiologica Scandinavica*, 49(2) (2005), pp. 170–6.

33. Okafor, U.V., H.U. Ezegwui and K. Ekwazi, 'Trends of different forms of anaesthesia for caesarean section in South-eastern Nigeria', *Journal of Obstetrics and Gynaecology*, 29(5) (2010), pp. 392–5.

34. Xu, H., et al., 'Comparison of cutting and pencil-point spinal needle in spinal anesthesia regarding postdural puncture headache: a meta-analysis', *Medicine (Baltimore)*, 96(14) (2017), p. e6527.

35. Kendall, J.M., et al., 'Haematoma block or Bier's block for Colles' fracture reduction in the accident and emergency department – which is best?', *Journal of Accident and Emergency Medicine*, 14(6) (1997), pp. 352–6.

36. de Lange, J.J., M.A. Cuesta and A. Cuesta de Pedro, 'Fidel Pagés Miravé (1886–1923). The pioneer of lumbar epidural anaesthesia', *Anaesthesia*, 49(5) (1994), pp. 429–31.

37. Pagés, F., 'Anestesia metamérica (Part 1)', *Revista de Sanidad Militar*, 11(12) (1921), pp. 351–65.

38. Pagés, F., 'Anestesia metamérica (Part 2)', *Revista de Sanidad Militar*, 11(13) (1921), pp. 385–96.

39. Pagés, F., 'Segmental anaesthesia' (translation of Pagés' 1921 paper 'Anestesia metamérica' in *Revista de Sanidad Militar*), *Surveys in Anesthesiology*, 5(3) (1961), pp. 326–38.

40. Dogliotti, A.M., 'A new method of block anesthesia: segmental peridural spinal anesthesia', *American Journal of Surgery*, 20(1) (1933), pp. 107–18.

41. Husemeyer, R.P. and D.C. White, 'Topography of the lumbar epidural space. A study in cadavers using injected polyester resin', *Anaesthesia*, 35(1) (1980), pp. 7–11.

42. Carrie, L.E.S. and G. O'Sullivan, 'Subarachnoid bupivacaine 0.5% for caesarean section', *European Journal of Anaesthesiology*, 1(3) (1984), pp. 275–83.

43. Russell, R., et al., 'Combined spinal epidural anaesthesia for caesarean section: a randomised comparison of Oxford, lateral and sitting positions', *International Journal of Obstetric Anesthesia*, 11(3) (2002), pp. 190–5.

44. le Roux, J.J., K. Wakabayashi and Z. Jooma, 'Defining the role of thoracic spinal anaesthesia in the 21st century: a narrative review', *British Journal of Anaesthesia*, 130(1) (2023), pp. e56–65.

45. Chakravarthy, M., et al., 'High thoracic epidural anesthesia as the sole anesthetic for redo off-pump coronary artery bypass surgery', *Journal of Cardiothoracic and Vascular Anesthesia*, 17(1) (2003), pp. 84–6.

46. Chakravarthy, M., et al., 'Conscious cardiac surgery with cardiopulmonary bypass using thoracic epidural anesthesia without endotracheal general anesthesia', *Journal of Cardiothoracic and Vascular Anesthesia*, 19(3) (2005), pp. 300–5.

6. Gases, Vapours and Injections

1. Wells, H., *A History of the Discovery of the Application of Nitrous Oxide, Ether, and Other Vapors, to Surgical Operations* (Hartford: J. Gaylord Wells, 1847), 25 pp.

2. Smith, T., *An Examination of the Question of Anaesthesia* (New York: John A. Gray, 1858), 154 pp.

3. Archer, W.H. and H. Wells, 'The history of general anesthesia: published in the Hartford (Conn.) Courant, Dec. 9, 1846', *Journal of the American Dental Society of Anesthesiology*, 7(2) (1960), pp. 12–14.

4. Haridas, R.P., 'Horace Wells' demonstration of nitrous oxide in Boston', *Anesthesiology*, 119(5) (2013), pp. 1014–22.

5. Macintosh, R., 'Modern anaesthesia, with special reference to the Chair of Anaesthetics in Oxford', in J. Rupreht et al. (eds), *Anaesthesia. Essays on Its History* (Berlin and Heidelberg: Springer-Verlag, 1985), pp. 352–6.

6. Beinart, J., *A History of the Nuffield Department of Anaesthetics, Oxford 1937–1987* (Oxford: Oxford University Press, 1987), 214 pp.

7. Atkinson, R.S., G.B. Rushman and J.A. Lee, *A Synopsis of Anaesthesia*, 10th edn (Bristol: IOP Publishing, 1987), 898 pp.

8. Mapleson, W.W., 'Kinetics', in M.B. Chenoweth (ed.), *Modern Inhalational Anesthetics* (Berlin, Heidelberg, New York: Springer-Verlag, 1972), pp. 326–44.

9. Dorrington, K.L., *Anaesthetic and Extracorporeal Gas Transfer*. Oxford Medical Engineering Series (Oxford: Clarendon Press, 1989), 274 pp.

10. Clover, J.T., 'On the administration of nitrous oxide', *The British Medical Journal*, 2(410) (1868), pp. 491–2.

11. Clover, J.T., 'Remarks on the production of sleep during surgical operations', *The British Medical Journal*, 1 (1874), pp. 200–3.

12. Calverley, R.K., 'J.T. Clover: a giant of Victorian anaesthesia', in J. Rupreht et al. (eds), *Anaesthesia. Essays on Its History* (Berlin and Heidelberg: Springer-Verlag, 1985), pp. 18–23.

13. Shlugman, D. and M. Ward, 'Early anaesthesia at the Radcliffe Infirmary Oxford', *Proceedings of the History of Anaesthesia Society*, 53 (2021), pp. 39–41.

14. Dorrington, K.L., 'Asystole with convulsion following a subanaesthetic dose of propofol plus fentanyl', *Anaesthesia*, 44(8) (1989), pp. 658–9.

15. Tramèr, M.R., R.A. Moore and H.J. McQuay, 'Propofol and bradycardia: causation, frequency and severity', *British Journal of Anaesthesia*, 78(6) (1997), pp. 642–51.

16. Clover, J.T., 'On an apparatus for administering nitrous oxide gas and ether, singly or combined', *The British Medical Journal*, 2(811) (1876), pp. 74–5.

17. Knight, P.R. and D.R. Bacon, 'An unexplained death: Hannah Greener and chloroform', *Anesthesiology*, 96(5) (2002), pp. 1250–3.

18. Nunn, R.S., 'Fatal effects of ether vapour in a case of lithotomy', *London Medical Gazette*, 39 (1847), pp. 414–15.

19. Anonymous, 'Fatal operation under the influence of ether', *The Lancet*, 1 (1847), pp. 340–2.

20. Levy, A.G., 'Sudden death under light chloroform anaesthesia', *Proceedings of the Royal Society of Medicine*, 7 (1914), pp. 57–84.

21. Killian, H., 'Narkosestatistik', in *Narkose zu operativen Zwecken* (Berlin and Heidelberg: Springer-Verlag, 1934), pp. 260–308.

22. Andrews, E., 'The oxygen mixture, a new anaesthetic combination', *Chicago Medical Examiner*, 9(11) (1868), pp. 656–61.

23. Boulton, T.B., 'The rise and fall of general anaesthesia in the dental chair', *Society for Advancement of Anaesthesia in Dentistry Digest*, 4(7) (1980), pp. 156–65.

24. Landes, D.P., 'The provision of general anaesthesia in dental practice, an end which had to come?' *British Dental Journal*, 192(3) (2002), pp. 129–31.

25. Ellis, R.H. (ed.), *The Case Books of Dr. John Snow* (London: Wellcome Institute for the History of Medicine, 1994), 633 pp.

26. Snow, J., 'Case of death from amylene', *Medical Times and Gazette*, 15 (1857), pp. 133–4.

27. Mendelson, C.L., 'The aspiration of stomach contents into the lungs during obstetric anesthesia', *American Journal of Obstetrics and Gynecology*, 52 (1946), pp. 191–205.

28. Edwards, G., et al., 'Deaths associated with anaesthesia: a report on 1,000 cases', *Anaesthesia*, 11(3) (1956), pp. 194–220.

29. Wilson, G.R. and K.L. Dorrington, 'Starvation before surgery: is our practice based on evidence?' *BJA Education*, 17(8) (2017), pp. 275–82.

30. Okabe, T., H. Terashima and A. Sakamoto, 'Determinants of liquid gastric emptying: comparisons between milk and isocalorically adjusted clear fluids', *British Journal of Anaesthesia*, 114(1) (2015), pp. 77–82.

31. Hillyard, S., et al., 'Does adding milk to tea delay gastric emptying?' *British Journal of Anaesthesia*, 112(1) (2014), pp. 66–71.

32. Rüggeberg, A. and E.A. Nickel, 'Unrestricted drinking before surgery: an iterative quality improvement study', *Anaesthesia*, 77(12) (2022), pp. 1386–94.

33. Schimmelbusch, C., *Anleitung zur aseptischen Wundbehandlung*, 2nd edn (Berlin: Hirschwald, 1893), vii, 210 pp.

34. 'Yankauer masks', Wood Library-Museum of Anesthesiology. www.woodlibrarymuseum.org/museum/yankauer-masks/

35. Wawersik, V.J., 'Die Geschichte der Chloroformnarkose', *Anaesthesiologie und Reanimation*, 22(6) (1997), pp. 144–52.

36. Epstein, H.G., 'Principles of inhalers for volatile anaesthetics', *British Medical Bulletin*, 14(1) (1958), pp. 18–26.

37. Macintosh, R.R. and W.W. Mushin, 'Anaesthetics research in wartime', *South African Medical Journal*, 19(1) (1945), pp. 249–50.

38. Dobson, M., *The Right Stuff. Anaesthetic Equipment and Techniques That Work Best in Low Resource Countries* (Oxford: MD Publications, 2017), 94 pp.

39. Johnstone, M., 'The human cardiovascular response to Fluothane anaesthesia', *British Journal of Anaesthesia*, 28(9) (1956), pp. 392–410.

40. Bryce-Smith, R. and H.D. O'Brien, 'Fluothane: a non-explosive volatile anaesthetic agent', *British Medical Journal*, 2(4999) (1956), pp. 969–72.

41. Mapleson, W.W., 'The elimination of rebreathing in various semi-closed anaesthetic systems', *British Journal of Anaesthesia*, 26(5) (1954), p. 323–32.

42. Bain, J.A. and W.E. Spoerel, 'A streamlined anaesthetic system', *Canadian Anaesthetists' Society Journal*, 19 (1972), pp. 426–35.

43. Dorrington, K.L. and J.R. Lehane, 'Minimum fresh gas flow requirements of anaesthetic breathing systems during spontaneous ventilation: a graphical approach', *Anaesthesia*, 42(7) (1987), pp. 732–7.

44. Dorrington, K.L. and J.R. Lehane, 'Rebreathing during spontaneous and controlled ventilation with T-piece breathing systems: a general solution', *Anaesthesia*, 44(4) (1989), pp. 300–2.

45. Mapleson, W.W., 'Fifty years after – reflections on '"The elimination of rebreathing in various semi-closed anaesthetic systems"', *British Journal of Anaesthesia*, 93(3) (2004), pp. 319–21.

46. McGain, F., et al., 'Environmental sustainability in anaesthesia and critical care', *British Journal of Anaesthesia*, 125(5) (2020), pp. 680–92.

47. Shine, K.P., 'Climate effect of inhaled anaesthetics', *British Journal of Anaesthesia*, 105(6) (2010), pp. 731–3.

48. Slingo, M.E. and J.M. Slingo, 'Climate impacts of anaesthesia', *British Journal of Anaesthesia*, 126(6) (2021), pp. e195–7.

49. Allen, C., A.F. Smith and M.H. Nathanson, 'What can anaesthetists do to help combat the global climate emergency?' *Anaesthesia*, 77(4) (2022), pp. 367–71.

50. Rowbotham, E.S. and I. Magill, 'Anaesthetics in the plastic surgery of the face and jaws', *Proceedings of the Royal Society of Medicine*, 14 (1921), pp. 17–27.

51. Alsop, A.F., 'Non-kinking endotracheal tubes', *Anaesthesia*, 10(4) (1955), pp. 401–3.

52. Macintosh, R.R., 'A new laryngoscope', *The Lancet*, 1(6233) (1943), p. 205.

53. Magill, I.W., 'An improved laryngoscope for anaesthetists', *The Lancet,* 207(5349) (1926), p. 500.

54. Guedel, A.E., 'A nontraumatic pharygeal airway', *Journal of the American Medical Association*, 100(23) (1933), p. 1862.

55. Brain, A.I.J., 'The laryngeal mask – a new concept in airway management', *British Journal of Anaesthesia*, 55(8) (1983), pp. 801–5.

56. van Zundert, T.C.R.V., et al., 'Archie Brain: celebrating 30 years of development in laryngeal mask airways', *Anaesthesia,* 67(12) (2012), pp. 1375–85.

57. Dorrington, K.L. and W. Poole, 'The first intravenous anaesthetic: how well was it managed and its potential realized?' *British Journal of Anaesthesia*, 110(1) (2013), pp. 7–12.

58. Magill, I.W., 'Nembutal as a basal hypnotic in general anaesthesia', *The Lancet*, 217(5602) (1931), pp. 74–5.

59. Sear, J.W., 'Clinical pharmacology of intravenous anesthetics', in A.S. Evers, M. Maze and E.D. Kharasch (eds), *Anesthetic Pharmacology* (Cambridge: Cambridge University Press, 2011), pp. 444–65.

60. Bennetts, F.E., 'Thiopentone anaesthesia at Pearl Harbour', *British Journal of Anaesthesia*, 75(3) (1995), pp. 366–8.

61. Pandit, J.J., et al., '5th National Audit Project (NAP5) on accidental awareness during general anaesthesia: summary of main findings and risk factors', *British Journal of Anaesthesia*, 113(4) (2014), pp. 549–59.

62. Cox, D., 'The hidden long-term risks of surgery: "It gives people's brains a hard time"', *Guardian*, 24 April 2022. www.theguardian.com/science/2022/apr/24/the-hidden-long-term-risks-of-surgery-it-give-peoples-brains-a-hard-time

63. Sprung, J., et al., 'Cognitive function after surgery with regional or general

anaesthesia: a population-based study', *Alzheimer's and Dementia*, 15(10) (2019), pp. 1243–52.

64. Miller, D., et al., 'Intravenous versus inhalational maintenance of anaesthesia for postoperative cognitive outcomes in elderly people undergoing non-cardiac surgery', *Cochrane Database of Systematic Reviews*, 8(8) (2018), pp. 1–130.

65. Patel, D., et al., 'Cognitive decline in the elderly after surgery and anaesthesia: results from the Oxford Project to Investigate Memory and Ageing (OPTIMA) cohort', *Anaesthesia*, 71(10) (2016), pp. 1144–52.

66. Bratzke, L.C., et al., 'Cognitive decline in the middle-aged after surgery and anaesthesia: results from the Wisconsin Registry for Alzheimer's Prevention cohort', *Anaesthesia*, 73(5) (2018), pp. 549–55.

67. Ostlere, G. and R. Bryce-Smith, *Anaesthetics for Medical Students*, 9th edn (Edinburgh: Churchill Livingstone, 1980), 144 pp.

68. Boyle, R., 'The usefulness of natural philosophy and sequels to spring of the air, 1662–3', in M. Hunter and E.B. Davis (eds), *The Works of Robert Boyle,* vol. 3 (London: Pickering & Chatto, 1999), pp. 324–9.

7. The Paddywhack

1. Flanders & Swann, 'First and Second Law', YouTube. www.youtube.com/watch?v=VnbiVw_1FNs

2. Meyer, M., 'Flanders, Michael Henry (1922–1975)', in *Oxford Dictionary of National Biography* (Oxford: Oxford University Press, 2004).

3. Warrack, J., 'Swann, Donald Ibrahim,' in *Oxford Dictionary of National Biography*. (Oxford: Oxford University Press, 2004).

4. Clausius, R., *'Ueber verschiedene fuer die Anwendung bequeme Formen der Hauptgleichungen der mechanischen Wärmetheorie'*, *Annalen der Physik und Chemie*, 125(7) (1865), pp. 353–400.

5. Roy, C.S., 'The elastic properties of the arterial wall', *Journal of Physiology*, 3(2) (1881), pp. 125–59.

6. Williamson, R., 'A photograph of Sir Charles Sherrington and Professor Charles Smart Roy and three letters by Sir Charles Sherrington', *Medical History*, 3(1) (1959), pp. 78–81.

7. 'Obituary, Charles Smart Roy, M.A., M.D., F.R.S.', *The British Medical Journal*, 2 (1897). pp. 1031–2.

8. Roy, C.S. and C.S. Sherrington, 'On the regulation of the blood-supply of the brain', *Journal of Physiology*, 11(1–2) (1890), pp. 85–158.

9. Roy, C.S., 'Mountain sickness. Based on notes by Mr. W. M. Conway of his experiences in the Karakoram Himalayas', *Science Progress*, 3(14) (1895), pp. 85–98.

10. Thomson, W., 'On the thermo-elastic and thermo-magnetic properties of matter', *Quarterly Journal of Pure and Applied Mathematics*, 1 (1857), pp. 57–77.

11. Sancton, J., *Madhouse at the End of the Earth: The Belgica's Journey into the Dark Antarctic Night* (London: W.H. Allen, 2021), 368 pp.

12. Bayley, P., 'Robert Boyle and Robert Hooke', *University College Record* (1965), pp. 322–3.

13. Inwood, S., *The Man Who Knew Too Much: The Strange and Inventive Life of Robert Hooke, 1635–1703* (London: Macmillan, 2002), 485 pp.

14. Dorrington, K.L. and W. Poole, 'Robert Boyle, the first intravenous anaesthetic, and the site of the Shelley memorial', *University College Record* (2012), pp. 128–43.

15. Turner, J. M.W., *View of Oxford High Street (1810)*. www.ashmolean.org/ turners-high-street#listing_157006_0

16. University College website, 'Shelley Memorial'. www.univ.ox.ac.uk/ college_building/shelley-memorial/

17. Jardine, L., *Going Dutch. How England Plundered Holland's Glory* (London: Harper Collins, 2008), 406 pp.

18. Adams, R. and L. Jardine, 'The return of the Hooke folio', *Notes & Records of the Royal Society of London*, 60 (2006), pp. 235–9.

19. Hooke, R., *Lectures de potentia restitutiva, Or of Spring Explaining the Power of Springing Bodies* (London: John Martyn, 1678), 56 pp.

20. Hooke, R., *A Description of Helioscopes, and Some Other Instruments* (London: (John Martyn, 1676), 32 pp.

21. Anonymous, 'Galileo's Anagrams and the Moons of Mars'. www.mathpages. com/home/kmath151/kmath151.htm. I am indebted to Professor Anna Marie Roos for drawing this example to my attention.

22. Robinson, H.W. and W. Adams (eds), *The Diary of Robert Hooke M.A., M.D., F.R.S. 1672–1680* (London: Taylor & Francis, 1935), 527 pp.

23. 'Espinasse, M., *Robert Hooke* (London: William Heinemann, 1956), 192 pp.

24. Jardine, L., *The Curious Life of Robert Hooke. The Man Who Measured London* (London: Harper Collins, 2003), 422 pp.

25. Griffing, L.R., 'The lost portrait of Robert Hooke?' *Journal of Microscopy*, 278(3) (2020), pp. 114–22.

26. Unknown (attributed to Sir Peter Lely), *Portrait of a Man*. open.smk.dk/ artwork/image/KMS4139?q=*&page=0&filters=artist per cent3ASir per cent2520Peter per cent2520Lely

27. Swane, L., 'Erhervelser af fremmed Kunst', 1939, Statens Museum for Kunst, Copenhagen.

28. Greer, R., Portraits of Robert Hooke. commons.wikimedia.org/wiki/ Category:Paintings_by_Rita_Greer

29. Hooke, R., *Micrographia or Some Physiological Descriptions of Minute Bodies Made by Magnifying Glasses with Observations and Inquiries Thereupon* (London: J. Martyn and J. Allestry, 1665), 246 pp.

30. Rhythm Bones Society. rhythmbones.com/

31. Flanders & Swann, 'All Gall', YouTube. www.youtube.com/watch?v=_uukBpYD9PU

32. Hoeve, C.A.J. and P.J. Flory, 'The elastic properties of elastin', *Journal of the American Chemical Society*, 80 (1958), pp. 6523–6.

33. Hoeve, C.A.J. and P.J. Flory, 'The elastic properties of elastin', *Biopolymers*, 13(4) (1974), pp. 677–86.

34. Ramsay, J.A., 'Obituary: Torkel Weis-Fogh', *Nature*, 258 (1975), p. 651.

35. Yoshino, H., 'Random walk online simulation'. /e.sci.osaka-cu.ac.jp/yoshino/download/rw/cdirect.shtml

36. Dorrington, K.L. and N.G. McCrum, 'Elastin as a rubber', *Biopolymers*, 16(6) (1977). pp. 1201–22.

37. Rauscher, S. and R. Pomès, 'The liquid structure of elastin', *eLife* (2017), e26526. doi.org/10.7554/eLife.26526.021

38. Ferreiro, L.D., *Measure of the Earth: The Enlightenment Expedition That Reshaped Our World* (New York: Basic Books, 2011), 353 pp.

39. de La Condamine, C.-M., *'Mémoire sur une résine élastique, nouvellement découverte à Cayenne par M. Fresneau; et sur l'usage des divers sucs laiteux d'arbres de la Guiane ou France équinoctiale'*, *Histoire de l'Académie Royale des Sciences*, (1751), pp. 319–33. ia800207.us.archive.org/33/items/histoiredelacad512acad/histoiredelacad512acad.pdf.

40. Hall, W.H., *The New Royal Encyclopaedia; or, Complete Modern Dictionary of Arts and Sciences on an Improved Plan*, vol. 1 (London: C. Cooke, 1788), 713 pp.

41. Ciferri, A., C.A.J. Hoeve and P.J. Flory, 'Stress–temperature coefficients of polymer networks and the conformational energy of polymer chains', *Journal of the American Chemical Society*, 83(5) (1961), pp. 1015–22.

42. Cohen, I.B., 'Newton, Hooke, and "Boyle's Law" (discovered by Power and Towneley)', *Nature*, 204 (1964), pp. 618–21.

43. Dorrington, K.L., 'The theory of viscoelasticity in biomaterials', in J.F.V. Vincent and J.D. Currey (eds), *The Mechanical Properties of Biological Materials* (Cambridge: Cambridge University Press, 1980), pp. 289–314.

44. Dorrington, K., W. Grut and N.G. McCrum, 'Mechanical state of elastin', *Nature*, 255 (1975), pp. 476–8.

45. Onisto, M., S. Garbisa and M. Spina, 'Lorenzo Gotte (1926–1991): a pioneer of elastin', *European Journal of Histochemistry*, 60(3) (2016), pp. 210–11.

46. Gotte, L., M. Mammi and G. Pezzin, 'Some structural aspects of elastin revealed by X-ray diffraction and other physical methods', in W.G. Crewther (ed.), *Symposium on Fibrous Proteins Australia 1967* (Sydney: Butterworths, Australia, 1968), pp. 236–45.

47. Dorrington, K.L., 'Skin turgor: do we understand the clinical sign?' *The Lancet*, 1(8214) (1981), pp. 264–5.

48. McGee, S., 'Hypovolemia', in *Evidence-Based Physical Diagnosis* (Elsevier, 2018), pp. 77–9.

49. Marx, G., et al., 'Intravascular volume therapy in adults: Guidelines from the Association of the Scientific Medical Societies in Germany', *European Journal of Anaesthesiology*, 33(7) (2016), pp. 488–521.

50. Aguilar, O.M. and M. Albertal, 'Poor skin turgor', *New England Journal of Medicine*, 338(1) (1998), p. 25.

51. Lockhart, R.D., *Living Anatomy. A Photographic Atlas of Muscles in Action and Surface Contours* (London: Faber and Faber, 1963).

52. Patterson, S.W. and E.H. Starling, 'On the mechanical factors which determine the output of the ventricles', *Journal of Physiology*, 48(5) (1914), pp. 357–79.

53. Roy, C.S., 'On the influences which modify the work of the heart', *Journal of Physiology*, 1(6) (1879), pp. 452–96.

54. Zimmer, H.-G., 'Who discovered the Frank–Starling mechanism?' *News in Physiological Sciences*, 17 (2002), pp. 181–4.

55. Han, J.-C., et al., 'Re-visiting the Frank–Starling nexus', *Progress in Biophysics and Molecular Biology*, 159 (2021), pp. 10–21.

8. Inhabited Ruins

1. Beadle, M., *These Ruins are Inhabited* (London: Robert Hale, 1963), 188 pp. Muriel Beadle's account of spending a year in Oxford with her Nobel Prize-winning husband has inspired the present chapter.

2. 'Hertford College', in H.E. Salter and M.D. Lobel (eds), *A History of the County of Oxford: Volume 3, the University of Oxford* (Victoria County History, 1954), pp. 309–19. British History Online: british-history.ac.uk/vch/oxon/vol3/pp309-319

3. Hutton, K., 'Learning from my mistakes', Our Hatfield. www.ourhatfield.org.uk/content/topics/schools_education/schools_of_yesterday/hatfield-school/learning-from-my-mistakes-kenneth-hutton

4. Norwood, C., 'The Norwood Report (1943). Curriculum and Examinations in Secondary Schools. Report of the Committee of the Secondary School Examinations Council appointed by the President of the Board of Education in 1941' (London: His Majesty's Stationery Office, 1943), 152 pp.

5. Simon, B., *Education and the Social Order 1940–1990*. Studies in the History of Education, vol. 4 (London: Lawrence and Wishart, 1991), 646 pp.

6. Skinner, D., 'Early years of Hatfield School', www.ourhatfield.org.uk/content/topics/schools_education/schools_of_yesterday/hatfield-school/early-years-of-hatfield-school-by-daphne-skinner

7. Hutton, K., *Chemistry: The Conquest of Materials* (London: Penguin Books, 1957), 228 pp.

8. Goldman, L., 'The "Tanner Scheme" at Hertford College. Widening Access, Reforming Oxford, 1965–85', p. 72. www.hertford.ox.ac.uk/wp-content/uploads/2019/10/The-Tanner-Scheme-Research-Project-PDF.pdf

9. Tanner, N., 'The Hertford Scheme' (1970), p. 4. www.hertford.ox.ac.uk/wp-content/uploads/2018/05/Neil-Tanner-speech.pdf

10. Hall, R., 'Drive for more student diversity paying off, says Oxford University', *Guardian*, 11 May 2021. www.theguardian.com/education/2021/may/11/drive-for-more-student-diversity-paying-off-says-oxford-university

11. Brockliss, L.W.B., *The University of Oxford: A History* (Oxford: Oxford University Press, 2016), 871 pp.

12. Dowling, L., *Hellenism and Homosexuality in Victorian Oxford* (Ithaca and London: Cornell University Press, 1994), 173 pp.

13. Bergel, D.H., 'The visco-elastic properties of the arterial wall'. PhD thesis in Physiology (University of London, 1960), p. 249.

14. Paterson, D., 'In piam memoriam: Dr Derek H. Bergel', University of Oxford Department of Physiology, Anatomy & Genetics (2021). www.dpag.ox.ac.uk/news/dr-derek-h-bergel

15. Dorrington, K.L., 'Rubber-like elasticity in the body'. DPhil thesis in Engineering Science (University of Oxford, 1977), p. 265.

16. Gillman, P. and L. Gillman, *Collar the Lot! How Britain Interned and Expelled its Wartime Refugees* (London: Quartet Books, 1980), 352 pp.

17. Mahler, R., 'Obituary: Ernest Foulkes', *Independent*, 7 July 1993. www.independent.co.uk/news/people/obituary-ernest-foulkes-1483614.html

18. Foulkes Foundation, 'The Foulkes Foundation Trust Deed 1974'. register-of-charities.charitycommission.gov.uk/charity-search/-/charity-details/265166/governing-document

19. St Catherine's College Oxford, 'College history'. www.stcatz.ox.ac.uk/about-us/college-history/

20. Kuper, S., *Chums. How a Tiny Caste of Oxford Tories Took Over the UK* (London: Profile Books, 2022), 209 pp.

21. Harding, A., 'Obituary: Dame Rosemary Rue', *The Lancet*, 365 (2005), p. 566.

22. Cook, C., 'Interview with Dame Rosemary Rue', *Journal of Public Health*, 26(3) (2004), pp. 220–9.

23. Rue, R., 'Employment of married women doctors in hospitals in the Oxford region', *The Lancet*, 1(7502) (1967), pp. 1267–8.

24. Swerdlow, A.J. and E.R. Rue, 'Part-time medical training: 15 years' experience in the Oxford region', *British Medical Journal (Clinical Research Edition)*, 283(6303) (1981), pp. 1371–3.

25. Lachish, S., et al., 'Factors associated with less-than-full-time working in medical practice: results of surveys of five cohorts of UK doctors, 10 years after graduation', *Human Resources for Health*, 14(1) (2016), p. 62.

26. Jones, D.S. and J.H. Jones, 'Sir Edward Penley Abraham CBE. 10 June 1913 – 9 May 1999', *Biographical Memoirs of Fellows of the Royal Society*, 60 (2014), pp. 5–22.

27. Smårs, L., 'Transformative donation to college', *Linacre News*, 57 (2022), p. 4.

28. Anonymous, 'Nuffield (Penicillin) Research Fellowships', *Nature*, 161 (1948), p. 16.

29. University of Oxford, 'Student numbers'. www.ox.ac.uk/about/facts-and-figures/student-numbers?wssl=1

30. Herbert & Gowers & Co., 'The Viscount Nuffield and Lincoln College Oxford Deed relating to the Nuffield (Penicillin) Research Trust Fund', (1948), p. 3.

31. Raw, J., 'The doctors' mess: the unsung resource', *British Medical Journal*, 327(7416) (2003), p. 689.

32. West, M. and D. Coia, 'Caring for doctors Caring for patients. How to transform UK healthcare environments to support doctors and medical students to care for patients', General Medical Council (2019), 149 pp.

33. Darwall-Smith, R., *A History of University College Oxford* (Oxford: Oxford University Press, 2008), 605 pp.

34. Adams, M., *Aelfred's Britain. War and Peace in the Viking Age* (London: Head of Zeus, 2017), 509 pp.

35. Cox, A.D.M., 'The French petition', *University College Record* (1952–3), pp. 14–24.

36. Smith, W., *The Annals of University-College. Proving William of Durham the True Founder: and Answering All Their Arguments Who Ascribe It to King Alfred* (Newcastle upon Tyne: John White, 1728), 376 pp.

37. Hone, C.R., *The Life of Dr. John Radcliffe 1652–1714. The Eminent Physician* (London: Faber and Faber, 1950), 150 pp.

38. Nias, J.B., *Dr John Radcliffe. A Sketch of his Life with an Account of his Fellows and Foundations* (Oxford: Clarendon Press, 1918), 148 pp.

39. Guest, I., *Dr John Radcliffe and his Trust* (Oxford: The Radcliffe Trust, 1991), 595 pp.

40. Green, V.H.H., *The Commonwealth of Lincoln College, 1427–1977* (Oxford: Oxford University Press, 1979), 746 pp.

41. Pittis, W., *Some Memoirs of the Life of John Radcliffe, M.D. Interspersed with Several Original Letters: His Two Speeches in Parliament, and a True Copy of his Last Will and Testament,* 2nd edn (London: E. Curll, 1715), 108 pp.

42. QS Top Universities, 'QS world university rankings by subject: anatomy & physiology' (2023). www.topuniversities.com/university-rankings/university-subject-rankings/2023/anatomy-physiology

PICTURE CREDITS

Figure 1. Public resource National Library of Medicine USA: resource.nlm.nih. gov/101441395

Figure 2. Photograph by Robin Darwall-Smith, courtesy of the Master and Fellows of University College, Oxford

Figure 3. Courtesy of Dr Luigi Camporota

Figures 4–7, 12, 13. Courtesy of the Department of Physiology, Anatomy & Genetics, Oxford

Figures 8. and 9. Courtesy of Professor David Paterson

Figures 10. and 18. Courtesy of the Chalet Trust

Figure 11. Courtesy of Agence France-Presse

Figure 14. Courtesy of John Wiley & Sons

Figure 15. Creative Commons CC-PD-Mark, Public Domain commons. wikimedia.org/wiki/File:Stephen_Hales_measuring_blood_pressure_in_a_ horse_(1705).png

Figure 16. Academy of Sciences of Turin, Public domain, via Wikimedia Commons https://commons.wikimedia.org/w/index.php?curid=108116342)

Figure 17. Creative Commons Attribution 3.0 commons.wikimedia.org/wiki/ File:Mont_rose_juil07.JPG

Figure 19. Diagram by the author

Figure 20. Courtesy of the Wellcome Collection CCBY4.0

Figure 21. Courtesy of the *New England Journal of Medicine*

Figures 22. (a) and (b) author's images

Figure 23. Courtesy of the Wellcome Collection, Creative Commons Attribution BY-4.0

Figures 24, 25, 33, 35, 36. Images by the author

Figure 26. Courtesy of Shutterstock

Figure 27. From *La Presse Médicale*, 1911

Figure 28. Photo: CC BY-SA3.0: it.wikipedia.org/wiki/Anestesia_subaracnoidea; artist: Poul Buckhöj)

Figure 29. Originally from Gray's *Anatomy*; Public Domain: commons.wikimedia. org/wiki/File:Gray_111_-_Vertebral_column-coloured.png

Figure 30. Courtesy of the Wellcome Library. commons.wikimedia.org/wiki/File:Portrait_of_Arthur_E_Barker_by_Anton_Mansch,_Medical_world_Wellcome_L0028316.jpg Creative Commons Attribution 4.0)

Figure 31. Courtesy of the Wellcome Collection wellcomecollection.org/works/vfc88tve

Figure 32. (commons.wikimedia.org/wiki/File:Diagram_showing_the_parts_of_the_pharynx_CRUK_334.svg Creative Commons Attribution BY 4.0

Figure 34. Courtesy of the Science Museum London. Wellcome Collection. wellcomecollection.org/works/epc69f5s Commons Attribution BY4.0

Figure 37. CC-PD-Mark, Public domain image: commons.wikimedia.org/wiki/File:Roy_Sherrington_1893_01.jpg

Figure 38. Courtesy of Colin Beesley

Figure 39. Courtesy of the Ashmolean Museum

Figure 40. Courtesy of the National Gallery of Denmark

Figure 41. Courtesy of Carolyn McCrum

Figure 42. Courtesy of Subherwal, July 2017, Creative Commons CC-BY-Attribution 2.0), https://commons.wikimedia.org/wiki/File:Bridge_of_Sighs_(35895233456).jpg

Figure 43. Photograph by Lotte Meitner-Graf, courtesy of Michael Hutton

Figure 44. Photograph: ©Norman McBeath

Figure 45. Courtesy of Tristan Surtel, Creative Commons CC-BY-SA-4.0 at commons.wikimedia.org/wiki/File:Christ_Church_Great_Quad_panoramic.jpg

Figure 46. Courtesy of the Warden and Fellows of Merton College

Figure 47. Courtesy of the Foulkes Foundation

Figure 48. National Portrait Gallery, Courtesy of Nick Sinclair

Figures 49. and 51. Courtesy of the Master and Fellows of University College, Oxford

Figure 50. Photograph by David Hartley, courtesy of the Master and Fellows of University College, Oxford

Figure 52. Photograph by Robin Darwall-Smith, courtesy of the Master and Fellows of University College, Oxford

ACKNOWLEDGEMENTS

Each of the seven areas of endeavour that I explore in this book is inhabited by colleagues to whom I am indebted for inspiration and support. I leave mention of them to the respective chapters. I am grateful to the archivist of University College Oxford, Robin Darwall-Smith, for inspiring conversations, help in mining the College's archive and for his own photographs of our shared alma mater. Like many academics in Oxford, I have enjoyed two bolt-holes from which to study and write: college and department. David Paterson, Head of the Department of Physiology, Anatomy & Genetics, has provided constant support. Help with images has come from Colin Beesley and Peter Belk. My long-standing laboratory colleague Peter Robbins has kept me scientifically on my toes with frequent discussions over coffee.

Archivists Lucy Rutherford at Hertford College and Lindsay McCormack of Lincoln College have helped me in the hunt for historical figures. I am indebted to Peter Jones and his team at Profile Editions for remarkable support.

My most immediate debt goes to Stephen Golding, who has read the manuscript with an eagle eye more than once and made his way through several red pens suggesting edits to my sometimes-jolting prose. He has frequently alerted me to perspectives that I had not considered. Given that I have spent several decades working in a women's hospital, the most suitable analogy I have is to think of him as the midwife of this book.

My wife, Marion, has entered a period of poor health as I have worked on this project. I am indebted to her for encouraging me to take time to see it to completion.

KLD *12 June 2023*

INDEX